BSAVA Manual of
Exotic Pet and
Wildlife Nursing

Editors:

Molly Varga
BVetMed DZooMed MRCVS
RCVS Recognised Specialist in Zoo and Wildlife Medicine
Cheshire Pet Medical Centre, Holmes Chapel, Cheshire CW4 8AB

Rachel Lumbis
MSc BSc PGCert CertSAN RVN FHEA
Royal Veterinary College, Department of Veterinary Clinical Sciences,
Hawkshead Lane, North Mymms, Hertfordshire AL9 7TA

and

Lucy Gott
VN Cert Vet Nursing Exotic Species
Small Animal Teaching Hospital, University of Liverpool,
Leahurst, Neston, Wirral CH64 7TE

Published by:

British Small Animal Veterinary Association
Woodrow House, 1 Telford Way, Waterwells
Business Park, Quedgeley, Gloucester GL2 2AB

A Company Limited by Guarantee in England.
Registered Company No. 2837793.
Registered as a Charity.

Illustrations 2.3, 4.3, 4.18 and 4.29 were drawn by S.J. Elmhurst BA Hons (www.livingart.org.uk)
and are printed with her permission.

A catalogue record for this book is available from the British Library.

ISBN   978 1 905319 35 0

The publishers, editors and contributors cannot take responsibility for information provided
on dosages and methods of application of drugs mentioned or referred to in this publication.
Details of this kind must be verified in each case by individual users from up to date literature
published by the manufacturers or suppliers of those drugs. Veterinary surgeons are reminded
that in each case they must follow all appropriate national legislation and regulations (for
example, in the United Kingdom, the prescribing cascade) from time to time in force.

Printed in India by Imprint Digital
Printed on ECF paper made from sustainable forests

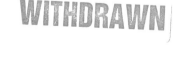

Other titles in the BSAVA Manuals series

Also from BSAVA

For information on these and all BSAVA publications please visit our website: **www.bsava.com**

Contents

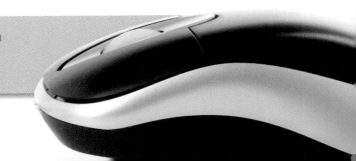

EPWN extra

For additional resources, including a range of client handouts, go to
www.bsava.com/EPWN-extra

Contributors

Wendy Bament BSc MSc RVN
Exotic and Wildlife Service, Hospital for Small Animals, Royal (Dick) School of Veterinary Studies, Easter Bush Veterinary Centre, Roslin, Midlothian EH25 9RG

Donna Brown VN CertVNES
Head Nurse, Edinburgh Zoo, Royal Zoological Society of Scotland, 134 Corstorphine Road, Edinburgh EH12 6TS

Suzetta Cameron BSc BVSc MSc MRCVS
Birch Heath Veterinary Clinic, Birch Heath Road, Tarporley, Cheshire CW6 9UU

Nick Carmichael BVSc BVM&S DCVS FRCPath DipECVCP MRCVS
RCVS Recognised Specialist in Veterinary Clinical Pathology
Veterinary Director, CTDS Ltd, Blacksmiths Forge, Brookfield Farm, Selby Road, Garforth LS25 1NB

John Chitty BVetMed CertZooMed CBiol MSB MRCVS
Anton Vets, Unit 11 Anton Mill Road, Andover SP10 2NJ

Judith Churm RVN
Daleside Veterinary Group, Main Road, Rhosrobin, Wrexham LL11 4RL

Jon Cracknell BVMS CertVA CertZooMed MRCVS
Director of Animal Operations, Longleat Safari and Adventure Park, Safari Park Office, Longleat, Wiltshire BA12 7NJ

Carli Dodd CertVNES RVN
Avian Veterinary Services, Manchester Road, Knutsford WA16 0SX

Sarah T. Flack BSc PGCE RVN
The Wylie Veterinary Centre, 196 Hall Lane, Upminster, Essex RM14 1TD

Emily Fletcher BVM&S CertZooMed MRCVS
Avian Veterinary Services, Manchester Road, Knutsford WA16 0SX

Lucy Gott VN CertVNES
Small Animal Teaching Hospital, University of Liverpool, Leahurst, Neston, Wirral CH64 7TE

Helen Heggie CertVNES RVN
Lawrie Veterinary Group, Kenilworth Court, North Carbrain Road, Cumbernauld, Glasgow G671BP

Richard Jones BVSc MSc MRCVS
Avian Veterinary Services, Manchester Road, Knutsford WA16 0SX

Emma Keeble BVSc DZooMed MRCVS
RCVS Recognised Specialist in Zoo and Wildlife Medicine
Exotic Animal Service, Department of Veterinary Clinical Studies,
Royal (Dick) School of Veterinary Studies, University of Edinburgh, Small Animal Hospital,
Easter Bush, Roslin, Midlothian EH25 9RG

Rebecca Lea VN
Sale, Cheshire M33 3LJ

William Lewis BVSc CertZooMed MRCVS
Wylie Veterinary Centre, 196 Hall Lane, Upminster, Essex RM14 1TD

Romain Pizzi BVSc MSc DZooMed MACVSc(Surg) FRES FRGS MRCVS
RCVS Recognised Specialist in Zoo and Wildlife Medicine
Royal Zoological Society of Scotland, Edinburgh Zoo, 134 Corstorphine Road, Edinburgh EH12 6TS;
Scottish SPCA National Wildlife Rescue Centre, Fishcross, Clackmannanshire FK10 3AN;
Special Lecturer in Zoo and Wildlife Medicine, University of Nottingham, Sutton Bonnington,
Leicestershire LE12 5RD

Matthew Rendle RVN
Zoological Society of London, Regent's Park, London NW1 4RY

Richard Saunders BSc BVSc MSB CBiol CertZooMed DZooMed MRCVS
Staff Veterinary Surgeon, Bristol Zoological Gardens Veterinary Department, Clifton, Bristol BS8 3HA

Lyndsey Stanton BSc CertVNES RVN
The Wylie Veterinary Centre, 196 Hall Lane, Upminster, Essex RM14 1TD

Lesa Thompson MA BVM&S DZooMed MSc MRCVS
RCVS Recognised Specialist in Zoo and Wildlife Medicine
Tokyo, Japan

Molly Varga BVetMed DZooMed MRCVS
RCVS Recognised Specialist in Zoo and Wildlife Medicine
Cheshire Pet Medical Centre, Holmes Chapel, Cheshire CW4 8AB

Emma Whitlock BSc VNS RVN
Senior Avian and Exotic Nurse, Great Western Exotic Vets, Unit 10 Berkshire House,
County Park Business Park, Shrivenham Road, Swindon, Wiltshire SN1 2NR

Foreword

When I worked in practice the care of the exotic patient, be it a pet or wildlife casualty, was rather hit and miss! Keep it warm and hydrated and hope for the best was a common maxim. Clinical practice has thankfully moved on and nowadays the nursing care of these species requires a significant level of knowledge and expertise.

The *BSAVA Manual of Exotic Pet and Wildlife Nursing* provides an invaluable point of reference for the veterinary nurse tasked with the nursing care of the less common species. It contains a wealth of information and its accessible presentation, for example the use of coloured text boxes and tables, ensures that the reader is able to locate relevant content easily and quickly. The book is laid out in a logical manner, starting with a chapter on the initial consultation and triage followed by chapters that discuss the biology and husbandry of mammals, birds and reptiles. The nursing care of the inpatient is then considered, with an introductory chapter which focuses on the individual requirements of each species before outlining specific nursing considerations. Chapters on diagnostic procedures, surgical management and anaesthesia follow, before returning to the consulting room with a chapter that outlines the points for consideration with respect to the running of exotic species nurse clinics and useful advice on client education. Each chapter contains self-assessment questions and uses numerous good quality images to support the factual content. The emphasis throughout is on the need to focus on the particular requirements of the species under treatment rather than extrapolation from the cat or dog, and the potential for risk from zoonotic disease is also considered where appropriate.

Although aimed at the veterinary nurse, the *BSAVA Manual of Exotic Pet and Wildlife Nursing* will prove an invaluable source of information for all clinical staff and students, and I am confident that it will quickly find a place on practice bookshelves.

Sue Badger VN CertEd
School of Veterinary Sciences, University of Bristol, Langford

Preface

In the last ten years, the range of animals presented for veterinary care has widened significantly, and the expectations regarding level of care have increased even more. This places a responsibility on both veterinary surgeons and veterinary nurses to apply their knowledge to the less familiar species. A seemingly familiar species such as a rabbit has significantly different nursing requirements to those of a cat or dog, and when species such as birds or reptiles are considered, the difference in requirements becomes even greater. With the advent of the new RCVS Code of Professional Conduct for Veterinary Nurses, it is now the responsibility of the individual nurse to ensure his/her competence prior to performing any treatment. This Manual aims to allow veterinary nurses with experience working with more familiar species to understand the varying issues involved in nursing exotic pets and wildlife, and to modify their skills and apply them to these less common species.

Written by veterinary nurses and veterinary surgeons with expertise in the field, the new *BSAVA Manual of Exotic Pet and Wildlife Nursing* discusses comparative nursing and supportive care of commonly kept exotic pets and frequently encountered species of wildlife. Patient care is discussed in a logical sequence, from the initial telephone call (including initial contact advice) through to consultation, admittance, hospitalization, and intervention.

This new Manual is designed to be practical and user-friendly, enabling the easy and direct application of theory to practice. The book is therefore an ideal resource for student and qualified veterinary nurses as well as other members of the veterinary healthcare team. A variety of useful tools including husbandry questionnaires, anaesthesia record forms and sample client handouts are also included, helping veterinary nurses to complete their duties easily and effectively.

We would like to take this opportunity to thank the authors and the BSAVA team for all their dedicated hard work in producing this Manual.

Molly Varga
Rachel Lumbis
Lucy Gott

August 2012

Veterinary Nurse e-Membership –

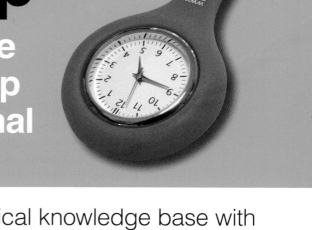

Join the BSAVA to become part of the UK membership association for small animal veterinary professionals

Further your career and expand your clinical knowledge base with support from BSAVA Veterinary Nurse e-Membership. Member benefits are designed to be practical and useful in day-to-day practice and provide access to the education and science you need

Veterinary Nurse e-Member benefits* include:

- Vet Stream lectures at Congress – only Veterinary Nurse e-Members can upgrade to attend Vet Stream lectures at Congress (non-member VNs can only attend Nursing Stream lectures)
- Discount on Veterinary Nurse CPD and Regional CPD
- Discount on all BSAVA Manuals
- Online access to the *Journal of Small Animal Practice*
- Subscription to **companion**
- Access to a growing range of online benefits such the BSAVA Health and Safety Resource and downloadable Client Information Leaflets
- A range of ancillary benefits

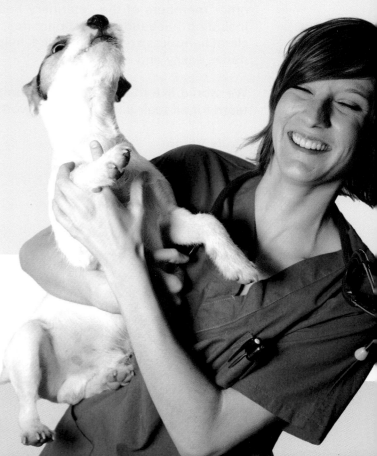

Find out more and join online at
www.bsava.com/vnmembership
or phone 01452 726700

*At October 2012. See website for current list of benefits

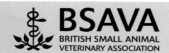

BSAVA
BRITISH SMALL ANIMAL
VETERINARY ASSOCIATION

Initial consultation

Emily Fletcher and Rebecca Lea

This chapter is designed to give information on:

- Telephone advice – how to identify emergencies and advise on the safe transportation of exotic pets and wildlife
- Strategies to reduce stress for exotic pets in the veterinary surgery environment
- The nurse's role in obtaining a history, including the use of client questionnaires
- Safe handling techniques
- Triage of emergency cases presented at the surgery
- Core principles of clinical examination

Telephone advice and transport

When a client contacts a veterinary practice, the first person they will speak to is the receptionist or veterinary nurse. This is the time at which a good impression must be made and the right advice given. Good telephone advice includes asking the right questions, giving correct information on transporting an animal safely, and identifying cases that constitute emergencies.

Exotic pets are becoming increasingly popular, and owners want to feel that they are going to a veterinary practice that understands the individual needs of their pet. Initial telephone advice is therefore more important now than it has ever been.

Small mammals

Rabbits

Owners should be advised to bring their rabbit into the practice as soon as possible if they report them to be showing one or more of the following clinical signs:

- Watery foul-smelling diarrhoea
- Acute collapse
- Bloated abdomen
- Myiasis (fly strike)
- Acute paralysis or head tilt
- Severe dyspnoea
- Heat stress
- Stranguria or dysuria
- Dystocia
- Seizures.

If in doubt as to whether a rabbit should be seen as an emergency it is best to be cautious and advise the owner to bring the animal to the practice as soon as possible. It is important to remember that rabbits are prey animals and so are skilled at masking signs of illness and pain. Subtle changes in their appetite, demeanour and faecal output can be important indicators that something is wrong. An animal that has not been seen to eat or defecate in a period of 12–24 hours should be considered an emergency and the owner should be told to bring them into the practice as soon as possible.

The following advice should be given to owners regarding the transport of their rabbit to the practice:

- Transport the rabbit using a dark cardboard box or a pet carrier
- Ensure the rabbit is secure and has adequate ventilation

- Consider lining the container with newspaper and hay to reduce soiling of the pet and to help ensure a comfortable journey (Figure 1.1)
- If bonded with another rabbit, bring both pets to the practice together to reduce the stress of being separated.

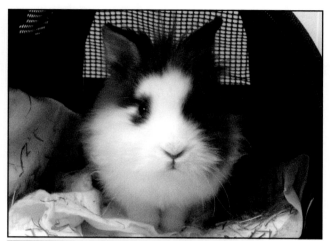

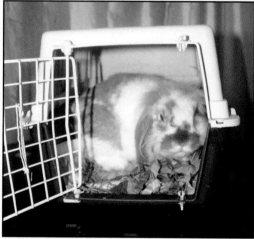

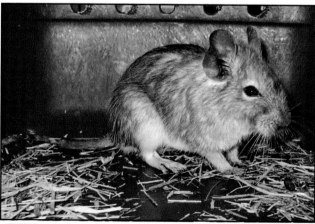

Species	Common reasons for emergency presentation
Mice and rats	Dyspnoea Trauma/dropped animal Diarrhoea Abscesses Wounds Neurological signs, e.g. sudden head tilt
Hamsters	Prolapsed eyes Diarrhoea Trauma Reluctance to move
Gerbils	Bloat Diarrhoea Seizures Trauma, e.g. fractures or tail degloving
Guinea pigs	Anorexia and gastrointestinal stasis Diarrhoea Dyspnoea Reluctance to move Dystocia Dysuria and stranguria
Chinchillas	Anorexia and gastrointestinal stasis Diarrhoea Dyspnoea Reluctance to move Dystocia Heatstroke Paraphimosis (fur ring) Fractures
Degus	Anorexia Dyspnoea Trauma, e.g. fractures or tail degloving (Figure 1.3) Diarrhoea Seizures Heatstroke
Chipmunks	Anorexia Dysuria Diarrhoea Reluctance to move Trauma, e.g. wounds or fractures Neurological signs, e.g. seizures Dyspnoea

1.1   A cat carrier can be used to transport rabbits. There is newspaper in the bottom, which can easily be replaced if it becomes soiled. A water dispensing bottle can be attached to the carrier door. (Courtesy of Sarah Pellett)

1.2   Common reasons for emergency presentation of rodent species.

Rodents

Common reasons for emergency presentation of rodent species are outlined in Figure 1.2. Owners should be advised to bring their pet into the practice as soon as possible if they report them to be showing one or more of these clinical signs. It should be borne in mind that most pet rodents belong to prey species and are therefore skilled at masking signs of pain and illness.

Rats and gerbils that are unwell or stressed can present with a red secretion at the nose and medial canthus of the eyes (Figure 1.4). This is a pigment called porphyrin, which is produced from the Harderian gland normally and builds up if the animal fails to wash it away when ill. If an owner reports the presence of this discharge they should be told to bring their pet to the practice as soon as possible.

1.3   A degu with a degloving injury. (Courtesy of E. Keeble).

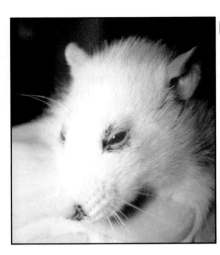

1.4 Porphyrin staining around the eyes and nose of a rat.

The following advice should be given to owners regarding bringing their pet to the practice:

- Transport the rodent using a secure pet carrier
- Smaller species such as mice should be transported in a small plastic container with a lid
- Ensure the rodent has adequate ventilation
- If using a larger carrier, consider lining this with newspaper; kitchen towel is a suitable alternative for smaller containers
- Gerbils, mice and hamsters will benefit from shredded paper or bedding material to hide in while being transported (Figure 1.5a)
- Gerbils and hamsters may be transported in their play balls (Figure 1.5b).

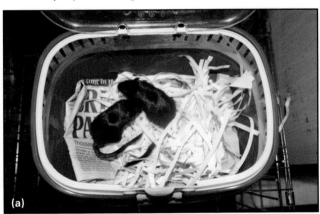

(a)

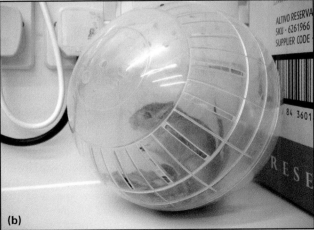

(b)

1.5 Gerbils may be transported **(a)** in a carrier or **(b)** in their exercise ball. (Courtesy of C. Dodd)

Ferrets

Ferrets are generally either very active or fast asleep. Due to their high surface area to volume ratio they can become hypothermic very quickly if collapsed. Owners should be advised to bring their ferret into the practice as soon as possible if they report them to be displaying one or more of the following clinical signs:

- Fainting or seizures
- Collapse
- Diarrhoea, especially if watery, bloody and foul-smelling and associated with ill health
- Dyspnoea
- Hyperthermia
- Hindlimb paresis or paralysis
- Vomiting
- Dysuria
- Discharges from eyes, nose or vulva
- Acute abdominal swelling.

Animals showing any of these clinical signs should be treated as urgent cases. If there is any doubt as to whether the animal constitutes an emergency it is best to be cautious and advise the owner to bring their pet to the practice as soon as possible.

Ferrets are often transported to the practice in pet carriers (Figure 1.6a). Owners should be advised to line the pet carrier with newspaper and to place a blanket or a ferret hammock in the carrier (Figure 1.6b); this provides the ferret with added comfort and a place to hide.

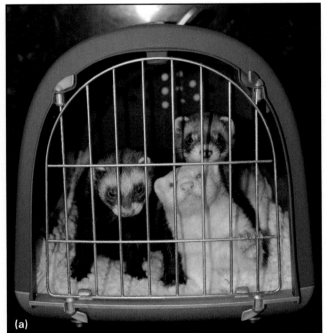

(a)

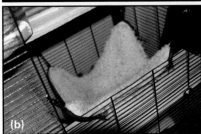

(b)

1.6 **(a)** Ferrets can be transported in a pet carrier. **(b)** This may contain a hammock. (Courtesy of Sarah Pellett)

Sugar gliders

Common reasons for emergency presentation of this species include:

- Weakness and ataxia
- Paralysis or paresis
- Seizures
- Traumatic incidents, e.g. wounds and fractures
- Diarrhoea
- Rectal prolapse
- Dysuria and stranguria.

Owners should be advised to bring their pet into the practice as soon as possible if they report them to be showing any of these clinical signs.

Sugar gliders are usually transported to the practice using a secure sleeping pouch; this is the least stressful method of transport for marsupials.

Birds

When a client telephones the practice to discuss a pet bird, the veterinary nurse or receptionist must first establish the urgency of the bird's condition. Birds tend to hide their illnesses because in the wild any signs of weakness would result in their being pushed out of the flock; a sick bird will attract predators. Birds will behave normally for as long as possible; therefore, by the time the client telephones, the bird has probably been ill for some time. Subtle signs are often unnoticed by the inexperienced or unknowledgeable owner, and ruffled feathers could mask the bird's weight loss (Figure 1.7).

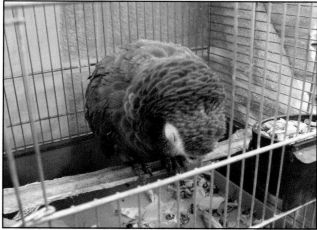

1.7 Ruffled feathers can mask weight loss. (Courtesy of C. Dodd)

The owner should be told to bring their pet bird to the practice immediately if any of the following signs are present:

- Sudden change in number or appearance of the droppings; yellow, rusty brown or tarry-black droppings could indicate internal bleeding, among other serious problems
- Sudden reduction in food intake; their extremely high metabolism requires adequate nutrition
- Sudden enlargement of any body part

- Personality or behavioural changes
- Abnormal respiratory sounds or difficulty in breathing, including mouth breathing whilst at rest
- Tail bobbing; repetitive and prolonged tail bobbing can be indicative of a respiratory infection
- Reduced vocalization
- Feathers 'fluffed up' for prolonged periods of time; this could indicate respiratory problems
- Bleeding or injury
- Regurgitation
- Nasal or ocular discharge or cloudy eyes
- Twitching/seizures/falling off perch.

Birds should be seen within 24 hours if the owner reports any of the following signs:

- Change in water consumption
- Change in weight or body condition
- Discharge from the bird's nares (nostrils) or redness and inflammation of the cere (Figure 1.8)
- Change in volume, number and appearance of droppings
- Decrease in food intake
- Decreased activity
- Dirty feathers; healthy birds are naturally hygienic animals, preening their feathers daily and bathing often.

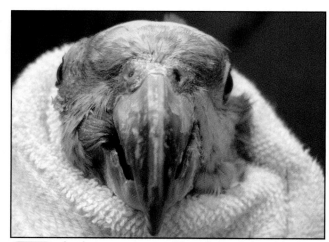

1.8 An Amazon parrot with unilateral sinusitis. Note the swollen cere, sinus and displaced globe on the parrot's right side. (Courtesy of C. Dodd)

A bird that has been bleeding must be classed as an emergency. The amount of blood lost may seem insignificant to the owner but the blood volume of a bird is extremely small and the percentage lost can therefore be quite high. If an owner has caused the bird to bleed by trying to clip its claws then a coagulant (e.g. flour) is recommended to stop the bleeding before the bird reaches the veterinary practice. A thorough clinical examination by the veterinary surgeon is still advised, even if the bleeding has stopped.

Once the urgency of the appointment has been established, a few facts should be sought. At the very least a minimal signalment should be established:

■ Species
■ Age
■ Sex.

As much information as possible about the injury or condition should also be obtained from the owner. Questions asked should include:

■ What signs is the bird showing?
■ Is it a traumatic injury or an illness?
■ How long has the bird been like this?
■ What was the bird like prior to you noticing the problem?

This information should then be passed on to the veterinary surgeon so that they are prepared for the patient's arrival at the practice.

Transport

Safe transport to the veterinary practice is essential. The following advice should therefore be given to owners.

■ Small birds should be transported in their own cages. This will allow the veterinary surgeon to examine the droppings in the bottom of the cage as well as to assess the cage and its accessories. Lead poisoning is not uncommon in psittacine birds, caused by the bird chewing its toys. Birds can suffer from zinc poisoning if they chew the cage bars.
■ Larger birds may need to be transported in a cat carrier if their cages are too large to manoeuvre. It is still important for the veterinary surgeon to evaluate the paper from the bottom of the cage and so this should be brought along separately.
■ Larger birds should not be brought to the practice on a harness or on the owner's shoulders. This is strongly discouraged because, although the bird may be tame for the owner at home, the veterinary practice is an unfamiliar setting and could potentially be very busy with other species that might scare the bird. This could result in an injury to the bird or to the owner, as the scared bird may bite. Escape is also a strong possibility.
■ If the bird is very poorly, its cage should be covered for darkness and warmth. Hot water bottles can be used to keep the bird warm during transportation. Owners should be advised that direct contact between the hot water bottle and bird could cause burns or overheating and, to prevent this, they should wrap the hot water bottle in a towel and place it in the carrier beneath another towel. When the bird arrives at the practice, it can be placed in a warm incubator or given supplemental oxygen if respiratory distress is evident.
■ All medications and supplements should be brought by the owner so that the veterinary surgeon can see what the bird has been given.
■ Birds of prey should be transported in raptor boxes; this dark environment helps to reduce stress levels during transportation. Raptors may also be brought to the practice on the falconer's arm 'hooded'. Birds of prey are sometimes trained to a hood. This covers the eyes but leaves the beak free and is useful for keeping the bird calm during transportation (Figure 1.9).
■ Chickens should be transported in a spacious cardboard box, lined with straw and with holes in the side for ventilation. A wire pet carrier could be used as an alternative but stress may be higher as the chicken can see its surroundings. Even though chickens generally get on well with other pets, an unfamiliar noisy waiting room may prove stressful.

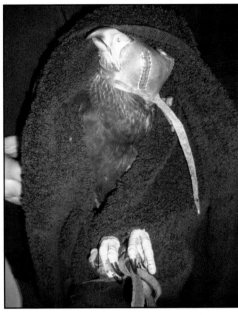

1.9

A hooded Harris' hawk.

Reptiles

The owner should be told to bring their pet to the practice as soon as possible if they report them to be showing one or more of the following clinical signs:

■ Acute collapse, not moving, unable to hold its head up
■ Dyspnoea, open-mouth breathing
■ Fluid coming from the mouth
■ Straining to pass faeces or unable to defecate/urinate
■ Prolapse from the cloaca
■ Traumatic injury, e.g. bitten by a dog or cage mate, road traffic accident
■ Seizures, twitching or has fallen from a branch
■ Bloody, foul-smelling, watery faeces.

If in doubt as to whether a reptile should be seen as an emergency, it is best to be cautious and advise the owner to bring the animal to the practice as soon as possible. It is, however, advisable to ascertain the species, size and any special considerations (e.g. whether it is venomous) before advising an urgent visit to the practice, in order for any specific requirements to be addressed. If the reptile is huge or venomous and the surgery is neither suitably equipped nor has specifically trained staff, the owner should be redirected to practitioners who can handle it.

An owner managing a common reptilian emergency should be given the following important advice:

- Keep the animal warm (except in the case of hyperthermia)
- Keep any wounds clean and apply pressure if actively bleeding
- Keep any prolapsed viscera clean and moist (apply petroleum jelly or keep in water)
- If the reptile is fitting, place it in a padded container to prevent injury during transportation.

When giving advice to owners, it is important to convey that the most important consideration when transporting a reptile is the maintenance of the correct environmental temperature. Most reptiles' optimal environmental temperature lies between 22 and 30°C. The use of hot water bottles should be recommended to owners in colder months or if long distances are being travelled. Owners should be advised to avoid burns or overheating by preventing direct contact between the hot water bottle and their reptile by, for example, wrapping the hot water bottle in a towel.

Transport

The appropriate method of transport will depend on the species of reptile:

- Smaller lizards should be transported in a clear plastic container with a ventilated lid (Figure 1.10a). Branches are an appropriate addition for arboreal species
- Larger lizards (e.g. iguanas) should be transported in large cardboard boxes. These must be secure and large enough to contain the tail
- Depending on size, appropriate transportation of snakes varies from the use of a clear plastic container with a secure ventilated lid to the use of a pillowcase or quilt cover for the larger breeds. This will need to be securely tied in a knot to prevent escape (Figure 1.10b).
- Tortoises should be transported in pet carriers (Figure 1.10c); these should ideally be lined with newspaper as tortoises have a tendency to urinate when handled.

Wildlife

A call from the public regarding wildlife is more often than not an emergency. Wild animals will naturally hide away from people and so will only be noticed and captured if badly injured or diseased.

Foxes and badgers

Callers reporting larger wildlife such as foxes or badgers should be told to exercise caution and to stay a safe distance away from the animal; foxes and badgers naturally fear humans, so approaching them can be unpredictable and dangerous. If the animal is in a secure setting, e.g. a garden or field, the caller should be told to contact the RSPCA, as they will have specialist training and equipment to handle and transport the animal. If the injured fox or badger is

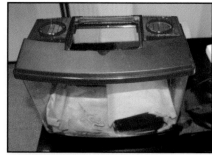
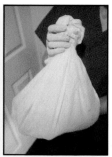
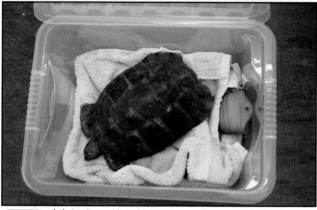

1.10 **(a)** A clear plastic transport box can be used to transport a leopard gecko. Kitchen towel (or similar) is a good substrate as it can easily be changed if it becomes soiled. Note the use of a wrapped heat pad. **(b)** A pillow case secured at the top can be used to transport small to medium-sized snakes. Larger snakes may require duvet covers. (Courtesy of Sarah Pellett) **(c)** Tortoises can be transported in open-topped plastic containers. Note the use of a hot water bottle, covered with a towel. (Courtesy of C. Dodd)

discovered in the road or on the roadside, the caller should be advised to move the animal at arm's length using a large blanket and with the use of heavy gloves. A 'fight or flight' response, however, could lead to the person getting bitten or scratched or the injured animal running back into the traffic. Transportation to the veterinary practice should be in a large pet carrier covered with a blanket to reduce stress and to keep noise to a minimum.

Common reasons for the emergency presentation of foxes and badgers are given in Figure 1.11. These animals are unlikely to allow capture unless seriously debilitated and will often avoid any unnecessary trips away from their earth or sett if debilitated. Any

Species	Common reasons for emergency presentation
Foxes	Road traffic collision (RTC) and associated trauma Mange Gunshot wounds and snare injuries Infectious diseases, e.g. leptospirosis 'Orphaned' fox cubs
Badgers	RTCs and associated trauma Territorial rump wounds and abscesses Myiasis Snare and trapping injuries Infectious diseases causing debilitation, e.g. tuberculosis

1.11 Common reasons for the emergency presentation of foxes and badgers.

animals that are captured are likely to be in the later stages of disease, unless they have sustained a traumatic injury that has left them in shock and unable to escape.

Hedgehogs

Hedgehogs are much slower than the majority of other wildlife and are therefore more likely to be brought in by a member of the public. They are nocturnal, so spotting them during the day can lead to the suspicion that they are injured. If a caller reports a hedgehog as having an obvious injury, they should be told to bring the animal into the veterinary practice. Callers should be told that it is advisable to wear gloves when handling hedgehogs (Figure 1.12), as they are a common carrier of ringworm. Placing them in a cardboard box lined with newspaper and hay should be advised.

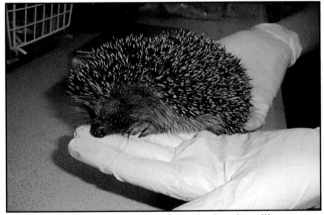

1.12 Wearing gloves is advised when handling hedgehogs.

Squirrels

Squirrels are exceedingly fast-moving creatures; if they have been rescued by a member of the public it is likely that they are badly injured or diseased. It is an offence for any person to release or allow to escape into the wild any animal included in Part 1 of Schedule 9 of the Wildlife and Countryside Act 1981 (which includes the grey squirrel). Special licences may be issued for up to 5 years to keep grey squirrels in captivity but certain specific conditions must be met. This licence is not required for care within the veterinary practice; however, the laws regarding release still apply (see further reading). The advice to the general public would be to leave the squirrel in the wild or bring it to the practice for euthanasia if badly injured.

Wild birds

Of the calls to veterinary practice regarding wildlife, reports of injured birds are the most common. Common reasons for emergency presentation of different groups of wild birds are given in Figure 1.13.

Birds such as pigeons and magpies often have injuries caused by cats or from flying into windows. If the caller reports that the bird has an obvious injury, they should be told to bring it to the veterinary practice for examination. If the bird is just suffering

Type of bird	Common reasons for emergency presentation
Garden birds	Found on ground – possibly due to trauma or weakness secondary to infection, e.g. *Trichomonas* or *Salmonella* infections Nestling/fledgling Traumatic, e.g. flew into window, attacked by a cat
Seabirds	Fishing hook or line attached to them Flown off track Oiled Traumatic
Raptors	Ocular damage Starvation Traumatic injuries, e.g. fractures, damage to feathers Unable to fly
Waterfowl	Botulism Bumblefoot Fishing hook and line injuries Toxins, e.g. lead poisoning, oil contamination (see Figure 1.46) Traumatic injuries, e.g. flown into powerlines

1.13 Common reasons for emergency presentation of different groups of wild birds.

from shock, the caller should be told to place the bird in a cardboard box high up on a wall; this will give it time to recover without the threat of being attacked by other animals such as cats. The caller should also be advised to offer the bird food and water.

Baby birds or fledglings are often found on the ground after falling from their nests. Callers reporting such incidents should be told to place the fledgling in a safe position, if possible away from any cats, near to where it was found, so that the parents can return and continue their care. Callers should be told not to bring baby birds to the veterinary practice unless badly injured and requiring euthanasia.

Callers reporting injured swans should be told to contact the RSPCA. They will have specialist equipment for restraint, e.g. the swan hook and bag (Figures 1.14 and 1.15), the use of which will avoid injury to the handler and the bird.

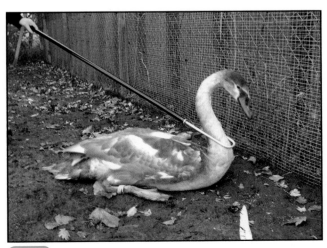

1.14 A swan hook in use.

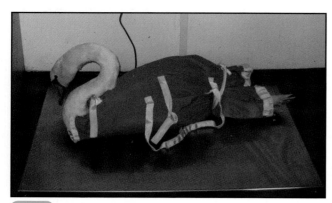

1.15 A swan bag.

Strategies for making the practice a less stressful place

All animals that are brought to the veterinary practice will be anxious due to the unfamiliar surroundings. To reduce the levels of anxiety, their time at the practice should be as stress-free as possible. The following general principles should be adhered to for all areas of the practice:

- For many species, including most birds and small mammals, stress levels can be reduced by subdued lighting and reduced noise
- Predator and prey species should be kept away from each other as much as possible.

The waiting room

- Certain species should be kept away from others. For example, ferrets should be kept away from rabbits. Ferrets are natural predators of rabbits and even their lingering smell can prove stressful for rabbits. Birds of prey should also be kept away from small mammal species due to their predatory nature.
- Having a separate waiting room for cats and dogs, away from exotic pets, is an ideal solution (Figure 1.16). If the waiting room door can be closed, the ambience can be maintained.

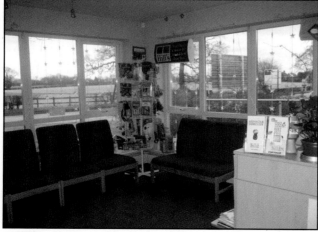

1.16 Having a separate waiting room for exotic pets will reduce stress levels.

The consulting room

- A different consulting room should be used if a ferret is due to be seen before a rabbit. Ideally they should be booked in at different times.
- Once the patient has been taken out of its cage/carrier, doors and windows should be kept closed to prevent it from escaping.
- Computer screens must be turned off in the consulting room when handling chipmunks due to this species' sensitivity to television, possibly due to the electromagnetic and ultrasonic radiation from the 15.6 kHz time-based oscillator.
- The stress levels of passerine birds can be reduced by dimmed lighting or by the use of red or blue lighting.
- Having the necessary equipment ready in the room will reduce the time of handling and therefore reduce stress levels.

The hospital ward

- Certain species should be housed separately from others. For example, raptors should not be positioned opposite or near prey species such as rabbits.
- Birds should be positioned in separate air spaces to avoid the transmission of diseases.

Assisting in obtaining a history

When the client arrives at the veterinary practice, a registration form must be completed plus a husbandry questionnaire. This will ascertain the history of the patient and can aid in the veterinary surgeon's diagnosis and treatment.

Client questionnaires

As much information as possible about the animal's normal home environment, husbandry and diet should be sought, as this forms a vital element in the diagnostic process, plan for nursing care and decisions regarding treatment. This is of particular importance in exotic species, where correct husbandry is crucial. Much of this information can be gained with the use of client questionnaires. The following is a list of the type of information that will be asked for in a client questionnaire, among more specific questions:

- Owner's details
- Pet's details
- Where the pet was sourced from
- Housing details
- Diet
- Duration of clinical signs
- Progression and type of clinical signs
- Treatments already given.

Examples of client questionnaires can be found at the end of this chapter.

Wildlife history

It is almost impossible to obtain the history of wildlife cases as most of these animals are brought into the practice with injury or illness and have never been observed in their natural habitat. In most cases the veterinary surgeon must therefore physically examine the animal for any information. However, if the animal has been in and around the client's garden then some information may be obtained, for example:

- Has the hedgehog been visible during the daytime? If so, for how long? (As a nocturnal creature this is not normal behaviour)
- Has the urban fox visibly lost weight or suffered from fur loss, indicative of mange or other diseases?

Any information that can be gathered might prove useful. The contact details of the person who found the animal and the location at which it was found are important pieces of information, both for when the animal improves enough to be released and for legal reasons.

Handling techniques

Small mammals

Rabbits

> **KEY POINT**
> Rabbits will be under increased stress if they pick up the scent of a predator species such as a ferret. Therefore, hand washing between patients, whilst always important when handling any species, is imperative. It may also be appropriate to change clothes between such species.

Rabbits must be restrained with extreme caution as they can react quickly and aggressively if frightened. The tame rabbit can be picked up by placing one hand under the chest and supporting the hindlegs with the other hand. The aggressive rabbit can cause damage to the handler with its claws and incisors. It can also cause damage to itself by 'thumping' with its hindlimbs and fracturing its spine. Handling an aggressive rabbit can be made easier by using a towel (Figure 1.17).

Once the rabbit has been captured it can be restrained in several different ways. Holding the rabbit in dorsal recumbency whilst it is wrapped securely in a towel with its head protruding enables syringe-feeding (Figure 1.18a) and medications to be administered. The advantage to this position is that the substances being administered are falling with gravity, so their loss is minimal. However, as a prey animal, this position can make the rabbit feel more vulnerable. Also, while this is a safe position to use in most rabbits (as they are obligate nasal breathers), it should not be used in other species (or in dyspnoeic rabbits) as there is a risk of aspiration.

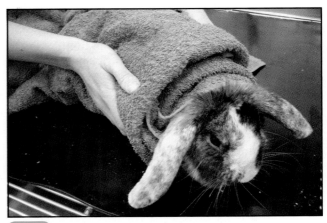

1.17 A rabbit wrapped securely in a towel.

Holding the rabbit in sternal recumbency with its head buried under the handler's arm and the body resting along the forearm and held closely to the chest is a more favourable position for the rabbit (Figure 1.18b). The hindlegs can then be held with the other hand to aid in blood sampling. It is important that the rabbit can breathe if the head is buried in the handler's arm and also that the rabbit does not overheat. Rabbits do not possess a significant number of sweat glands and do not naturally pant; overheating can therefore lead to fatalities.

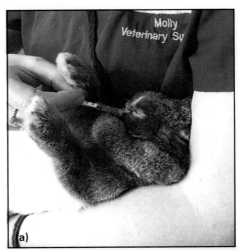

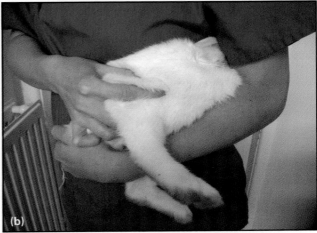

1.18 (a) Restraint of a rabbit in dorsal recumbency for syringe-feeding. (b) Restraint of a rabbit in sternal recumbency for blood sampling.

Rodents

Rodents should be handled firmly, gently and with confidence. It is advisable to examine them close to the tabletop so that if the patient jumps or is dropped it will reduce the chance of an injury. Placing the rodent on the table will encourage it to release its grip if it does happen to bite.

Mice

Mice are renowned for biting, especially if being handled by a stranger in unfamiliar surroundings. Grasping the tail near to the base and positioning the mouse on to a non-slip surface is recommended (Figure 1.19a). To avoid being bitten, the scruff should be grasped firmly between thumb and forefinger (Figure 1.19b). Mice can be difficult to catch and examine without scruffing.

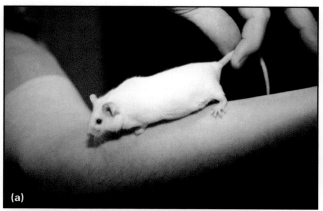

(a)

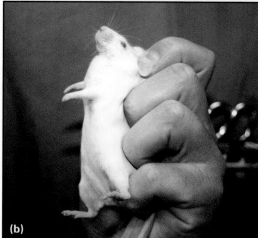

(b)

1.19 **(a)** Mice can be restrained by lifting them by the base of the tail, supporting the forelimbs once lifted. **(b)** Scruffing may occasionally be required.

Rats

Rats are less likely to bite due to their increased socialization, but as they are nocturnal it is advisable to check the animal is awake before trying to pick it up. They should be grasped around the shoulders, holding the hindfeet with the other hand to support their weight (Figure 1.20). If the rat needs more restraint, the base of the tail can be grasped before scruffing with thumb and forefinger.

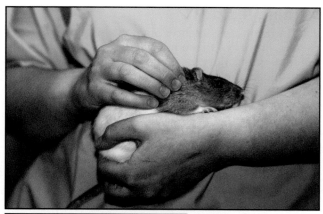

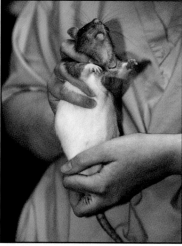

1.20 Rats can be restrained by grasping them around the shoulders, with the other hand holding the hindfeet.

Hamsters

Hamsters characteristically bite. Like rats, they are nocturnal and so it is advisable to ensure the patient is awake before trying to handle it. The Russian hamster is more aggressive than other breeds. A tame hamster can be cupped between the hands. The aggressive hamster should be placed on to a non-slip surface, and gentle but firm pressure placed on to the scruff with the finger and thumb of one hand. Scruffing (Figure 1.21) should only be used on an aggressive patient or for administering medications as there is a risk that the eyes may prolapse.

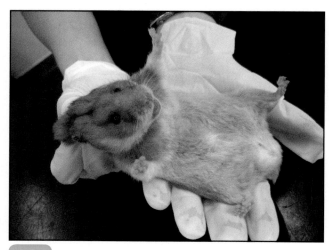

1.21 Scruffing a hamster.

Gerbils

Gerbils rarely bite but can jump if frightened. They can be handled like the hamster using the cupping technique. The more aggressive patient should be grasped by the scruff between the thumb and forefinger of one hand. Gerbils should never be lifted by the tail as degloving injuries may occur.

Guinea pigs

Guinea pigs are fairly easy to restrain once caught. They move at high speeds, especially if they are in unfamiliar surroundings and have been separated from their companions. The risk of spinal damage can be reduced by grasping the guinea pig firmly around its shoulders while supporting the hindquarters (Figure 1.22). Putting pressure on the guinea pig's large abdomen should be avoided. The chest and shoulders should be raised if the dorsal recumbency position is to be used.

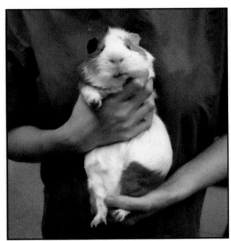

1.22 Supporting the hindquarters of a guinea pig will prevent spinal damage.

Chinchillas

Chinchillas are fast-moving like guinea pigs but, again, once capture is successful the restraint is minimal. Subdued lighting and reduced noise will aid in their capture. They should be held gently around the chest, just behind the forelegs, while the other hand supports the hindlegs (Figure 1.23). Grasping the base of the tail and supporting the body with the other hand is an alternative restraint technique. Scruffing

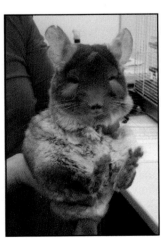

1.23 Chinchillas should be held gently around the chest and be supported around their pelvis and hindlegs. (Courtesy of J. Hedley)

the chinchilla will result in fur loss, known as 'fur slip', and so must never be attempted; this would result in a bald patch, which could take weeks to re-grow.

Degus

Restraint of degus is similar to that of chinchillas. They should be examined on a non-slip surface and weighed in a container, as they can bite and jump off the scales.

Chipmunks

Chipmunks are extremely 'highly strung' and have the potential to bite. A lightweight, dark net should be used to catch the chipmunk initially; it can then be quickly scruffed or carefully grasped around the shoulders. Degloving injuries can occur if a chipmunk is held by the tail. Occasionally, it may be possible for hand-reared chipmunks to be cupped in the hands.

Ferrets

Ferrets that are tame and used to being handled can be picked up by placing one hand around the chest and using the other hand under the hindlimbs as support (Figure 1.24). The more aggressive, hunting ferret should be scruffed firmly at the back of the neck, using the other hand to hold around the pelvis. They can be distracted easily using food treats if a simple procedure is being performed.

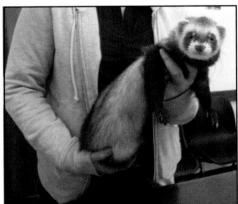

1.24 Handling a tame ferret.

Sugar gliders

A sugar glider can be restrained by grasping the scruff of its neck and holding it in a towel (Figure 1.25). Handlers must be aware that sugar gliders may twist around to bite.

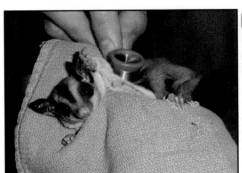

1.25 Restraint of a sugar glider using a towel.

Birds

> **KEY POINT**
> The veterinary surgeon or nurse should not attempt to handle a bird until a thorough history has been obtained from the owner. The bird should be observed in its carrier while the history is being taken. This will avoid any surprises if the bird is very poorly and the owner can be warned of the possibility that the stress of handling may lead to a fatality.

When attempting to restrain birds, dimming the lights or shutting the curtains will calm those that are diurnal in nature. Reducing noise levels is also advisable when dealing with birds. To speed up the capture and to reduce stress levels, all objects should be removed from the transport box. If this is the bird's cage then toys, perches and water and food bowls should all be removed. This will make the capture easier and safer for the bird and the veterinary surgeon. All equipment needed for the examination must be ready to reduce the time needed for restraint, and questions from the clients should be answered after the examination so as not to increase the time spent handling the bird.

Psittacine birds

Restraint of psittacine birds such as macaws should be focused on the extremely powerful hooked beak. The extreme power is due to the kinetic joint, a hinge mechanism that is present where the upper beak joins the skull. The use of a towel is advised for medium to larger parrots, e.g. the Amazon parrot and the African grey (Figure 1.26). For smaller species, such as the budgerigar, a duster or handkerchief will suffice.

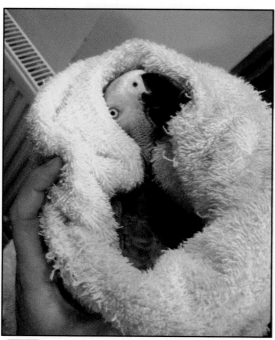

1.26 Restraint of an African grey parrot in a towel.

> **How to restrain a parrot**
> 1. Approach the parrot with confidence and without hesitation. If the perches have been removed then the parrot will be on the floor or sides of the cage.
> 2. Place the towel over the bird and restrain it firmly but gently around its neck.
> 3. Position the thumb and forefingers underneath the lower beak and push upwards to prevent biting. In smaller birds, hold the neck between the index finger and middle finger. The thumb and forefinger can then be used for manipulating the legs or wings.
> 4. Once the bird's neck has been restrained, wrap the towel around the wings and claws to prevent the bird from damaging itself and the handler.

Quite often parrots, especially the Amazon breed, will prevent capture by lying on their backs with their feet in the air, preventing the handler from grasping their neck. Tipping the cage on to its side should encourage the bird to grab the cage sides with its beak, thereby allowing capture from behind.

> **KEY POINT**
> Once a bird has been captured, restraint must be gentle as it requires the outward movement of the ribcage for inspiration. The lungs of all bird species have a rigid structure and there is no functional diaphragm present. Air is drawn into the lungs by inflating the air sacs; overzealous handling will prevent this from happening and may result in a fatality.

Passerine birds

Restraint of passerine birds such as the mynah bird is very similar to that of psittacine birds. Their beaks are less powerful but may still cause damage.

Raptors

When the falconer arrives at the practice, the bird will usually be hooded (see Figure 1.9). The hood covers the eyes but leaves the beak free and is useful for keeping the bird calm. They will either be transported in a raptor box or brought in on the falconer's arm using leather gauntlets. Many raptors will also have jesses on their legs; these are leather straps attached to their ankles which allow the bird to be restrained while on the falconer's arm. To encourage the bird to step on to the gauntleted arm, it must be placed in front of and slightly raised from the surface the bird is already standing on, as they naturally step up on to surfaces. The jesses are then held between the thumb and forefinger to prevent the bird flying away.

Restraint of raptors such as the Harris' hawk is focused on the feet. The talons are very powerful and sharp, as they are used in the wild for catching prey and then ripping the meat. They can do serious damage to the inexperienced handler. The beak can also be dangerous in larger species such as eagles.

To 'cast', the bird's shoulders are grasped from behind using a towel, holding the wings against the body with the thumbs and first two fingers of each hand (Figure 1.27). The remaining fingers restrain the legs as far down as possible and must be placed between the legs to avoid the bird grasping itself and injuring its legs or feet. If a hood has not been placed then the towel can be used to reduce the light and stress levels. Again, as with psittacine birds, the restraint must be gentle to allow sternal movement for breathing and therefore avoid suffocation.

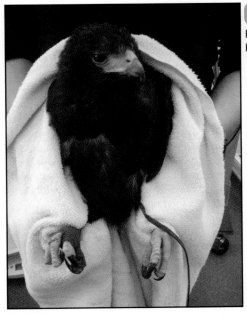

1.27 Restraint of a Harris' hawk.

Owls

Restraint of the owl is fairly similar to that of the other raptors. However, because they are nocturnal, hoods and dimly lit rooms will have no effect in reducing stress. They can be relatively docile so restraint in these circumstances is generally kept to a minimum (Figure 1.28). Some owls can be aggressive and will scratch and bite, especially feisty wild tawny owls and the larger eagle owls. These will require more restraint.

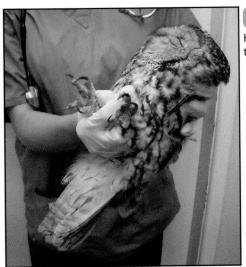

1.28 Handling a tawny owl.

Waterfowl

Occasionally ducks (Figure 1.29), geese and swans are brought to the veterinary practice. Geese and swans are very strong birds and may flap their wings and bite. Swans in particular can be very dangerous if able to flap their very powerful wings. To restrain a goose or swan, a cloth or towel can be placed over the body to contain the wings to avoid damage to the bird and handler, then the bird can be 'scooped up' and its body held against the handler's body tucked under one arm. Gently hold around the neck just below the head to prevent biting. A cloth gently placed over the head may have a calming effect. Smaller ducks can be handled in much the same way as chickens (see below).

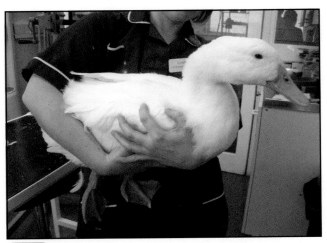

1.29 Restraint of an Aylesbury-cross duck.

Pigeons

Restraint of pigeons needs to be fairly gentle. Their peck is not painful, so restraint of the head is not necessary. Placing both hands around the body dorsally will keep the wings safely against the bird's body. The 'racing pigeon hold' involves placing the feet through the gap between the index and middle finger of one hand that is also supporting the breast and holding the wings (Figure 1.30).

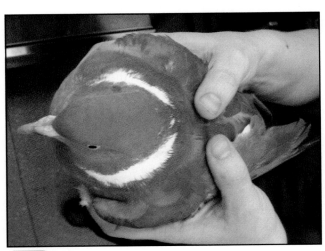

1.30 Gentle handling of a pigeon.

Poultry

Restraint of the chicken is quite gentle and quick movements must be avoided. Both hands are used to take a firm hold of the body, holding the wings against the body so that they cannot flap. Holding the chicken against the handler's body and supporting the chicken's weight with one hand is advised (Figure 1.31).

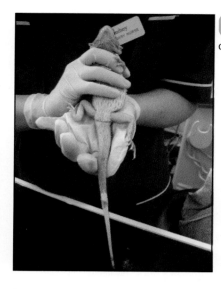

1.32 Handling a bearded dragon.

Iguanas

The green iguana can be quite aggressive and, in addition to the dangers of its teeth and claws, it can also use its tail like a whip to lash out at the handler. The use of a large towel can aid in the capture before restraining as described for bearded dragons and geckos (Figure 1.33).

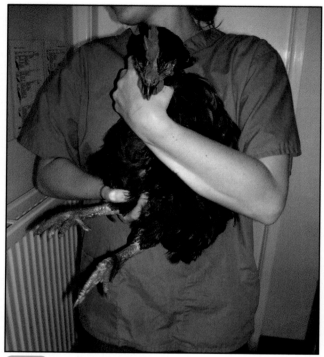

1.31 Restraint of a chicken.

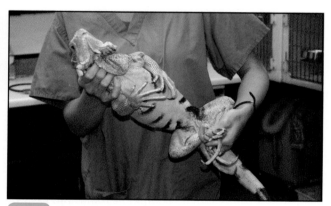

1.33 Handling an iguana.

Reptiles

Lizards

Claws and teeth are the two danger zones when handling a lizard. Control of the head will prevent the animal from biting, and covering the head will have a calming effect. Restraint of the limbs will prevent scratching and can be achieved by bringing one hand around the chest and restraining one forelimb with the forefinger and thumb and the other between the third and fourth finger. The other hand must grasp the lower back, again controlling one hindlimb with the thumb and forefinger and the other with the third and fourth finger. The lizard can then be held upright for blood sampling from its tail. The tail of a large lizard can be placed underneath the handler's arms.

Bearded dragons and geckos

These are generally docile lizards and need minimal restraint (Figure 1.32), with the exception of the tokay gecko, which can give a painful bite. They can be picked up by the handler cupping the hands under their abdomen, placing the index finger up towards their neck between their forelegs, and resting their rear end on the handler's arm. Day geckos are extremely fragile and are best examined in a clear plastic container and not handled.

The vasovagal reflex may be utilized to subdue the aggressive lizard. By placing cotton-wool pads over the eyes and securing them with a bandage (Figure 1.34), the pressure applied stimulates the parasympathetic autonomic nervous system. Heart rate, blood pressure and respiration rate reduce and procedures such as radiography can be performed. Stimuli such as noise and touch will return the lizard back to its normal state.

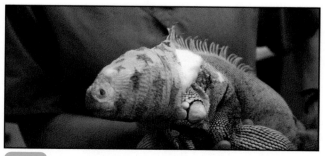

1.34 The vasovagal reflex used in the iguana.

Points to remember when handling lizards

- Wear gloves and then wash your hands, as *Salmonella* is present on reptile skin.
- Never restrain a lizard by its tail; 'autotomy' (shedding of the tail) will result. This is done in the wild to confuse the attacker and offer an easy meal. The tail will re-grow eventually but will never look as good as the original. The green iguana will only re-grow its tail as a juvenile, up to 3 years old.
- Overzealous restraint can lead to serious injury if the lizard is suffering from metabolic bone disease and therefore has a fragile skeleton, liable to spontaneous fracture.
- Like birds, lizards lack a diaphragm. This can result in the digestive system encroaching into the lung space and increasing inspiratory effort if handled inappropriately.

Snakes

Restraint of snakes concentrates on the head, as the main danger is their bite. By placing the thumb over the back of the skull and curling the fingers under the chin, the head can be controlled (Figure 1.35). The rest of the snake's body should be supported in a number of places along its length.

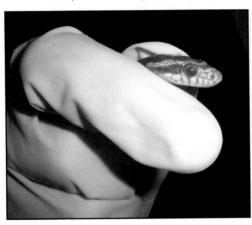

1.35 The head of the snake must be restrained.

Larger snakes

Several handlers must be present for snakes over 2 metres long, e.g. the boa constrictor and the Burmese python. Asphyxiation is a potential danger, as the snake can wind itself around the handler's chest or neck. Unwinding the snake must be done from the tail end.

Venomous snakes

It is very important to obtain as much information as possible about the species prior to handling in order to best assess risk factors. Handling should be performed by at least two personnel who are competent and well experienced with reptiles. It is important to be prepared; an agreed emergency protocol and training of all staff could prove to be life-saving if a venomous bite occurs. Preparation should also include research into healthcare and contact details for zoo professionals experienced in treating venomous bites, who can be a point of contact in an emergency and can provide an antivenom if needed. Practices in areas where venomous snakes are indigenous may have antivenom on site.

Restraint of a poisonous snake should be carried out using a snake hook, which is a steel rod with a blunt shepherd's crook at one end. Snake hooks are used to loop under the body of the snake in order to move it into a container at arm's length. The handler can use the hook to trap the head flat on the floor and can then grasp it with their hand. (NB Venomous lizards such as the beaded lizard and Gila monster can be restrained using the same method.)

If a snake is presented in a bag, large gripping tongs (longer than arm's length) should be used to manipulate the bag to prevent bites through the material. Clear plastic tubes are very useful for restraint; the head and cranial portion of the snake can be safely contained in the tube, leaving the rest free for examination.

If there are any doubts regarding the practice's capabilities of handling venomous species, such animals should be referred directly to another practice that can handle them appropriately.

Tortoises

Most tortoises are easily handled using both hands to hold both sides of the shell behind the front legs (Figure 1.36). Tortoises should never be left on a tabletop as they can move quickly and so may end up on the floor. The only danger presented when handling the larger tortoises is that they can retract their legs into their bodies, leading to trapped fingers between the tortoise's legs and its shell.

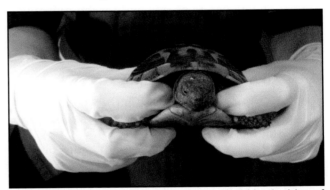

1.36 Both hands should be used to hold both sides of the tortoise's shell, behind the front legs.

Turtles and terrapins

These can be restrained as for tortoises but more care is needed as they are renowned for biting due to their mobile necks. A net can be used to remove aquatic turtles from the water. Soft-shelled and aquatic species are best handled with soft cloths or gloves so as not to mark the shell.

Amphibians

Due to the sensitivity of amphibians' skin to the oils in human hands, handling must be kept to a minimum. Amphibians should be moved using clean, rinsed hands or latex gloves. They can also be moved by using fine fish nets. Larger amphibians may need to be sedated for safe transportation to the practice.

Wildlife

Foxes

The fox's head needs immediate restraint when handling. The teeth are very sharp and can lead to a nasty bite. A large towel must be thrown over the fox and the neck grasped with both hands. Care must be taken with handling because the frame of a fox resembles that of a cat rather than a dog, and fractures of limbs or ribs are possible from rough handling.

Badgers

Restraint of the badger is achieved most successfully with the use of a 'dogcatcher' pole snare. Badgers have extremely powerful jaws, which can cause serious damage to an inexperienced handler. They can also use their claws to scratch. A thick towel and heavy gloves can be used to restrain the badger, applying pressure to either side of the neck region just in front of the shoulders. Unless the patient is severely debilitated, manual restraint is limited and the use of chemical restraint is essential for examination. Tuberculosis is a potential zoonotic risk to the handler.

Hedgehogs

Restraint of the hedgehog is minimal as they are rarely aggressive. Their defence mechanism is to curl up in a ball and it can be quite difficult to coax them out of this position. Wearing gloves is advisable for protection against its spines and for the prevention of the spread of ringworm, which they commonly carry on their skin and spines.

How to uncurl a hedgehog

- Place it on the floor and wait for it to show an interest in the surroundings, uncurl and walk around; or
- Bounce it gently in your (gloved) hands or stroke its spines firmly from neck to rump. This should make it begin to uncurl. Once the hedgehog has uncurled, allow its front feet to come into contact with a surface (preferably with some grip). Grip its hindfeet gently as if to 'wheelbarrow' it around. This allows good inspection of the head, ventrum and legs.

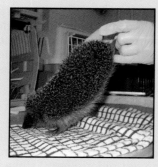

The 'wheelbarrow' approach used for examining hedgehogs.

Squirrels

Restraint of the squirrel involves scruffing the neck with one hand, whilst the other hand supports the hindlimbs. They have a tendency to bite so the use of heavy gloves or a thick towel is recommended. Subdued lighting will aid capture, as squirrels are diurnal. Like the gerbil, a squirrel should never be restrained by the tail as a degloving injury may occur. There is a risk of catching leptospirosis from the squirrel, which can be reduced by wearing gloves, careful hand hygiene and avoidance of bites.

Bats

Restraint of the bat must concentrate on the head as bats can bite with their sharp teeth. Placing a thumb underneath the chin pushes the lower jaw upwards and reduces the chances of being bitten.

 WARNING
Gloves must be worn when handling bats as they may carry the lyssavirus, which is closely related to the rabies virus.

Wild birds

Wild birds such as pigeons and magpies are probably the most common wild animals brought into the veterinary practice. Handling and restraint will be the same as for the bird species brought in as pets (see earlier).

Swans are the most difficult to restrain due to their long necks. Restraint must initially be of the head, achieved by grasping the upper neck from behind, curling the fingers around the neck and supporting the back of the neck with the thumb. A swan hook can also be used to catch the neck high up under the bill (see Figure 1.14). Once captured, the wings must be restrained using a large towel wrapped around the sternum. Swan cradle bags are also often used to contain the body and wings, leaving the head, neck and feet free (see Figure 1.15).

Triage

On arrival at the practice, animals should be assessed to determine the priority and urgency of treatment based on the seriousness of their condition, particularly if an urgent appointment had been arranged following a telephone call to the surgery. Triage can greatly increase the chance of a positive outcome.

Small mammals

Determination and interpretation of vital signs in small mammals

Determination of vital signs in mammalian exotic and wildlife species is comparable to that of the more familiar domestic animals. Assessment of respiratory and heart rate should be carried out prior to handling. Normal respiratory and heart rates for mammalian species can be found in ▶

Chapter 2. Thoracic auscultation using a paediatric stethoscope will allow assessment of the heart rate and character, and of the lung fields. Pulses can be monitored using the femoral artery in smaller species and can be felt in the auricular arteries of rabbits.

Rectal temperature should be obtained at the start of the examination. A rabbit's temperature should be 38.5–40°C, and most rodents should have temperatures between 36 and 39°C. A ferret's temperature can range from 37.8 to 40°C.

Rabbits

Initial assessment

On arrival at the practice, a quick assessment of the patient by a nurse can be useful in determining how ill the animal is. It can be difficult to assess this, as some rabbits that are presented for routine consultations will be alert, looking around, standing on their hindlegs and keen to interact, whereas other more nervous animals will huddle in the corner of their carrying box trying to hide from view. Any animal that is obviously bloated, lying in lateral recumbency, passing watery diarrhoea or open-mouth breathing should be brought to the attention of the veterinary surgeon as soon as possible.

Physical examination

A quick physical examination can be very useful. This should include the following:

- Measure the heart rate
- Measure the respiratory rate
- Assess the mucous membrane colour and measure the capillary refill time
- Assess the hydration status (best done using the hairless skin in the inguinal region or the inside of the pinna)
- Assess the body condition
- Measure the rectal temperature
- Assess the abdomen for bloat.

Stabilization

It is important to assess any immediate life-threatening problems so that they can be addressed as quickly as possible, to improve the chances of a positive outcome (Figure 1.37).

Oxygen therapy

Most rabbits presented as emergencies will benefit from oxygen therapy. Oxygen chambers can be constructed by wrapping the animal's carrier in plastic bags or clingfilm. Purpose-designed incubators or plant propagators may also be used. Alternatively, an Elizabethan collar can be placed on the rabbit and clingfilm then stretched across the front. Oxygen can then be supplied into the collar to create an individual oxygen chamber.

Clinical sign	Action
Bloat	Start fluid therapy and pain relief (meloxicam dose of 0.6 mg/kg s.c. q12h or q24h). Place in oxygen-enriched environment
Diarrhoea	Assess hydration status and start fluid therapy as soon as possible
Dyspnoea	Place in oxygen-enriched environment. Give oxygen via facemask or directly from anaesthetic circuit if not too stressful. Increasing humidity can help to act as a mucolytic
Hyperthermia	Mild increases in rectal temperature can occur through stress. Any rabbit presenting with a temperature above 41°C should be cooled by spraying with cool water, wrapping in wet towels and giving cooled fluids
Hypothermia	Can occur in shocked animals. Increase the rabbit's temperature by placing in a warmed environment, e.g. an incubator, or by wrapping in towels, using hot water bottles or microwavable pads and wrapping bubble wrap around extremities. Be careful not to overheat the rabbit. Make sure any hot water bottles, etc. are not directly touching the rabbit's fur or skin as these can lead to thermal burns in collapsed animals
Myiasis	Clip and clean wounds; remove larvae manually. Initiate fluid therapy and pain relief (meloxicam dose as above)

1.37 Common emergency presentations and initial stabilization techniques for rabbits.

Fluid therapy

Dehydration is common on presentation. In anorexic rabbits with gut stasis, fluid therapy is essential to the initial treatment. See Chapter 6 for more information.

Rodents

Rodents that are commonly kept as pets in the UK include rats, mice, hamsters, gerbils, guinea pigs, chinchillas, degus and chipmunks. These are primarily prey species and, as such, hide signs of illness well, and often present in a collapsed state.

The general principles of assessment and treatment are similar for all rodents; however, techniques and decisions regarding their treatment will differ depending on the species, socialization, etc.

Initial assessment

Initial assessment of a rodent can provide a great deal of information, and should start with an assessment of the animal's general demeanour.

- Mice are generally very lively when in good health and will scurry around the carrying box trying to hide. Rats are usually slower moving and easier to handle than mice. Both rats and mice should be interested in their surroundings, alert and responsive to stimuli.
- Hamsters are nocturnal and are therefore likely to be asleep when presented at the practice. If suddenly awoken or startled a hamster can react

aggressively and possibly bite, so it is important to rouse them gently prior to handling. Once awake, a hamster should be alert and show interest in its new environment, walking around and sniffing.

- Gerbils and degus should normally be bright, alert and responsive when awake, especially in a new environment.
- Guinea pigs will often try to hide from view under the substrate in their carrying box, run around and vocalize. Most animals, apart from those that are very well handled, will vocalize when being lifted up and examined.
- Chinchillas are usually fairly lively animals. They will move around the carrying box to avoid being caught and can be wriggly to handle.
- Chipmunks are easily stressed animals and, unless they are in a torpid state on presentation or are well handled and used to human contact, they are unlikely to allow a thorough clinical examination without an anaesthetic. In their carrying box or cage they should be alert and show interest in their new surroundings.

General signs of ill thrift include slow movement, a dull, starey coat (greasy and unkempt, which implies a lack of grooming due to illness or injury) and a lack of interest in the surroundings. A rodent that is sitting still, reluctant to move once awake, hunched up with its eyes closed or breathing heavily is either very ill, cold or in a lot of discomfort or pain. In extreme circumstances these animals will be presented almost comatose, lying on their side or fitting.

Physical examination

A preliminary physical examination to assess the patient should be carried out while it is awake if possible. This should include the following:

- Measure heart rate – this is often difficult to count in smaller species but listening to the rhythm can be useful
- Measure respiratory rate and assess respiratory character
- Assess mucous membrane colour and capillary refill time – the colour of the feet (Figure 1.38) or tail can be useful as mucous membrane colour can be difficult to assess. Often an animal in respiratory distress or with cardiac disease will have pale extremities or a blue cyanotic tinge in extreme circumstances
- Assess hydration status
- Assess body condition
- Measure rectal temperature
- Check that the eyes are bright and alert with no discharge
- Assess abdomen for bloat.

Stabilization and fluid therapy

Any small mammals that are presented as emergency cases will benefit from being placed in a warm (20–26°C), oxygen-enriched environment, preferably in a dark quiet area, away from predators. It is important not to overheat these patients as they cannot sweat.

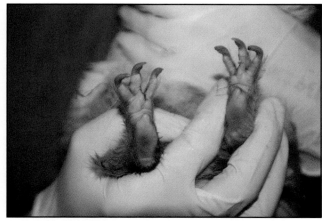

1.38 It is useful to look at the colour of the feet in rodents such as guinea pigs, as assessing mucous membrane colour can be difficult. (Courtesy of Sarah Pellett)

If small enough, a mouse, gerbil or hamster can be placed in a facemask to administer oxygen at high concentrations; however, this can have a considerable cooling effect.

The individual case assessment and the experience of the clinician are both important factors in assessing which route is most suitable for administration of fluids (see Chapter 6 for more information).

Species-specific problems

- **Hamsters** will hibernate if the environmental temperature drops below 10°C, so if it is difficult to rouse them (and for the majority of sick hamsters), it is beneficial to place them in a warm (20–25°C), oxygen-enriched environment.
- **Guinea pigs and chinchillas:**
  - Bloat, dyspnoea, hypothermia, hyperthermia and diarrhoea should be managed in the same way as for rabbits
  - Paraphimosis or fur ring is caused by an accumulation of matted fur that constricts around the penis inside the prepuce, leading to swelling of the penis (Figure 1.39). Gentle removal of the fur and re-placement of the

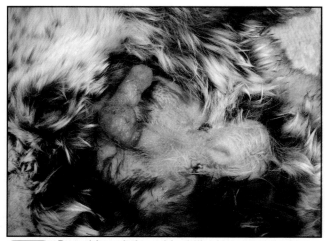

1.39 Paraphimosis in a chinchilla. Note the swollen penis distal to the constriction. (Courtesy of C. Dodd)

penis as soon as possible is recommended to prevent long-term damage and necrosis

- Any ill or hospitalized guinea pig should be given an exogenous source of vitamin C at 10 mg/kg/day orally, increasing to 30 mg/kg/day during pregnancy.

■ **Chipmunks** can enter a state of torpor during prolonged cold weather. They will be unresponsive to touch but, provided there is no underlying disease, will respond well to fluid therapy and gradual warming up.

Ferrets

Initial assessment

Ferrets normally sleep for prolonged periods of time and may well be asleep upon arrival at the practice. They should be allowed to wake up in their own time so that their normal behaviour can be assessed. Healthy animals will rouse and respond relatively quickly to noises, especially unfamiliar voices, and gentle movement of the bedding. They are usually keen to investigate their new surroundings and will be alert and interactive. If the animal is known to be collapsed or if they are unresponsive to their new surroundings, recumbent and unwilling to be roused, with profuse diarrhoea, or open-mouth breathing they should be regarded as emergencies and seen as soon as possible.

Physical examination

A physical examination should be carried out that includes the following:

■ Measure the heart rate and assess the heart rate character
■ Measure the respiratory rate and assess the respiratory character (best achieved before handling)
■ Assess mucous membrane colour and measure capillary refill time
■ Assess hydration status
■ Assess body condition
■ Measure rectal temperature.

Stabilization

■ Any collapsed ferret, unless suffering from hyperthermia, will benefit from being placed in a warm, oxygen-enriched environment.
■ If dehydrated or hypovolaemic, fluid therapy should be instigated as soon as possible to correct deficits.
■ Fitting, salivating and pawing at the mouth are all signs that can be associated with hypoglycaemia in ferrets; this is corrected very quickly by administration of sugar or glucose orally, or glucose solutions intravenously. Ideally, a blood glucose measurement should be taken prior to the administration of glucose.
■ Animals that are hyperthermic should be cooled gradually using wet cloths (not cold, as marked changes in temperature can induce shock), cool fluids and fans.

■ Status epilepticus seizures can usually be controlled by inducing anaesthesia.
■ Dyspnoeic animals will benefit from oxygen therapy and increased humidity. Nebulization is very useful initially and for long-term therapy.

Fluid therapy

Dehydration is a common finding on examination of most cases seen as emergencies. Fluids should always be warmed to body temperature prior to administration except in cases of hyperthermia. See Chapter 6 for more information.

Sugar gliders

Sugar gliders are small marsupials that require a large living area, to promote natural behaviour, and a specific diet that emulates their natural one of sap and gum of eucalyptus and acacia trees. It is particularly important that these dietary requirements are met, with most animals presented for diseases that have occurred secondary to poor diet and husbandry.

Sugar gliders are nocturnal and can enter a torpid state during the day (or if they get very cold), from which they can be difficult to rouse. With the correct restraint they should be amenable to conscious handling and examination. If they are well socialized they are likely to be inquisitive at the practice, but shy animals will attempt to hide away from view. They can be quite vocal, especially when alarmed or scared.

Before handling a sugar glider, it should first be observed to see how it moves around its carrying box. Healthy animals should be very agile. While sugar gliders may move slowly when cold, if they are still struggling to move normally once warmed this could be a sign of underlying musculoskeletal disease. A preliminary clinical examination should include measurement of heart rate, respiratory rate and rectal temperature, and assessment of mucous membrane colour (if possible), hydration status and body condition.

Any animal presented as an emergency will benefit from being placed in a warm (20–25°C) oxygen-enriched environment in a quiet, darkened room. For fluid requirements please refer to Chapter 6.

Birds

Initial assessment

On arrival at the practice, a quick assessment of the bird can be essential for determining how sick it is. A great amount can be learned by observing a bird from a distance for a few minutes when it arrives at the practice. Aside from critical patients, most birds will try to look as healthy as possible in new surroundings. Their guard can lapse after a few minutes, or sometimes leaving the bird alone and using remote observation can help to determine the true extent of a bird's illness; an alert bird can revert to looking fluffed up and lethargic when it is unaware of being watched.

Determination and interpretation of vital signs in birds

Normal respiratory and heart rates for various avian species can be found in Chapter 3. Birds in respiratory distress or circulatory failure may exhibit shallow breathing at a faster rate than normal. They can also be seen to open-mouth breathe or show marked inspiratory effort with obvious 'abdominal' involvement or 'tail bobbing' while perching. Any evidence of respiratory distress or depressed demeanour could indicate severe underlying disease. Although a quick diagnosis is often the key to a good recovery in many of these cases, this should be weighed up against how suitable a patient is for restraint for examination, anaesthesia and investigation.

Heart rate can be difficult to determine in small birds as it is often too fast to count. However, listening to the heart should not be overlooked as it can be useful in picking up arrhythmias and murmurs. Measuring heart rate in the larger psittacine birds, raptors and waterfowl is usually possible as the rate is generally slow enough to count. A stethoscope should be used to auscultate the heart, listening either over the pectoral muscles or dorsally.

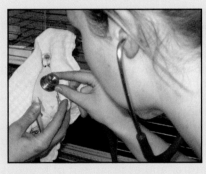

Using a paediatric stethoscope to listen to the heart of a budgerigar during clinical examination. (Courtesy of C. Dodd)

The pulse can be assessed easily in an anaesthetized bird and in larger species. It should be assessed for strength and any deficits in collapsed patients. The easiest place to assess the pulse is the brachial artery, which runs across the patagium just above the elbow joint. Gentle pressure should be applied as it can easily be occluded in smaller and collapsed patients.

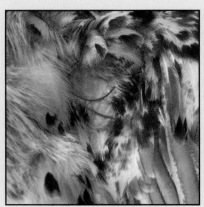

Position of the brachial artery (red line) and vein (blue line) with respect to the elbow joint in a chicken.

Blood pressure can be measured using either the wing or the leg. A paediatric cuff and Doppler ultrasound probe can be used. Systolic blood pressure has been found to range from 108 to 220 mmHg depending on the species.

Cloacal temperature can be assessed; however, reliable data have not been established for individual species or sizes of bird. Normal readings should be 41–44°C for most species. Readings significantly above or below this should be treated appropriately.

Stabilization

■ Collapsed, fluffed-up birds sitting on the bottom of their cages and those in respiratory distress should be placed immediately into a warm (30–40°C), oxygen-enriched critical care cage in a quiet, dimly lit area.
■ Unnecessary handling should be avoided until essential fluids, drugs, equipment and personnel have been gathered in preparation to carry out emergency treatment.
■ It may be safer to carry out emergency procedures in stages, allowing the bird to rest in between times.
■ Stabilization of a severely collapsed patient is likely to be essential prior to collecting diagnostic samples.
■ If the patient is bleeding, pressure should be applied to the wound until the bleeding has been stemmed.
■ If the bird is having a seizure, it should be placed in a padded cage, given drugs as instructed by a veterinary surgeon, e.g. calcium or diazepam, and should possibly be anaesthetized to stop the seizure.

Fluid therapy

Many birds presented as emergencies are likely to have been subclinically ill for some time. These birds may be hypovolaemic, dehydrated and in a negative energy balance. Fluid replacement is essential. The condition in which a patient presents will determine which route is most appropriate to administer fluids. Please refer to Chapter 6 for more information.

Crop tubing is an essential technique for all nurses dealing with hospitalized birds; it is the quickest way of administering fluids.

Crop tubing

1. Wrap the bird in a towel, or ask an assistant to hold the bird for you.
2. Where safe to do so, place a finger in the commissure of the beak to hold it open, allowing you to see the glottis at the back of the tongue. It is difficult to see the glottis in psittacine birds as they have a large fleshy tongue. A metal purpose-made crop tube, a soft piece of drip tubing or a wide-bore intravenous catheter (depending on the size and type of patient) can then be passed from ▶

the left of the bird over the back of the tongue, avoiding the glottis, down the oesophagus (on the right side of the neck) and into the crop. It should be possible to palpate the tube in the crop to ensure it is in the right place.

3. Watch for regurgitation at all times and stop straight away if noticed.

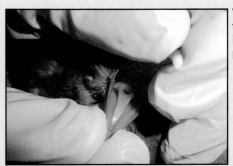

View of the glottis in a wood pigeon.

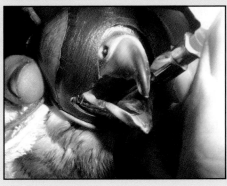

Placement of a crop tube in a red-naped shaheen.

Anorexic birds rapidly reach a negative energy balance and can quickly become very weak. Specialized oral avian fluids are available that will provide essential sugars and amino acids. Dehydration must be addressed on initial presentation but when this has been corrected, nutritional support must be started. Unless a bird begins eating on its own once it is rehydrated, feeding should be initiated by crop tubing (see Chapter 6). An easily absorbed food requiring minimal digestion should be chosen, ideally an avian hand-rearing food or recovery formula.

Intracoelomic (equivalent to intraperitoneal) fluids are not safe for use in birds, as their coelomic cavity involves a series of interconnecting air sacs, which are needed for respiration. Fluid placed into these areas would interfere with the respiratory system and in large volumes could potentially lead to death.

Hypothermia

Anorexic birds rapidly become hypothermic. Maintaining a normal body temperature can use vital energy. Placing all critical avian patients in a warm cage or incubator can help them conserve much needed energy. They should ideally be kept between 30 and 40°C (normal body temperature is 41–44°C).

Oxygen therapy

An oxygen-enriched environment will help most avian emergencies, especially dyspnoeic patients, to stabilize more rapidly. Providing oxygen via a facemask can be useful, although it may be stressful.

Reptiles

Initial assessment

Due to most reptiles' rather stoical nature, illness and disease often go unnoticed for long periods of time. Many patients that are presented in an acute state of collapse may have been suffering for a lengthy period of time and so may actually be in the terminal stages of an illness. These cases need initial stabilization, which is often the same, independent of the underlying cause of illness.

On arrival at the practice it is often useful for the animal to be brought into the treatment room or assessed by a nurse as soon as possible. If a veterinary surgeon is not immediately free and the reptile is stable then it should be placed in a warmed vivarium or incubator. If an animal is in a collapsed state then a quick physical examination should be carried out, paying particular attention to the vital signs:

- Is this animal alive? Assessment of whether a reptile is alive can be challenging. If a Doppler ultrasound probe is available this can be used to detect a heart beat or pulse. The glottis should also be checked (Figure 1.40). At rest the glottis should be closed. If it is found to be open and not moving then the animal is likely to be dead but this should be confirmed using a Doppler ultrasound probe. Many practices have these as part of blood pressure monitoring equipment. Alternatively, auscultation with a stethoscope is possible. Noise from movement of skin scales may be reduced by placing a thin, damp cloth between the stethoscope and the skin.
- Is there a heart beat? What is the heart rate?
- Is the animal breathing? What is the respiratory rate?
- What is the mucous membrane colour? This can be difficult to assess as there may be a great variation in pigmentation, even in animals of the same species
- What is the animal's weight and body condition?

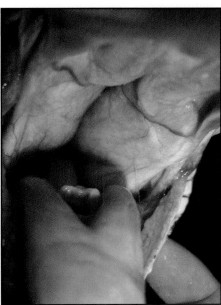

1.40

View of an open glottis in an iguana. This is comparable with other reptilian species. (Courtesy of C. Dodd)

Determination and interpretation of vital signs in reptiles

Respiratory rate should always be assessed prior to handling a patient. Normal respiratory and heart rates for reptiles can be found in Chapter 4. Excessive rib movements and open-mouth breathing might be seen in lizards and snakes with respiratory disease. Dyspnoeic tortoises show exaggerated limb movements in and out of their shell in order to move air as efficiently as possible through their lungs. Excess respiratory secretions may be seen either at the nose or in the mouth.

Heart rate and character is best assessed using a Doppler ultrasound probe, although auscultation can be carried out in snakes and lizards. In snakes the heart is located in the cranial third of the body and can be seen and palpated in thin individuals. In most lizards the heart is located cranially in the thoracic cavity and the stethoscope or Doppler ultrasound probe is best placed between the front limbs. In monitor lizards it is found more caudally. Auscultation is difficult in chelonians due to their shells. Using a Doppler ultrasound probe placed at the thoracic inlet should enable the heart to be assessed.

Cloacal temperatures is not a useful clinical parameter as these animals are ectothermic and readings will vary depending on the environmental temperature at the time of presentation.

Stabilization

Emergency procedures should be started if necessary. These can include:

- Resuscitation
- Placement of an endotracheal tube (ETT) (Figure 1.41) to commence intermittent positive pressure ventilation (IPPV)
- Removal of respiratory fluids using gravity
- Application of pressure to actively bleeding wounds and cleaning if contaminated.

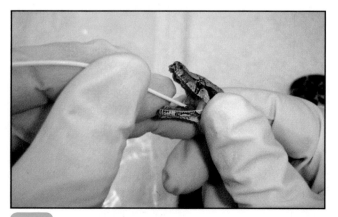

1.41 Intubation of a snake. (Courtesy of C. Dodd)

These procedures may need to be carried out prior to taking a detailed history.

Thermoregulation

A collapsed reptile should be warmed up slowly if it is cold on presentation. If it is suffering from hyperthermia it should be cooled down slowly using tepid water, cool towels and by placing it in an environment at the cool end of its preferred optimum temperature range (POTR).

> ⚠️ **WARNING**
> **Do not place a collapsed reptile directly under or on top of a heat source as it may not be able to move away and could end up with hyperthermia or burns.**

Fluid therapy

Many reptiles presented as emergencies have been subclinically ill for some time, and will often have substandard husbandry conditions that can lead to severe dehydration over prolonged periods. This can lead to hypovolaemia and renal damage. Providing circulatory support as soon as possible is therefore essential (see Chapter 6).

Re-feeding syndrome

A malnourished reptile should be re-introduced to nutritional support slowly. This is to prevent re-feeding syndrome, a condition that can cause life-threatening hypophosphataemia and hypokalaemia as the cellular uptake of phosphate and potassium ions is suddenly increased due to insulin stimulation. To avoid this, animals that are anuric (have not urinated in the previous 10 days) should be given only water initially, by mouth, until they urinate. Fluids should also be given by the intraosseous or epicoelomic routes, with total fluid rates of up to 4 ml/100 g/day until urination occurs, dropping to 2 ml/100 g/day after urination but until potassium and uric acid levels in the blood decrease. Once a reptile has urinated, the levels of nutrition should be increased slowly, starting with for example, half-strength Critical Care Formula (Vetark). Monitoring blood levels of uric acid and potassium and also urine output is recommended throughout the initial recovery period of any malnourished reptile. See Chapter 6 for more information.

Wildlife

Veterinary practices have a moral obligation to take in wildlife from members of the public. During practice hours, small wild mammals and wild birds should be treated free of charge if they are brought to a veterinary practice. Veterinary surgeons are obliged by their professional code to provide any necessary pain relief or euthanasia. However, the extent of treatment given depends on the individual practice, with some giving only emergency treatment while others will carry out surgical procedures either free of charge or at minimal cost. The RSPCA will contribute to the cost of the initial emergency treatments or euthanasia of cases brought in out of practice hours, or if a larger wild animal is involved, e.g. a deer. The RSPCA's contribution will only be approved if a veterinary surgeon, not a member of the public, calls the RSPCA before the treatment is undertaken. The veterinary surgeon must obtain an incident number, and treatment will be agreed on a case-by-case basis. The only avian species that this applies to are swans, geese and raptors.

Wildlife cases can often be transferred to specialist centres that will treat and rehabilitate them once they have been stabilized. The initial stabilization can be life-saving and very rewarding to carry out.

With any wildlife emergency the most important piece of information to establish as quickly as possible is whether the animal is going to recuperate to be fit for release and have an equal chance of survival compared with any other of the same species. This does not necessarily mean that it will be in perfect physical condition at the time of release but that it should be fit to carry out normal daily activities such as finding food and shelter, with respect to the species that is being dealt with and the way in which it carries out these functions. Prior knowledge of an individual species' natural history can be useful when deciding whether it will meet these criteria, but is certainly not essential for carrying out simple life-saving procedures.

Determination and interpretation of vital signs in wild mammals

The principles of determination and interpretation of vital signs in wild mammal species are as for small mammal species (above). This is also true of wild birds and pet birds. Determination of vital signs in some wildlife species can be limited in the conscious animal, depending on its demeanour at presentation.

Foxes and badgers

When a fox or badger is first presented it is important to assess its level of awareness and whether it can be examined whilst conscious. Gentle but firm pressure should be applied around the animal's head and neck with a broom or other long-handled object to see what response is provoked. If there is little response and the animal is comatose then it may be safe to place a towel over its head and scruff. A muzzle can be placed to aid safe examination. If in any doubt as to whether the animal is conscious, it should be sedated before examination, as badgers and foxes can give nasty bites and are very strong.

The preliminary examination should be similar to that for a dog.

- Measure heart and respiratory rate and assess character. Pulses can be monitored using the metatarsal or metacarpal arteries.
- Assess body condition.
- Assess mucous membrane colour and hydration status.

The examination should include a check for any wounds and fractures. If wounds are present, the surrounding fur should be clipped and the wound then cleaned with diluted disinfectant and checked for evidence of myiasis. Dressings should be applied as necessary. Splints can be applied to fractured legs. Most injured animals will benefit from fluid therapy, which is easiest to administer intravenously via the cephalic vein. Warmth should be provided either via a heat lamp or by placing the animal in an incubator. Heat pads and wires are likely to be chewed once the animal's demeanour has improved. Analgesics and antibiotics should be administered to badgers and foxes as necessary, at the same doses as for dogs.

Foxes with fractured limbs may need to be euthanased by a veterinary surgeon, as the length of time taken to rehabilitate them makes reintroducing them to the wild very difficult; they are territorial animals and are likely to be ousted from their group. Humanized cubs and foxes with chronic mange in poor body condition are also poor candidates for rehabilitation.

Older debilitated badgers that may have been displaced from their sett due to age or disease tend to be in poor body condition, with worn teeth and territorial rump wounds. They are unlikely to survive in the wild once rehabilitated and are likely to be euthanased by a veterinary surgeon on humane grounds.

Hedgehogs

Hedgehogs are most likely to be presented for the following reasons:

- People have found them wandering outside during the day
- Traumatic incidents, e.g. strimming injuries, dog bites, road traffic collisions, burns from bonfires (Figure 1.42)
- Skin disease
- Myiasis.

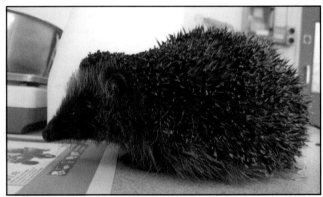

1.42 Hedgehog with burnt spines after being caught in a bonfire. (Courtesy of D. Hunter)

It is very important to examine hedgehogs thoroughly as soon as possible. Many will not uncurl if they are very unwell or injured. In such situations, the use of gaseous anaesthesia may encourage the hedgehog to relax and uncurl without damage.

Wounds should be bathed and cleaned, as many may be old and contaminated. The ears, eyes, mouth and perineum, along with any wounds, should be checked for myiasis, especially in warmer weather. It is common to see fly eggs laid in the mouth, especially in juveniles. Any eggs or maggots should be physically removed. Antibiotics and analgesics should be started as necessary as advised by the veterinary surgeon.

Warmed subcutaneous fluids should be given to any hedgehog that is presented. Maintenance fluid requirements are 100 ml/kg/day. There is a large subcutaneous space, so fairly large boluses of 20–30 ml/kg can be given. Many animals that are presented will be hypothermic, so providing a warm environment (20–25°C) will be essential to recovery (Figure 1.43).

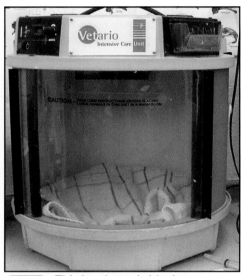

1.43 This incubator is ideal to create a warm environment for hypothermic animals.

Hedgehogs with only one eye will cope well, but are best kept in a sheltered environment if possible. Forelimbs should not be amputated as this will leave the hedgehog unable to dig for food; however, they could also be kept in a sheltered environment. Hindlimb amputees will cope better in the wild, although the author (EF) has seen animals presented that have lost a hindlimb and have been subsequently unable to scratch and remove ectoparasites from that side, causing a considerable build-up. It is questionable whether it is ethical to keep wild animals in enclosed spaces; nevertheless, hedgehogs that are still able to carry out most normal functions can be kept for long periods in this way.

Squirrels

Squirrels will most commonly be presented with traumatic injuries due to road accidents or bite wounds. Parapoxvirus disease is commonly seen in red squirrels and, despite intensive supportive care, these patients rarely survive.

Most animals will benefit from warmth and fluid therapy. Subcutaneous fluids are easily administered between the shoulder blades at volumes of up to 10 ml. Severely debilitated animals will benefit from intravenous fluids via the femoral vein, and subdued individuals may be held for oral administration of fluids and medications. Pain relief and antibiotics should be given as necessary.

It should be noted that it is illegal to keep or release grey squirrels without a licence to do so (as mentioned previously); therefore many of these animals should be euthanased upon admission.

Bats

Bats will most commonly be presented for traumatic injuries, including wing bone fractures, wing tears and cat bite injuries. Due to their small size, any injury is likely to lead to secondary dehydration and malnutrition very quickly. Bats with large soft tissue wounds or open fractures are likely to be euthanased. Most other wounds will heal well. Wing tears will mostly heal well, irrespective of size or whether the wing edge is involved (Figure 1.44).

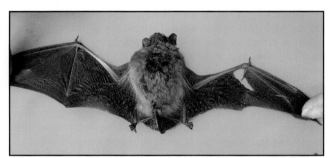

1.44 A tear in the wing of a pipistrelle bat. Despite the large size of this wing tear, it is likely to heal on its own in a matter of weeks. (Courtesy of Sergio Silvetti)

Torpid animals will benefit from gentle heat to warm them slowly. A torpid bat should be placed in an escape-proof container, with paper towels draped along the sides, which the bat can use to climb should it become active.

Subcutaneous fluids are easily administered at a site on the dorsal thorax, although many bats will take fluids from a syringe via an intravenous catheter sheath or nasolacrimal irrigating cannula. Warmed Hartmann's solution or an amino acid, electrolyte and dextrose solution (e.g. Duphalyte, Fort Dodge) are both suitable preparations to give subcutaneously at 0.1 ml per 5 g bat.

Wild birds

Avian cases will range from tiny sparrows and finches to seabirds (Figure 1.45), raptors and waterfowl (Figure 1.46). On initial presentation, it is important to assess whether the animal has any obviously life-threatening wounds or injuries, e.g. a contaminated open long bone fracture. The bird is likely to be in shock, traumatized, in pain and dehydrated on presentation. An initial brief examination should be carried out to check for life-threatening injuries before supportive fluids are given.

The examination should include the following:

1. Check the eyes for haemorrhage, rupture or other signs of trauma.
2. Check the beak for softness, fractures and trauma (Figure 1.47).
3. Check the inside of the mouth for white plaques or bloody discharge.

4. Check each wing separately by holding at the carpus and gently extending. This will allow the patagial ligament to be examined (this ligament extends from the shoulder to the carpus and is essential for flight).
5. Feel down each bone when the wing is extended for any soft tissue swelling or crepitus.
6. Feel the keel bone or sternum and palpate the pectoral muscles to either side to assess body condition score.
7. Palpate down the length of each leg for any soft tissue swelling or crepitus.
8. Assess both the dorsal and plantar surfaces of the feet for any wounds, fractures or signs of bumblefoot.

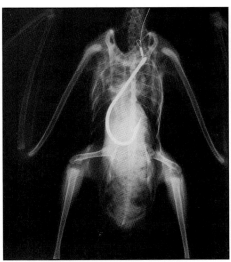

1.45 Radiograph of a fishing hook swallowed by a herring gull. (Courtesy of D. Hunter)

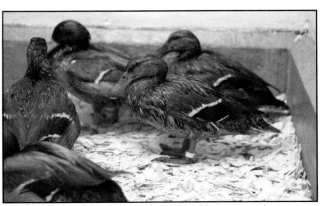

1.46 A group of oiled mallards. (Courtesy of D. Hunter)

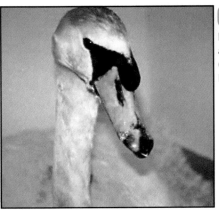

1.47 Mute swan with a fractured beak. (Courtesy of D. Hunter)

If there are no obvious life-threatening injuries on initial examination, fluids should be administered as soon as possible. Stressed birds are unlikely to feed themselves. The easiest way to administer fluids is by crop tubing. If there are any signs of trauma, birds will benefit from a dose of meloxicam at 0.1–0.2 mg/kg i.m. q24h.

Larger waterfowl tolerate intravenous drips very well. Fluids are given via the medial metatarsal vein (Figure 1.48), which is the most efficient way of administering fluids in severely debilitated animals.

Placing the bird in a warm oxygen-enriched environment in a quiet room away from any predator species and humans is ideal.

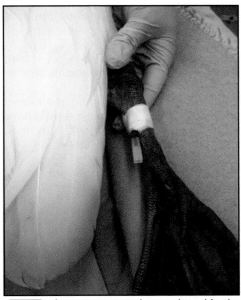

1.48 Intravenous catheter placed in the medial metatarsal vein of a swan.

Core principles of clinical examination

Clinical examination techniques carried out in domestic species can be applied to many exotic and wildlife species. Any clinical examination should consist of a systematic evaluation of an animal's organs, senses and behaviour.

As previously discussed, observing many of these species either in their own environment or giving them opportunity to exhibit 'normal' behaviour is very important for distinguishing whether the animal is genuinely feeling bright and alert or whether they are 'putting on a show' in their new surroundings. Most exotic pet and wildlife species that will be brought to the practice are prey animals and so will initially try to look healthier than they are actually feeling. It is also important to learn to distinguish a shy and nervous animal from one that is feeling unwell. The owner should be able to provide information about their pet's normal behaviour.

A systematic clinical examination should involve examining all body systems in turn so that nothing is missed that could aid diagnosis. This type of examination is carried out once the animal has been stabilized. This author (EF) prefers to carry out a clinical examination starting at the cranial end of the animal and working backwards along the body.

Mammals

Mammalian clinical examination should be based upon that for a dog or cat. However, in rabbits and rodents, differences in dentition and digestive systems will need to be taken into consideration; for example, listening to gut sounds is a very important part of the clinical examination.

Birds

Respiratory rate should be counted prior to handling for further examination. Thoracic auscultation, both ventrally and dorsally, can be useful to listen for any adventitious lung or air sac noises.

Heart rate is very difficult to count in most bird species but listening to the rhythm and character is important.

Most birds will be stressed by being restrained and those that are collapsed or dyspnoeic should have only a minimal examination carried out. The head should be examined first:

- **Eyes:** Any discharges, bleeding or periocular swelling, which can indicate sinusitis and infection (see Figure 1.8)
- **Ears:** Any discharges
- **Nares:** Any discharges or build-up of dead cells that can cause rhinoliths, especially in birds with hypovitaminosis A (Figure 1.49a)
- **Mouth:** Damage to the tongue and discharge from the choana (the opening in the roof of the mouth that communicates with the sinuses).

It is difficult to assess mucous membrane colour as many birds' mouths are pigmented. Capillary refill time measurement is not possible in most species. However, in species with combs these can be used to assess anaemia, dehydration and cyanosis if they are pale, flaccid or have a blue tinge, respectively.

Body condition scoring is carried out by feeling the sternum or keel bone and the pectoral muscles to either side. Weighing birds is very important as, if the bird has lost weight despite seeming to eat normally, this is often the first sign that something is wrong. Most raptor owners will weigh their birds on a daily basis and will be able to tell you exactly what their weight is. However, parrot owners rarely do this and are often shocked to learn that their bird is either obese or underweight. Daily weight records of hospitalized birds should be kept, preferably at the same time each day prior to any assisted feeding or administration of medication.

Hydration status can be assessed by skin tenting, but this is limited in bird species as there is generally not a lot of spare skin. Eyes can look sunken in dehydrated birds but this is often a subjective measurement, with haematological parameters being the most accurate way of assessing dehydration in birds.

The feathers should be given a general check, in the same way that the skin of a mammal is checked. Feather dust, a white powder made up of minute particles of keratin shed by the powder down feathers, is normal in many species. Examination of feathers could reveal evidence of self-trauma (i.e. feather chewing; Figure 1.49b) or plucking, which could be an indication of behavioural issues or an underlying medical condition; or the presence of feather mites, and may also provide information regarding nutritional status and deficiencies.

Each wing should be checked by gently extending each side in turn, paying particular attention to the feathers, feeling the patagial ligament for any swelling or wounds, and feeling each of the bones in a similar method to that adopted when examining mammalian limbs.

The legs and feet should be checked, feeling down the length of each bone and examining each surface of the foot, especially the plantar surface, for evidence

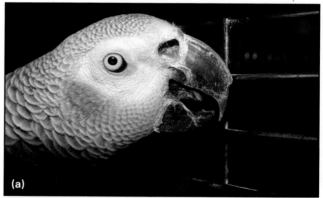

(a)

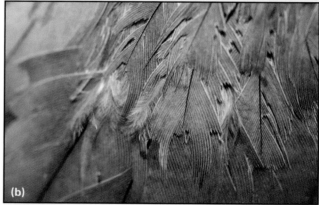

(b)

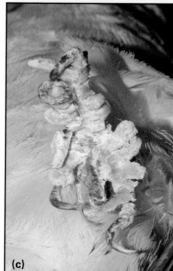

(c)

1.49 The physical examination of bird patients can be very helpful in making a diagnosis. **(a)** Vitamin A deficiency can cause rhinoliths to form. **(b)** An example of feather chewing or barbering in an African grey parrot. **(c)** Hyperkeratosis caused by vitamin A deficiency in an Amazon parrot. (Courtesy of A. Humphries)

of any bumblefoot lesions; these could indicate problems with the surfaces on which the bird is standing. Unilateral bumblefoot is often a sign that the bird is favouring that particular foot, indicating that there may be an underlying problem in the opposite leg that is causing the bird some discomfort.

Reptiles

Respiratory rate should be counted prior to examination, along with the depth and character of breaths. Any open-mouth breathing should be noted. The heart can be auscultated using a stethoscope through a cloth but a Doppler ultrasound probe is preferred (Figure 1.50); this can be used to listen to the heart or jugular pulse (this produces an audible representation of the beat). Lung auscultation has limited use.

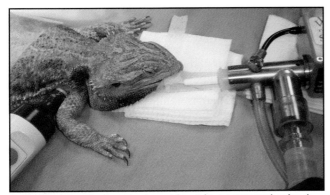

1.50 Monitoring the heart beat in an anaesthetized bearded dragon using a Doppler ultrasound probe. (Courtesy of J. Hedley)

Physical examination should begin at the head:

- **Eyes:** Discharges, periocular swelling and/or sunken appearance
- **Nostrils:** Patency, surrounding discoloration (especially in tortoises), discharges or bubbles being produced
- **Mouth** (Figure 1.51): Mucous membrane colour, ulceration, caseous lesions and discharges. Capillary refill time will be difficult to check in most species. Teeth in lizards and snakes should be checked for colour, swellings of the gums, fractures or discharges
- **Tympanic membranes** (Figure 1.52): Any bulging or trauma.

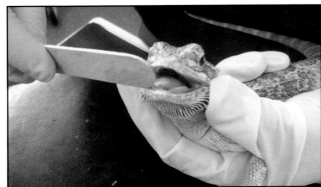

1.51 Using a tongue depressor to open the mouth of a bearded dragon to allow oral examination.

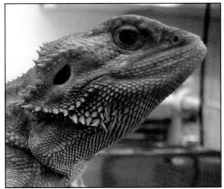

1.52 A normal tympanic membrane on the side of the head in a bearded dragon.

Body condition scoring in lizards should be based on how easily the spine and pelvic bones can be palpated and seen, and the amount of fat that is laid down on either side of the tail base (Figures 1.53 and 1.54). In snakes the body condition scoring should be based on how easy the spine and ribs are to see and feel; they should be prominent enough that they can be felt but they should not be so prominent that they can be obviously seen. In tortoises the author (EF) prefers to use palpation around the shoulders, pre-femoral fossa and pelvis to assess body condition. Weighing a reptile every time it is presented at the practice, or on a regular basis at home, is important to keep a record of trends in weight gain or loss. This can be especially useful in tortoises as owners tend not to notice weight loss as quickly as in other species.

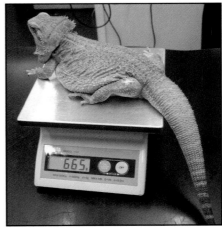

1.53 Weighing an overweight bearded dragon. Note the wide tail due to fat deposited here.

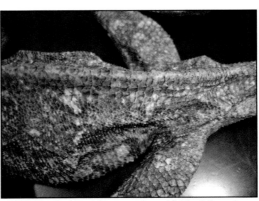

1.54 A severely emaciated frilled lizard. Note the prominent spine and pelvic bones. (Courtesy of C. Dodd)

KEY POINT

The Jackson's ratio calculation is a useful tool when assessing bodyweight in Hermann's and spur-thighed tortoises but it should be interpreted with caution as other factors such as egg binding, follicles or ascites may give misleading results. The ratio should be used in combination with a body condition score and should never be used in individuals with shell deformities.

Hydration status can be assessed subjectively by looking at the skin condition and how sunken the eyes are; it can be assessed more accurately by looking at haematology and increases in certain biochemical values, e.g. uric acid, urea and sodium. Monitoring weight, urine pH and specific gravity are also useful indicators of hydration status. The eyes can also look sunken due to severe weight loss, leading to depletion of the retrobulbar fat pad.

The skin should be examined for signs of dysecdysis (problems in shedding), scars, burns, wounds, discoloration, parasites and infections.

Each limb and joint should be examined for swellings, crepitus and pain; the toes should be inspected for signs of dysecdysis causing constriction and necrosis of the digits. The cloaca should be checked for prolapse (Figure 1.55) or discharge.

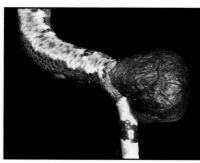

1.55 Cloacal prolapse in a snake. Note the desiccation of the tissues. (Courtesy of C. Dodd)

References and further reading

Association of Avian Veterinarians (2012) *AAV Client Education Brochure: Signs of Illness in Birds.* AAV Publications Office, Denver

Donoghue S and Langenberg J (1996) Nutrition. In: *Reptile Medicine and Surgery*, ed. DR Mader, pp. 148–153. WB Saunders, Philadelphia

Keeble E and Meredith A (2009) *BSAVA Manual of Rodents and Ferrets.* BSAVA Publications, Gloucester

Lumeij JT and Ritchie BW (1994) Cardiology. In: *Avian Medicine: Principles and Application*, ed. BW Ritchie *et al.*, p. 696. Wingers Publishing, Florida

Maclean B and Raiti P (2004) Emergency care. In: *BSAVA Manual of Reptiles, 2nd edn*, ed. SJ Girling and P Raiti, pp. 63–70. BSAVA Publications, Gloucester

Meredith A and Flecknell P (2006) *BSAVA Manual of Rabbit Medicine and Surgery, 2nd edn.* BSAVA Publications, Gloucester

Meredith A and Johnson-Delaney C (2010) *BSAVA Manual of Exotic Pets, 5th edn.* BSAVA Publications, Gloucester

Mitchell M (2006) Therapeutics. In: *Reptile Medicine and Surgery, 2nd edn*, ed. DR Mader, pp. 631–642. Saunders Elsevier, St. Louis

Mullineaux E, Best D and Cooper JE (2003) *BSAVA Manual of Wildlife Casualties.* BSAVA Publications, Gloucester

Paul J and Windham W (2009) *Keeping Pet Chickens.* Interpet Publishing, Dorking

Quesenberry KE and Carpenter JW (2003) *Ferrets, Rabbits and Rodents: Clinical Medicine and Surgery, 2nd edn.* Saunders Elsevier, St. Louis

Raftery A (2005) The initial presentation: triage and critical care. In: *BSAVA Manual of Psittacine Birds, 2nd edn*, ed. N Harcourt-Brown and J Chitty, pp. 35–49. BSAVA Publications, Gloucester

Useful websites

Advice and legislation relating to red squirrels: www.naturalengland.org.uk/ourwork/regulation/wildlife/species/redsquirrels.aspx#licence

Handling the Avian Emergency: www.exoticpetvet.net/avian/avianer.html

Wildlife and Countryside Act 1981: www.defra.gov.uk

Self-assessment questions

1. Which animals should never be restrained by the tail due to the risk of a degloving injury?
2. What type of animal would wear 'jesses'?
3. Which infection can a bat potentially pass to humans?
4. Which animal has a sensitivity to television?
5. Which animal can suffer from 'fur slip'?
6. What is the most important thing to do when an exotic pet is presented at the practice to get an idea of how critical the patient is?
7. Describe the technique of crop tubing an avian patient.
8. If a Doppler ultrasound probe is unavailable to assess the heart beat or pulse, how else can you tell whether a reptile is dead or alive?
9. What are the main routes used for fluid administration in a tortoise?
10. What would you do with a rabbit that was presented on a hot summer day with a rectal temperature of 42°C?
11. What would you do to prepare for a collapsed hamster that was being brought to the practice?
12. Describe how to carry out a brief clinical examination of a sparrowhawk brought in by a member of the public.
13. What is the 'wheelbarrow' technique used for with hedgehogs and what does it allow you to do?
14. How would you assess the hydration status of a bearded dragon?
15. Where is it easiest to feel a bird's pulse?
16. How would you most easily assess the heart beat of a reptile?

Client questionnaires ▶

Small mammal admission questionnaire

DETAILS

Owner's details..

Pet's details...

Species .... Breed .... Age...................................... Sex *(M/F/unknown)* ....

SOURCED FROM

[　] Breeder　　[　] Pet shop　　[　] Other *(please specify)* ....

How long has the pet been in the owner's possession?...

HOUSING DETAILS

[　] Cage　　[　] Hutch, indoors　　[　] Hutch, outdoors　　[　] Tank

Substrate used...

Housed separately or in a pair/group?...

DIET

Type of food offered ....

Amount offered .... Amount eaten ....

How is drinking water offered?

[　] Bowl　　[　] Bottle

Has there been an increase in thirst?..

Any vitamin and mineral supplements used? ....

DURATION OF CLINICAL SIGNS

How long has the pet been ill for?..

PROGRESSION AND TYPE OF CLINICAL SIGNS

List clinical signs ....

List any disease history of this pet...

List any disease history of any in-contact pet ....

TREATMENTS ALREADY GIVEN

List treatments already prescribed ....

An example of a client questionnaire for admitting a small mammal.

Bird admission questionnaire

DETAILS

Owner's details..

Pet's details..

Species .... Breed .... Age.................................... Sex *(M/F/unknown)* ....

ORIGIN OF BIRD

[   ] Captive bred   [   ] Wild bred

How long has the pet been in your possession? ....

SOURCED FROM

[   ] Breeder   [   ] Dealer   [   ] Pet shop   [   ] Other *(please specify)* ....

HABITAT

[   ] Cage   [   ] Aviary   [   ] Free indoors   [   ] Outdoors   [   ] Other *(please specify)* ....

EXPOSURE TO OTHER BIRDS

Are there other birds in the house?...

Are the other birds sick? Have any died?..

DIET

Type of food offered?..

Any vitamin and mineral supplements used? ....

Recent dietary changes by you or the bird?..

DURATION OF CLINICAL SIGNS

How long has the bird been ill? _____

PROGRESSION AND TYPE OF CLINICAL SIGNS

List clinical signs, e.g. faecal changes, increased thirst, increased respiratory effort, changes in vocalization or behaviour

....

TREATMENTS ALREADY GIVEN

List treatments already prescribed ....

An example of a client questionnaire for admitting a bird.

Bird of prey admission questionnaire

DETAILS

Owner's details..

Pet's details...

Species .... Breed .... Age.................................. Sex *(M/F/unknown)* ....

ORIGIN OF BIRD

[   ] Wild caught   [   ] Domestic bred

How long has the bird been in your possession?..

SOURCED FROM

[   ] Private owner   [   ] Breeder   [   ] Other *(please specify)* ....

EXPOSURE TO OTHER BIRDS

Do you keep other birds?..

If yes, are any other birds sick? Have any died? ....

HUSBANDRY

[   ] Aviary   [   ] Tethered   [   ] Flying bird, last flown?..   [   ] Breeding only

DIET

Diet fed and how much food given? ....

Source of food: wild quarry (shot or caught) or farmed?..

Is casting fed? ....

When did the bird last cast? Was it normal?..

Any vitamin and mineral supplements used? ....

WEIGHT

Normal flying weight?..

Normal moulting weight?...

Weight normal for level of feeding?...

FLYING

Is the bird keen to fly? ....

Is it tiring easily? ....

DURATION AND TYPE OF CLINICAL SIGNS

How long has the bird been ill? ....

List of clinical signs/injuries, mute appearance...

TREATMENTS ALREADY GIVEN

List treatments already prescribed ....

An example of a client questionnaire for admitting a raptor.

Reptile admission questionnaire

DETAILS

Owner's details ....

Pet's details ....

Species .... Subspecies............................. Age.................................. Sex *(M/F/unknown)* ....

SOURCED FROM

[ ] Breeder   [ ] Importer   [ ] Pet shop   [ ] Other *(please specify)* ....

NATURAL HABITAT

[ ] Arboreal – vertically arranged environment   [ ] Terrestrial – horizontally arranged environment

[ ] Desert – dry environment   [ ] Rainforest – high humidity   [ ] Aquatic

SPECIFICATIONS FOR ENCLOSURE

Size of enclosure: Length .... Depth.................................. Width..................................

Substrate used..

Lighting provided including UV..

Temperature: Daytime range..................... Nighttime range................ Day length..........................

Humidity: Daytime............................. Nighttime...........................

EXPOSURE TO OTHER REPTILES

Have there been any other reptiles sharing the vivarium in the last 6 months? ....

Have any been sick or died?...

DIET

Type of food offered ....

Amount offered .... Amount eaten .... Frequency of feeding..............................

How is drinking water offered?

[ ] Bowl   [ ] Spray   [ ] Other *(please specify)* ....

Any vitamin and mineral supplements used? ....

DURATION OF CLINICAL SIGNS

How long has the reptile been ill? ....

PROGRESSION AND TYPE OF CLINICAL SIGNS

List clinical signs ....

List any disease history of this reptile ....

List any disease history of any in-contact reptile...

TREATMENTS ALREADY GIVEN

List treatments already prescribed ....

An example of a client questionnaire for admitting a reptile.

Mammals: biology and husbandry

Emma Keeble and Helen Heggie

This chapter is designed to give information on:

- Species and common breeds of commonly kept exotic pet mammals, less commonly kept exotic pet mammals and native UK wild mammals
- Natural history and normal behaviour
- Basic anatomy and biology (where this differs from that of cats and dogs), with clear descriptions of sexing
- Specific dietary and housing requirements (including the requirements of wild mammals in captivity), to enable the veterinary nurse to accommodate the needs of any hospitalized mammal patient as well as provide correct advice to owners

---

Commonly kept pet species

Rabbits

Common breeds

A number of breeds of the domestic or European rabbit are popular in the UK (Figure 2.1), varying in size from the small dwarf breeds (0.8–1 kg) and the commonly kept lop breeds (1.5–3 kg), to the large continental giant breeds (6–10 kg). More information can be obtained from the British Rabbit Council website (www.thebrc.org).

Natural history and normal behaviour

The domestic rabbit was introduced to Europe by the Romans over 2000 years ago. It has become the third most popular pet in the UK and can be kept either as an outdoor pet or as an indoor 'house rabbit'.

Rabbits are naturally curious animals that actively explore their surroundings. Owners should be reminded, especially if they have decided to keep the rabbit indoors, that their pet will happily chew and dig household objects. Rabbits will jump on and off

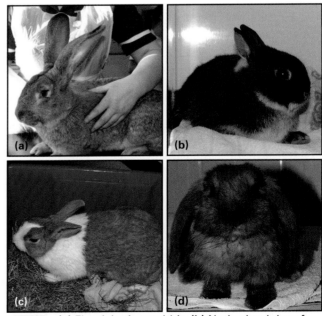

2.1 (a) Flemish giant rabbit; (b) Netherland dwarf rabbit; (c) tortoiseshell Dutch rabbit; (d) dwarf lop rabbit. (Courtesy of Alistair Lawrie)

furniture, run quickly across an open area and may also chase their owner. While exploring their surroundings, rabbits mark their territory from small glands situated under their chin. Entire males and females will also spray urine to mark their territory.

Rabbits are generally quiet animals, which makes them good household pets. They will, however, stamp their hindfeet if they perceive danger and may also emit a high-pitched scream if frightened. A rabbit that does not want to be disturbed will grunt and rush towards an intruder, which can be quite intimidating.

Anatomy and physiology

Biological data for the domestic rabbit are given in Figure 2.2.

Average life expectancy (years)	7–10
Bodyweight (kg)	0.8–10
Heart rate (beats/min)	180–250
Respiratory rate (breaths/min)	30–60
Body temperature (°C)	38.5–40

2.2 Biological data for the domestic rabbit.

Eyes

Rabbits have a wide field of vision that covers 190 degrees for each eye. Their sensitivity to light is eight times greater than that of humans, due to their wide pupillary dilation. They possess a double retinal system of rods and cones, which readily detect motion and are sensitive to the blue and green light present at twilight.

Ears

Rabbits have excellent hearing. The external ears are large vascular organs, which serve as heat regulators as well as sensory organs. They are often the site of preference for intravenous access.

Teeth

Rabbits have open-rooted teeth that grow continuously. The dental formula is I2/1, C0/0, PM3/2, M3/3. They have three pairs of incisors (2 × upper, 1 × lower). The incisors are not used in prehending food, which means they can be removed in severe cases of incisor malocclusion. The gap between the incisors and the molars is called the diastema. The premolars and molars work together as one unit, and are often called cheek teeth. Malocclusion results from an insufficiently fibrous and abrasive diet.

Upper respiratory tract

Rabbits have sensory pads at the entrance to each nostril. The nostrils can twitch between 20 and 150 times per minute when the rabbit is alert or excited and are still when the rabbit is relaxed. Rabbits have a long tongue, a narrow oropharynx and a small glottis. Intubation is possible, although may be difficult, and laryngospasm can be a common complication when attempting intubation.

Thorax

The thorax is small compared with the abdomen. A large thymus gland is present in adults; it is situated ventral to the heart and extends forward into the thoracic inlet. The lungs are made up of cranial, middle and caudal lobes. The caudal lobe on the left side is smaller than that on the right due to the presence of the heart. Rested respiration consists of muscular contractions of the diaphragm. Rabbits do not use their intercostal muscles for respiration.

Digestive system

Rabbits are herbivores and possess a large hindgut. They are non-ruminants; caecotrophy (the practice of eating the soft faeces or caecotrophs to enhance nutrient extraction from a nutrient-poor diet) and browsing behaviour allow them to achieve high food conversion (Figure 2.3). Normal browsing behaviour in rabbits consists of selection of young, succulent plant material. This allows rabbits to maintain a high metabolic rate. Coarse fibres are ingested to stimulate gut motility.

The stomach lies to the left-hand side of the abdomen and is thin walled. The cardia is located in the centre of the lesser curvature. Due to this positioning, rabbits are unable to vomit; pre-anaesthesia fasting is therefore unnecessary. Food, fluid and hair are found normally in the stomach.

The small intestine is short and makes up 12% of the gastrointestinal volume. It is responsible for digestion and absorption of sugars and proteins from food, as well as vitamins, fatty acids and proteins from the caecotrophs. High-carbohydrate diets inhibit secretions of motilin (a peptide secreted by the endocrine cells of the duodenum and jejunum, which helps with stimulation of gastrointestinal motility), leading to gut stasis problems.

Rabbits possess the largest caecum of all animals relative to their size. The caecum is thin-walled, coils in on itself in three gyral folds, and terminates in a blind-ended, thick-walled tube called the vermiform appendix. Caecotrophs are formed from fine fibre particles and fluid, which are retained in the caecum to form high-nutrient particles.

The goblet cells of the colon produce mucus, which coats the particles; they resemble grape-like clusters. The colon consists of two sections: proximal and distal. The proximal colon has a fusus coli, which is unique to lagomorphs. The fusus coli is a 6–8 cm length of thickened muscle, which is lined by a thick mucosa. It has a heavy supply of ganglion cells and is influenced by aldosterone and prostaglandins. It acts as the pacemaker for colonic motility.

Urinary system

Rabbits pass copious amounts of urine, as they are less able than other mammals to concentrate their urine. Calcium is excreted via the kidneys into the urine, unlike other mammals in which it is excreted in bile. Rabbits that are fed a high-calcium diet are more susceptible to the precipitation of solutes and to urolithiasis, due to the combination of excess calcium in the urine and an alkaline pH (Figure 2.4).

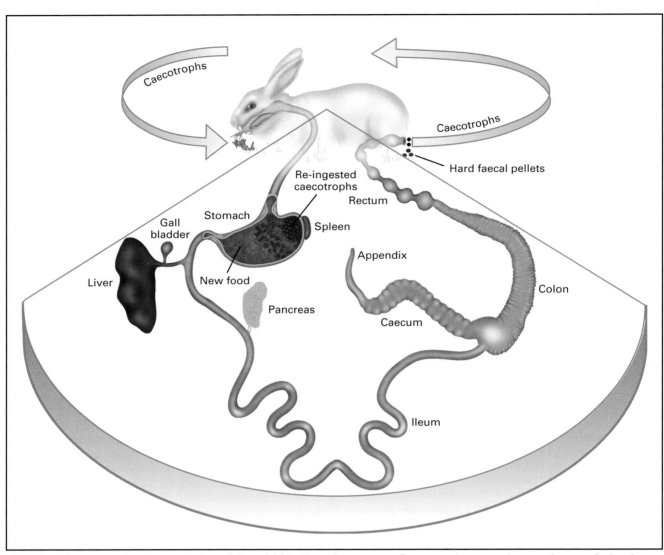

2.3 Diagrammatic representation of the rabbit's digestive system. Caecotrophs are re-ingested to maximize the use of nutrients. (Reproduced from the *BSAVA Manual of Rabbit Medicine and Surgery, 2nd edition*)

Urine colour	Tends to be turbid due to calcium excretion. Colour can be white, orange/brown, yellow or red
Urine pH	7.5–8.8 (alkaline)
Urine specific gravity	1.003–1.036
Urine volume (ml/kg/day)	20–350

2.4 Urinalysis for the domestic rabbit.

Urine colour can vary. Plant pigments can cause the urine to turn a bright red, which can be confused with haematuria. Due to calcium being excreted in the urine, it will also take on a creamy appearance. When the urine is centrifuged, or 'spun down', the calcium sediment is very evident.

Reproduction

Reproductive data for the domestic rabbit are given in Figure 2.5.

Age at sexual maturity (months)	4–5
Oestrous cycle	Induced ovulation. No regular oestrous cycle, receptive every 5–6 days
Gestation period (days)	31–32
Litters per year	Average 3–5
Average litter size	4–12
Post-partum oestrus	Within 24 hours of kindling (giving birth)
Birth weight (g)	40–50
Birth characteristics	Altricial (undeveloped), with sealed eyelids and ear canals
Age at weaning (days)	16–21

2.5 Reproductive data for the domestic rabbit.

Sexing

The prepuce has a circular orifice and the anogenital distance is longer in males than it is in females (Figure 2.6). The penis can be fully extruded by applying gentle digital pressure in a craniocaudal direction along the prepuce. The vulva has a slit-shaped orifice and cannot be fully everted. Sexing young, immature rabbits can be more difficult.

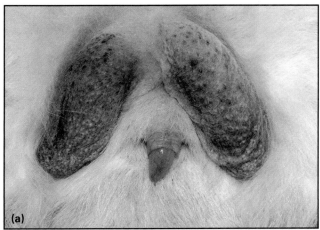

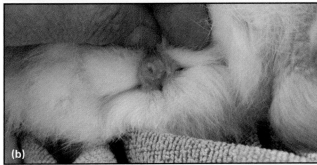

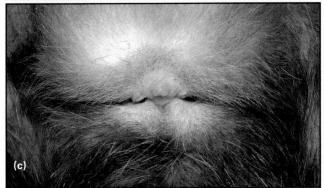

2.6 **(a)** Entire male rabbit. **(b)** Castrated male rabbit. **(c)** Female rabbit genitalia.

Diet

It is essential that rabbits are fed a high-fibre, low-carbohydrate diet in order to maintain normal gut motility and caecotrophy. Increased caecal retention time is brought about by a low-fibre diet. This leads to hypomotiliy of the gut and a decrease in the amount of caecotrophs being produced. High carbohydrates in the diet provide a medium for bacteria (e.g. *Escherichia coli* and *Clostridium spiroforme*) to colonize, which leads to a drop in the gut pH, inhibiting normal flora.

The diet of a rabbit should consist of:

- Good quality hay, e.g. Western Timothy
- Fresh grazing – access to grass and weeds (grass cuttings should not be fed)
- Fresh leafy dark green vegetables
- Fresh root vegetables (small amount)
- A small amount of dried grass pellets (1 tablespoon per day for dwarf/standard breeds; 2 tablespoons per day for giant breeds)
- Fresh, clean water, which should always be provided in a small, heavy ceramic bowl (research has shown that rabbits drink more via this route); a dropper bottle may also be used, to provide an additional source of water.

Housing

Rabbits housed outside should be provided with a large hutch (at least 1.8 square metres and high enough for the rabbit to rear up on its hindlegs). The hutch should be raised at least 45 cm off the ground. This will deter the advances of wild rabbits and in particular help prevent infestation from their fleas (which can leap at least 18 cm). There should be a separate sleeping compartment, which should be packed with straw for insulation. The hutch should be situated in a dry, draught-free area.

Indoor rabbits should be provided with as large a cage as possible. There should be a covered section that the rabbit is able to retreat to (Figure 2.7).

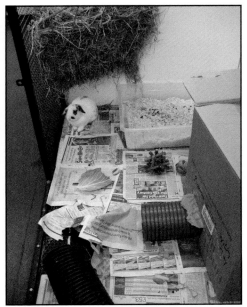

2.7 An indoor rabbit set-up. A hide area, tunnels for bolt holes, a hay rack and a litter tray have been provided. As large an area as possible should be provided, to allow the rabbit to exercise fully.

Rodents

There are over 2000 different species of rodent, divided into five suborders. These include the myomorphs (mouse-like rodents), hystricomorphs (porcupine-like rodents) and sciuromorphs (squirrel-like rodents).

Myomorphs

Species

Mice and rats belong to the Muridae family. Hamsters (Syrian and dwarf species) (Figure 2.8) and Mongolian gerbils belong to the Cricetidae family (the burrowing rodents). There are four commonly kept species of dwarf hamster: the Chinese hamster, the Roborovski hamster, the Russian dwarf Campbell hamster and the Russian dwarf winter white hamster. There are several different varieties of pet mice, rats and Syrian hamsters, depending on coat type, colour and markings.

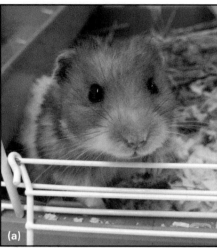

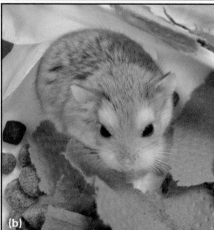

2.8
(a) Syrian hamster.
(b) Roborovski dwarf hamster.

Anatomy and physiology

Biological data for myomorphs are given in Figure 2.9.

- **Eyes:** Albino rats have poor vision and rely on their vibrissae (whiskers) for navigation.
- **Teeth:** The word 'rodent' comes from the Latin verb *rodere*, meaning 'to gnaw'. Rodents have sharp, chisel-shaped, orange/yellow to white open-rooted, constantly growing incisors. There is a large diastema and the mandible is wider than the maxilla. The molar teeth are rooted in myomorphs. The dental formula is Il/l, C0/0, PM0/0, M3/3.
- **Digestive system:** A rodent digestive tract comprises a simple stomach, a large sacculated caecum and an elongated colon. Hamsters have two parts to the stomach: a non-glandular forestomach and a glandular region, separated by muscular folds. Coprophagy is common among rodents. Myomorph rodents cannot vomit or regurgitate due to a muscular ridge between the lower oesophagus and the stomach. Hamsters possess large paired cheek pouches for food storage.
- **Urinary system:** Gerbils are desert species in the wild and so are able to concentrate their urine and drink very little water.
- **Reproduction:** Female rodents have separate vaginal and urethral orifices, with the vaginal opening remaining closed until oestrus. Myomorphs are prolific breeders and dystocia is rare. After mating, a vaginal plug is formed. All species (except chipmunks) show a post-partum oestrus within about 24 hours of parturition; males and females should be separated unless a constant state of pregnancy or lactation is desired. Young are altricial (blind and without hair). Reproductive data for myomorphs are given in Figure 2.10.
- **Coat and scent glands:** Yellowing of the coat is common in older male rats. Hamsters have pigmented scent glands located either side of their flanks. Gerbils have a normal large ventral scent gland mid-abdomen, used to mark their territory.
- **Adaptation to adverse environments:** Gerbils are able to withstand large temperature fluctuations. Gerbils normally have high levels of serum cholesterol and a short red blood cell lifespan (10 days). It is normal for red cells to show basophilic stippling on blood smears. Dwarf hamsters do not hibernate, whereas Syrian hamsters do. All hamsters are nocturnal; however, it is not uncommon to find Roborovski hamsters out during the daytime.

	Mice	Rats	Hamsters (Syrian)	Gerbils
Average life expectancy (years)	1–2.5	3	1.5–2	1.5–2.5
Bodyweight (g)	20–40	225–500	100–200	70–130
Body temperature (°C)	37.5	38	38 (hibernates)	38
Heart rate (beats/min)	500–600	260–450	280–412	300–400
Respiratory rate (breaths/min)	100–250	70–150	33–127	90–140

2.9   Biological data for myomorphs.

	Mice	Rats	Hamsters (Syrian)	Gerbils
Age at sexual maturity (weeks)	3–4	6	6–10	10–12
Gestation period (days)	19–21	20–22	15–18	24–26
Average litter size	5–12	6–12	3–7	3–6
Age at weaning (days)	21	21	21–28	21–28
Comments				Form monogamous pairs. Male helps rear the young.

2.10 Reproductive data for myomorphs.

Sexing

The anogenital distance is greater in males and testicles are obvious in the scrotal area of intact males (Figure 2.11). In females the distance is much shorter, with visible nipples evident. In mature male hamsters, testicular bulges are visible when viewed from above (Figure 2.12).

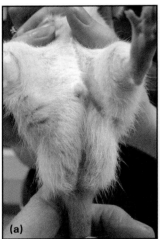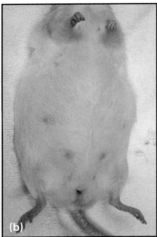

(a)   (b)

2.11 Male (**a**) and female (**b**) rat genitalia.

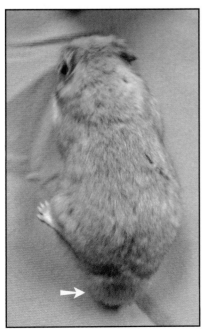

2.12 A male hamster with testicular bulges (arrowed).

Diet

- Rats and mice are omnivorous opportunists and have a tendency to obesity if given a high-sugar or high-fat diet. Ideally, a commercial rodent cereal mix or complete rodent pellet should be fed, supplemented with a small quantity of fruit, vegetables and occasional household scraps or dog biscuits. Scatter feeding will encourage foraging behaviour. *Ad libitum* fresh water should be provided daily in drinking bottles.
- Hamsters and gerbils should be fed rodent mix or pellets, with fruit and vegetables and occasional insects and animal protein as a treat. Hamsters store food in their nest boxes and old food should be removed regularly. A small amount of good quality hay should also be offered.

Housing

Myomorphs should be housed indoors in metal- or plastic-based cages. Some commercially available cages consist of a system of plastic tunnels, interconnecting nesting areas and a main exercise area (Figure 2.13). These provide a more natural tunnel-based environment, although can be difficult to clean and have reduced ventilation. Shredded paper or hay should be used for nesting material; hay should be dust-free, to reduce the risk of respiratory disease. Cotton-, nylon- or cellulose-based materials should be avoided as these may cause cheek pouch impactions in hamsters or become entangled around limbs. Hamsters and gerbils require deep

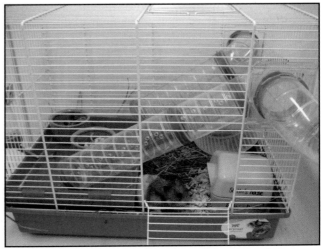

2.13 Typical hamster housing, with access door open.

substrate for burrowing; wood shavings are the best for this, although peat, wood pulp, paper-based and corn cob materials may also be used. Nest boxes and hide areas should be provided as well as branches, tubes, ladders and exercise wheels (solid rather than open to prevent injuries). Exercise is particularly important for hamsters as in the wild they travel vast distances, and exercise balls can also be used. Sand baths should be provided for gerbils. Wood- and paper-based products such as cardboard rolls and boxes to gnaw are also enjoyed. Animals should be kept out of direct sunlight. Cages should be cleaned out twice weekly, to ensure good hygiene and to prevent high levels of ammonia accumulating, which could predispose animals to respiratory disease.

Mice, rats and gerbils are highly social animals and should be kept in single-sex groups (although males may fight) or as breeding pairs. Syrian hamsters should be housed singly. Dwarf hamsters are sociable and should ideally be kept in same-sex pairs or breeding groups.

Hystricomorphs

Species and common breeds

Guinea pigs, chinchillas and degus belong to the Hystricomorpha suborder (porcupine-like rodents). Guinea pigs (also known as cavies) belong to the Caviidae family. Chinchillas belong to the Chinchillidae family. Degus (also known as brush-tailed rats) belong to the Octodontidae family, meaning 'eight-toothed rodent' referring to the figure-of-eight pattern on the surface of their molar teeth.

The most common breeds of guinea pig are the English (or American in the USA), which has a short coat (Figure 2.14a), the Abyssinian, which has a rosetted coat (Figure 2.14b), and the Peruvian, which is longhaired (Figure 2.14c). There are many different varieties with a range of coat colour, markings and hair type. Chinchillas have different colour varieties (white, brown velvet, black velvet, charcoal, and pastels); however, the natural colour is a bluish-grey with a white underside. Degus are naturally brown over the dorsum, with a cream underside and lighter-coloured circles around the eyes (Figure 2.15).

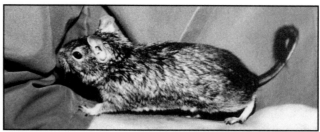

2.15 A degu. (Reproduced from the *BSAVA Manual of Exotic Pets*)

Natural history and normal behaviour

All three species originate from South America, where they live in family groups in burrows high in the mountainous regions of the Andes. Guinea pigs are farmed for meat in Peru and chinchillas were originally bred in captivity for their fur. Guinea pigs are crepuscular (active at dawn and dusk), chinchillas are nocturnal and degus are diurnal.

Guinea pigs make excellent children's pets as they are easy to handle, rarely bite, have little odour and are sociable. Guinea pigs and degus are highly vocal and communicate using a range of sounds.

Anatomy and physiology

Biological data for hystricomorphs are given in Figure 2.16.

- **Eyes:** Degus have excellent eyesight.
- **Ears:** All three species possess excellent hearing and have well developed tympanic bullae.
- **Teeth:** Hystricomorphs have the dental formula I1/1, C0/0, PM1/1, M3/3. They differ from myomorphs in that their incisors and cheek teeth are open-rooted and continuously growing, which often results in dental problems when they are given diets lacking in fibre.
- **Digestive system:** Hystricomorphs are hindgut fermenters, with a simple stomach and a large caecum occupying the left side of the abdomen. They are coprophagic.
- **Reproduction:** Male guinea pigs have large seminiferous vesicles extending from the pubis into the abdomen. Female hystricomorphs have separate vaginal and urethral orifices, with the vaginal opening usually non-patent until oestrus.

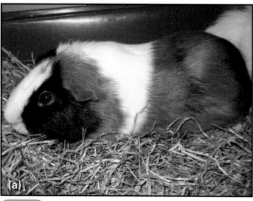
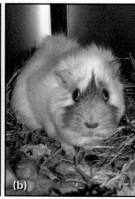
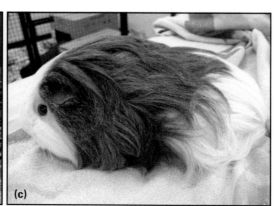

2.14 (a) English guinea pig; (b) Abyssinian guinea pig; (c) Peruvian guinea pig.

	Guinea pigs	**Chinchillas**	**Degus**
Average life expectancy (years)	4–7	10–15	7
Bodyweight (g)	750–1000	400–500	170–300
Body temperature (°C)	38–39	38–39	37.9
Heart rate (beats/min)	190–300	200–350	274[a]
Respiratory rate (breaths/min)	90–150	40–80	123[a]

2.16 Biological data for hystricomorphs. [a] Long, 2007.

	Guinea pigs	**Chinchillas**	**Degus**
Age at sexual maturity	Female: 4–5 weeks Male: 8–10 weeks	8 months	6 months
Gestation period (days)	63	111	90
Average litter size	2–6	1–4	6–8
Age at weaning (weeks)	3	6–8	4
Comments	Polyoestrous, with oestrus every 15–17 days. Young are precocial (relatively mature and developed)	Large vaginal plug is present after mating. Young are precocial	Breed at any time of the year; induced ovulators in presence of the male. Eyes of young open at 2–3 days old

2.17 Reproductive data for hystricomorphs.

In the pregnant guinea pig, the pubic symphysis gap widens 24–36 hours before parturition to approximately 2 cm. However, this symphysis fuses at around 12 months of age, causing dystocia if breeding is allowed after this age. Reproductive data for hystricomorphs are given in Figure 2.17.

- **Coat, tail and scent glands:** Guinea pigs have no tail and a well developed sebaceous gland on the dorsal rump area, used for marking their territory. Chinchillas have very dense coats, with each follicle growing up to 90 hairs. Degus have long tails with brush-like hair at the tip.

Sexing

Male guinea pigs have a round preputial orifice. The penis can be extruded by gentle pressure cranial to the prepuce (Figure 2.18a). Females have a V-shaped vulva (Figure 2.18b). Both sexes have two inguinal nipples.

In chinchillas, the anogenital distance is greater in males. Males have no scrotum and the testes are in or near the inguinal canal (Figure 2.19a). Females have a large urethral process above the slit-like vulva, which can easily be confused with a penis (Figure 2.19b).

Degus can be sexed as for chinchillas.

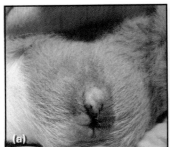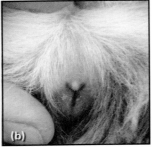

2.18 Male (a) and female (b) guinea pig genitalia.

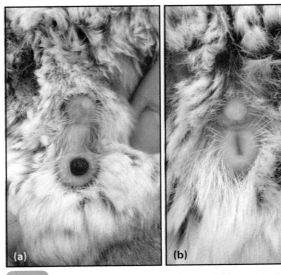

2.19 Male (a) and female (b) chinchilla genitalia.

Diet

- Guinea pigs have an absolute mimimum dietary requirement for vitamin C of 10 mg/kg per day, rising to three times this amount in pregnancy. Commercial guinea pig diets are often supplemented with vitamin C, but the shelf-life is short, and cool, dark storage conditions must be provided. The diet of guinea pigs should include a limited amount of commercial grass-based pellets plus large quantities of good quality hay or grass and a variety of greens (e.g. groundsel, dandelion, cow parsley and broccoli). Water should be provided in a drinking bottle and/or water bowl, and this should be changed daily.

■ Chinchillas and degus should be fed a small amount of grass-based chinchilla pellets and good quality hay *ad libitum*, supplemented with small amounts of vegetables. Sugar-rich treats should be avoided, as these can lead to dental caries.

Housing

Guinea pigs should be housed in wooden hutches or in wire cages with plastic bases (Figure 2.20). If outdoors, they should be raised from the ground to prevent exposure to draughts and should be out of direct sunlight, as they are very susceptible to extremes of temperature. Wood shavings and hay are suitable bedding materials. Regular daily exercise and grazing should be provided. A movable run or ark or a permanent outdoor pen is ideal, covered to prevent predation and with shelter (e.g. a box or a piece of drainpipe). Guinea pigs should be kept in single-sex groups, pairs or harems. Rabbits tend to bully guinea pigs and can transmit infections, e.g. *Bordetella bronchiseptica*, so they should not be kept together as companions. The two also have different dietary requirements.

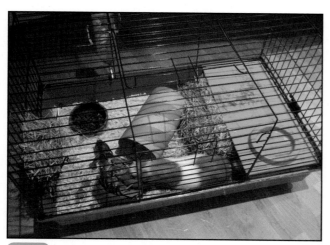

2.20 Indoor guinea pig housing.

Chinchillas must be housed indoors. A large wire cage (at least 2 m × 2 m × 1 m) is ideal, with a nest box, branches to gnaw and shelves at different heights to climb. A dust bath should be provided daily to keep the fur in good condition. Females are aggressive to each other so must be keep alone or in a breeding pair.

Degus should be housed as for chinchillas, with the addition of a deep substrate for burrowing, tunnels and an exercise wheel. They should be housed in groups or pairs.

Sciuromorphs

Species

Siberian chipmunks are often seen in captivity in the UK. The wild type has five black and white characteristic stripes along the back and tail; however, different colour varieties exist in captivity such as albino and piebald.

Natural history and normal behaviour

Chipmunks are diurnal, burrowing rodents that live in loose colonies with individual burrows in the wild. They will go into a state of torpor if the ambient temperature drops. Chipmunks do not tolerate domestication well and remain essentially wild in captivity. They are difficult to handle and very easily stressed.

Anatomy and physiology

Biological data for the Siberian chipmunk are given in Figure 2.21.

■ **Teeth:** Chipmunks have the dental formula I1/1, C0/0, PM2/1, M1/3.
■ **Digestive system:** They have cheek pouches for carrying food back to the nest. They are coprophagic.
■ **Reproduction:** Chipmunks do not show a post-partum oestrus. Females will abandon the young if stressed. Reproductive data for the Siberian chipmunk are given in Figure 2.22.

Average life expectancy (years)	3–5
Bodyweight (g)	80–150
Body temperature °C	38 (torpor may occur)
Heart rate (beats/min)	264–296
Respiratory rate (breaths/min)	75

2.21 Biological data for the Siberian chipmunk.

Age at sexual maturity (months)	12
Gestation period (days)	28–32
Average litter size	2–6
Age at weaning (weeks)	6–7
Comments	Females in oestrus every 13–14 days and will chirp to the male. Young are altricial and very vocal in the first 2 weeks of life

2.22 Reproductive data for the Siberian chipmunk.

Sexing

The anogenital distance is greater in males, with an obvious prepuce present. Testes are seasonally enlarged during the breeding season (March to September).

Diet

Chipmunks are omnivorous and will eat seeds, grains, nuts, eggs, fruit, vegetables and insects. They will also eat any mice that venture into their enclosure. A commercial pelleted diet for rats and mice should be given to chipmunks in captivity, with occasional day-old chicks, mealworms, cooked animal protein and boiled eggs. Pregnant or lactating females can be given supplementary protein, e.g. cooked chicken.

Housing

Housing is best outside in large aviary-like enclosures (Figure 2.23). Chipmunks should be kept in pairs or harems. They are very active and will exhibit stereotypic behaviour in small cages. Nest boxes, branches, pipes, rocks and an exercise wheel should be provided, with a soil, sand or bark-chipping floor. A double safety door on the enclosure is advisable as chipmunks are very fast movers. If kept indoors, the enclosure must be away from television sets, as the sound frequencies emitted cause intense stress.

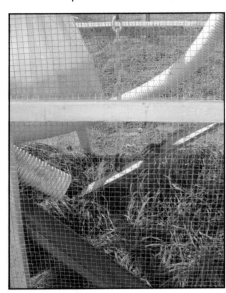

2.23

A Siberian chipmunk in an outdoor aviary-like enclosure.

Ferrets

Species

Ferrets are true carnivores of the order Carnivora and family Mustelidae. Ferrets are related to weasels, otters and badgers.

Natural history and normal behaviour

Ferrets have been used by humans for hunting rabbits and rats for over 2000 years and were domesticated from the wild polecat. Nowadays many ferrets are kept as house pets.

It is common for ferrets to sleep for up to 18 hours a day, which may make lethargy difficult to assess in an individual. Typically they show short energetic bouts of activity, followed by deep sleep. Seasonal weight loss is also common during the summer months, with as much as 40% bodyweight reduction. Ferrets are intelligent hunters. They will tolerate other carnivores (cats and dogs) but will assume that all other species are prey.

Anatomy and physiology

Biological data for the domestic ferret are given in Figure 2.24.

Ferrets are anatomically and biologically similar to dogs and cats, with the heart situated relatively caudally over the sixth to eighth rib. Ferrets have elongated bodies with a highly flexible spine, and so are adapted for running in tunnels and cavities.

Average life expectancy (years)	6–8
Bodyweight (kg)	Adult male (hob): 1–2 Adult female (jill): 0.5–1
Body temperature (°C)	37.8–40
Heart rate (beats/min)	180–260
Respiratory rate (breaths/min)	33–36

2.24 Biological data for the domestic ferret.

- **Teeth:** The dental formula is I3/3, C1/1, PM3/3, M1/2.
- **Upper respiratory tract:** Ferrets are nasal breathers like rabbits, although oral respiration is possible.
- **Reproduction:** In males, testicular descent occurs by 6 weeks of age and the inguinal rings close after this. The prostate is the only accessory sex gland in males. The female reproductive tract is similar to that of the bitch. Gestation lasts for 42 days and pregnant females should be separated from males. Dystocia is rare. If unmated, females will remain in oestrus (with an obviously swollen vulva; Figure 2.25) and high levels of oestrogen will result in oestrogen-dependent bone marrow suppression (anaemia, immunosuppression) and a hormonal alopecia. This is not seen in the USA due to neutering of pet ferrets at an early age before sale. Vasectomized hobs may be run with females as 'teasers' but mating is violent and can result in injuries and pseudopregnancy; this is therefore not recommended for pet or show ferrets. Current recommendations are *not* to neuter ferrets but to use hormone therapy such as proligestone in females, or GnRH implants (deslorelin) every 18–24 months in both males and females. Proligestone injections are associated with side effects such as skin reactions, pyometra, pseudopregnancy and breakthrough oestrus, and owners should be made aware of this. Neutering can lead to adrenal gland disease. Neutered males are known as 'hobbles'. Implantation of neutered ferrets will prevent adrenal gland disease. Testes

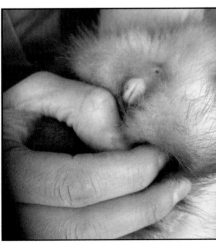

2.25

Swollen vulva of a female ferret (jill) in oestrus.

Age at sexual maturity (months)	6–9
Gestation period (weeks)	42
Average litter size	2–10
Age at weaning (weeks)	8
Comments	Reflex ovulation. Seasonally monoestrous from February to September in the UK. Oestrus can last 6 months if unmated and will lead to ill-health. Kits are altricial

2.26 Reproductive data for the domestic ferret.

descend only during the breeding season (February to August in the UK). Reproductive data for ferrets are given in Figure 2.26.

- **Skin and coat:** Ferret skin is extremely tough, and seasonal alopecia is common during the summer, with a thicker coat developing over winter. Colour varieties range from polecat or 'fitch' through to sandy and albino. Sebaceous glands in the skin produce the characteristic ferret odour and may excrete a brownish-yellow substance, which discolours the fur. It is the skin secretions rather than the anal glands that impart the characteristic smell; 'de-scenting' is therefore not possible.

Sexing

The anogenital distance is greater in males, with an obvious prepuce on the ventral abdomen and an os penis. Females have a shorter anogenital distance.

Diet

Ferrets are obligate carnivores and even pet ferrets maintain a basic hunting instinct. Commercial dry pelleted ferret diets are available which, when combined with weekly baths, help to minimize ferrets' musky smell. Fresh water should always be made available with a dry food diet. As this type of diet may result in boredom, food can be scattered or hidden to provide enrichment. Occasional treats may also be given, such as raw eggs, dead chicks, mice and rabbits. However, obesity is common and so the amount of food given should be carefully monitored. Ferrets may also stash food and this should be removed regularly.

Housing

Ferrets can be housed in a large hutch (Figure 2.27) outdoors during the summer months and moved into an outbuilding over the winter. Direct sunlight should be avoided as ferrets are prone to heat stress. Wood shavings, shredded newspaper and straw are suitable bedding materials. Ferrets are clean animals and will use a litter tray. Large secure exercise areas should be regularly available, or ferrets can be taken for walks on a harness and lead. They are social and can be kept in single-sex or mixed-sex pairs or in larger harems. House ferrets should have a secure cage where they can be kept when the owner is absent. Environmental enrichment is important and a variety of tubes, boxes and climbing platforms can be used to provide this.

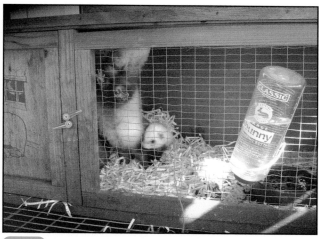

2.27 Typical outdoor ferret housing.

Less commonly kept pet species

Skunks

Species

The striped skunk is sometimes encountered in captivity (Figure 2.28). It belongs to the family Mephitidae.

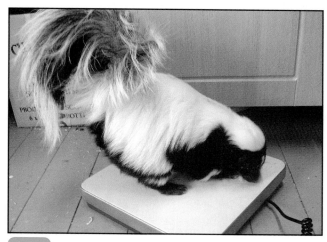

2.28 A striped skunk.

Natural history and normal behaviour

Skunks are native to North America, where their habitat ranges from desert areas and woodland to grassy plains and suburbs. Skunks do not hibernate but may become dormant during cold winters. They are solitary but come together for mating; males may mate with several females in the wild. They are most active at dawn and dusk.

Skunks are curious and inquisitive animals. They are also friendly and like playing, but may become more aggressive with maturity. They enjoy digging and foraging for food, and plenty of environmental enrichment should be provided. They are generally not recommended by the authors as pets.

Anatomy and physiology

Biological data for the striped skunk are given in Figure 2.29.

- Skunks have poor short-range vision.
- Anal scent glands are situated one on either side of the anus. Muscles surrounding these glands enable the contents to be sprayed a considerable distance, and the highly offensive smell acts as a deterrent for attackers. The smell is irritant and may cause temporary blindness.
- Reproductive data for the striped skunk are given in Figure 2.30.

Average life expectancy (years)	Captivity: 8–10 Wild: 3
Bodyweight (kg)	0.75–4
Body temperature (°C)	37–38.9
Heart rate (beats/min)	140–190
Respiratory rate (breaths/min)	35–40

2.29 Biological data for the striped skunk.

Age at sexual maturity (months)	12
Gestation period (days)	62–66
Average litter size	4–7
Age at weaning (weeks)	8
Comments	Seasonally polyoestrous. Induced ovulators with delayed implantation. One litter per year. Kits are born blind and deaf. Eyes open at 3 weeks.

2.30 Reproductive data for the striped skunk.

Sexing

Sexing is easy, based on external genitalia: males have a greater anogenital distance, with obvious testes and scrotal sac.

Diet

Skunks are omnivores, feeding on berries, grasses, roots, leaves, nuts, insects, grubs, small mammals, birds' eggs and amphibians in the wild. They may also scavenge for food. In captivity they should be fed a mix of dry dog food, tuna, chicken, vegetables and occasional fruit, with added vitamin/mineral supplements. Obesity and hepatic lipidosis are common in skunks, especially if they are fed cat food.

Housing

Skunks should be housed in secure wire cages at night. They require a large area to exercise and a hide area for sleeping in. They are extremely inquisitive and are good at climbing. Toys should be provided. Bedding should consist of wood shavings or newspaper to allow some digging behaviour. They are easy to litter train. Skunks can be kept on their own or with neutered littermates.

Raccoons

Species

The raccoon (Figure 2.31) is a member of the Procyonidae family, related to coatis, olingos and kinkajous.

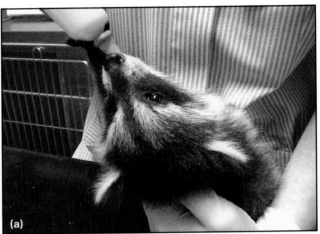

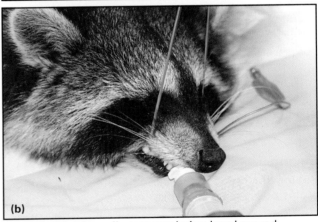

2.31 **(a)** A juvenile raccoon being hand-reared on milk formula. **(b)** An adult raccoon anaesthetized for castration. (Courtesy of Jo Hedley)

Natural history and normal behaviour

Raccoons are native to North America, where their habitat includes streams, coastal marshes, farmland, open forest and suburbs. Raccoons are nocturnal animals and are usually solitary. In the wild they inhabit hollow trees and logs and use the ground burrows of other animals for raising young or for sleeping in during the coldest part of the winter months. They weigh their heaviest in the winter, when they can double in weight. They are good swimmers and can climb trees.

Vocalization is common, particularly between a mother and her kits. Raccoons may act unpredictably and aggressively, particularly during the mating season. In some states in the USA keeping raccoons as pets is forbidden or may require a permit. They do not make good pets in the opinion of the authors.

Anatomy and physiology

Biological data for the raccoon are given in Figure 2.32.

Average life expectancy (years)	Captivity: 20 Wild: 1.5–3
Bodyweight (kg)	3.5–9
Body temperature (°C)	39.3
Heart rate (beats/min)	78 [a]
Respiratory rate (breaths/min)	24 [a]

2.32 Biological data for the raccoon. [a] Values obtained under general anaesthesia (Vogler *et al.*, 2010).

Raccoons are highly intelligent, with a good long-term memory. Their coat comprises almost 90% dense underfur, which insulates against cold weather. They have extremely dexterous front paws, which they use for foraging for food.

Reproductive data for the raccoon are given in Figure 2.33.

Age at sexual maturity (months)	Male: 24 Female: 12
Gestation period (days)	63–65
Average litter size	2–5
Age at weaning (weeks)	16
Comments	In the wild, young are born between April and May. Kits are born deaf and blind; eyes open after 23 days

2.33 Reproductive data for the raccoon.

Sexing

Sexing for raccoons is as for skunks (see earlier). Males possess an os penis.

Diet

Raccoons are omnivorous. In the wild they feed on fruit, nuts, grubs, crickets, small mammals, birds' eggs and nestlings, aquatic animals, cultivated crops and grains. They are known for their habit of 'washing' their food in water, using long slender digits. Wildlife biologists believe that raccoons have very sensitive fingers and, as they forage for food in water (for crayfish, tadpoles, frogs, etc.), they feel what they are doing rather than see what they are about to eat. In captivity, racoons should be given the same diet as for skunks (see earlier). Obesity is common, associated with poor diet and a lack of exercise in captivity.

Housing

Housing for raccoons should be as for skunks (see earlier).

African pygmy hedgehogs

Species

The African pygmy hedgehog (Figure 2.34) is a member of the family Erinaceidae. It is also known as the 'white-bellied' or 'four-toed hedgehog'.

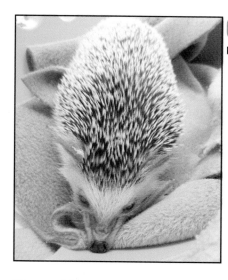

2.34 An African pygmy hedgehog.

Natural history and normal behaviour

African pygmy hedgehogs originate from Central and Eastern Africa, where they live in savannah grassland or scrub in burrows. They are nocturnal animals and are highly territorial and solitary, except during courtship and when raising young. Extremes of temperature will produce a torpid state, but they do not undergo a true hibernation. 'Self-anointing' is common (see later).

Anatomy and physiology

Biological data for the African pygmy hedgehog are given in Figure 2.35.

Average life expectancy (years)	Captivity: 5–7
Bodyweight (g)	Adult male: 500–600 Adult female: 250–400
Body temperature (°C)	36.1–37.2
Heart rate (beats/min)	180–280
Respiratory rate (breaths/min)	25–50

2.35 Biological data for the African pygmy hedgehog.

The dorsum is covered in spines. Contraction of the muscular ring called the orbicularis muscle enables African pygmy hedgehogs to roll up into a ball as a defence mechanism.

Reproductive data for the African pygmy hedgehog are given in Figure 2.36.

Age at sexual maturity (weeks)	8
Gestation period (days)	34–37
Average litter size	3–5
Age at weaning (weeks)	4–6
Comments	Polyoestrous all year round; oestrous cycle 3–17 days. Cannibalism of young is common; do not disturb female around parturition

2.36 Reproductive data for the African pygmy hedgehog.

Sexing

Males have a mid-abdominal prepuce/large anogenital distance. The testes are intra-abdominal. Males have large intra-abdominal accessory sex glands. Females have a very short anogenital distance, with the vulva directly below the anus.

Diet

African pygmy hedgehogs are insectivores/omnivores and in the wild will primarily eat insects, as well as worms, snails, slugs, spiders, birds' eggs, small vertebrates and some fruit. In captivity, their diet should consist of one to two tablespoons of high quality low-fat dry cat food per day, together with half a teaspoon of boiled egg or low-fat cottage cheese, half a teaspoon of chopped fruit (e.g. grapes, bananas, apples or pears) or vegetables (e.g. cooked carrots, peas, tomatoes or leafy greens) per day and occasional treats (mealworms, waxworms and crickets). Special hedgehog insectivorous diets are also commercially available. A daily vitamin/mineral supplement should also be given. Care should be taken to avoid obesity.

Housing

African pygmy hedgehogs should be housed singly (as they are solitary in the wild) or in same-sex pairs raised together. They are active animals and so require large cages (0.6 × 0.9 m minimum floor space). They can climb and so their cage must be secured with a lid. A hide area and exercise wheel should be provided. Soft substrate such as shredded newspaper, hay and wood shavings is ideal. The cages must be artificially heated to maintain a temperature between 24 and 29°C, using a heat mat or ceramic bulb and lighting (10–14 hours per day). African pygmy hedgehogs can be litter trained.

Slender-tailed meerkats

Species

The slender-tailed meerkat (Figure 2.37) is a member of the Herpestidae family.

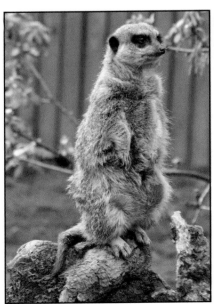

2.37 A slender-tailed meerkat. (Courtesy of Alistair Lawrie)

Natural history and normal behaviour

Slender-tailed meerkats originate from South Africa. In the wild they live in dry, open plains with hard or stony ground. Meerkats are very social and live in large colonies, averaging 15–30 members. Most meerkats in the group are siblings or offspring of the alpha pair.

Anatomy and physiology

Biological data for the slender-tailed meerkat are given in Figure 2.38.

Average life expectancy (years)	12–14
Bodyweight (g)	680–900
Body temperature (°C)	36.3–38.8 [a]
Heart rate (beats/min)	[a]
Respiratory rate (breaths/min)	[a]

2.38 Biological data for the slender-tailed meerkat. [a] Values follow a marked daily rhythm, with rectal temperature, respiratory rate and heart rate lowest at night (Müller and Lojewski, 1986).

- Meerkats are longsighted and will often miss food that is directly in front of them.
- They have the unique ability to close their ears; this is to keep dirt out while they burrow.
- They often depend on their sense of smell to find food.
- Both males and females share a similar physical appearance, including short hair and grey or tan markings. The markings along their backs are unique. Meerkats have dark brown or black bands around their eyes, which are thought to reduce glare from the sun; this enables them to spot predatory birds while looking directly into the sun.
- All four of a meerkat's feet possess a very sharp, curved non-retractable claw, used to dig their burrows.
- Reproductive data for meerkats are given in Figure 2.39.

Age at sexual maturity (years)	1–2
Oestrous cycle	Can breed all year round
Gestation period (days)	70
Average litter size	2–5
Birth weight (g)	25–36
Age at weaning (weeks)	7–9

2.39 Reproductive data for the slender-tailed meerkat.

Sexing

Male meerkats have a greater anogenital distance than females, with a small scrotal sac and testicles (Figure 2.40). The prepuce is located on the midline ventral abdomen. The vulva is evident in females.

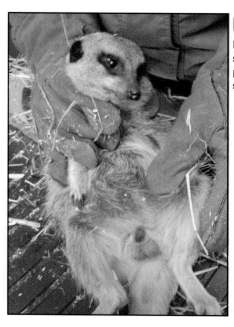

2.40 Male meerkat, showing prepuce and scrotal sac.

Diet

Roughly 85% of the diet should be comprised of insects and small vertebrates, with chopped fruit, hardboiled egg and commercial ferret food making up the remainder of the diet.

Daily food requirements:

- Insects, e.g. mealworms, waxworms, crickets, locusts
- Dead mice and/or day-old chicks
- Fruit, e.g. apples, grapes, pears
- Hardboiled egg, fed once or twice a week
- Commercial ferret food (biscuits)
- Vitamin and mineral supplement.

Housing

There should be access to both an indoor and outdoor enclosure. For one pair of meerkats, the indoor surface area should be at least 8 m². The outdoor enclosure should be at least 16 m² (52 square feet); the larger the group, the more surface area required. The enclosures should be furnished, with communal sleeping areas in which there should be nest/den boxes. There should also be areas to hide or shelter. Other relevant features of meerkat enclosures are lookouts and basking spots. Due to the hierarchical structure of meerkat groups, visual barriers such as rocks, tree trunks, etc. should be provided to allow the subordinate members of the group to escape from constant monitoring by the more dominant individuals. Sand or sandy material should be chosen as the substrate for meerkats; this will allow natural digging behaviour. Rocks and stones should also be provided to help maintain good nail condition and length. All substrate should be removed at least once a year to allow the enclosure to be cleaned and disinfected thoroughly. Enclosure fencing should be buried deeply to prevent meerkats from tunnelling out.

Marsupials

Sugar gliders

Species

The sugar glider belongs to the species *Petaurus breviceps* (Figure 2.41).

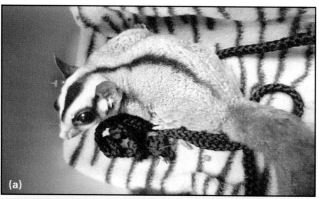

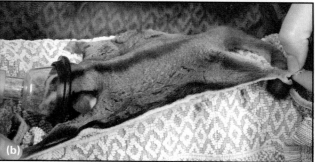

2.41 (a) A sugar glider. (b) An anaesthetized sugar glider, showing the extent of the patagium.

Natural history and normal behaviour

Sugar gliders are Native to Australia and New Zealand. They are social animals that live in groups of up to 12 individuals in the wild.

Anatomy and physiology

Biological data for the sugar glider are given in Figure 2.42.

Average life expectancy (years)	12–14
Bodyweight (g)	Male: 115–160 Female: 95–135
Body temperature (°C)	Average 32
Heart rate (beats/min)	200–300
Respiratory rate (breaths/min)	16–40

2.42 Biological data for the sugar glider.

- Sugar gliders have blue/grey fur, with a black line extending from the nose to the lower back. To allow them to glide, they have a patagium, which extends from the lateral aspect of the forelimb to the tarsus.
- They have five digits on each foot; the second and third digits on the hindfeet are partially fused to aid climbing.

- Sugar gliders have a cloaca into which the gastrointestinal tract, urogenital tract and reproductive tract all empty.
- Reproductive data for the sugar glider are given in Figure 2.43.

Age at sexual maturity (months)	Male: 12–14 Female: 8–12
Oestrous cycle	Polyoestrous
Gestation period (days)	16
Litters per year	May have 2
Average litter size	1–2
Birth weight	0.19 g (joey weighs 5–8 g once emerged from the pouch, fully furred)
Age at weaning	Joey leaves pouch at approx 70 days, independent at 17 weeks but may remain in parental nest

2.43   Reproductive data for the sugar glider.

Sexing

Males have a bifurcated penis and a pendulous scrotum, which is located cranial to the penis. They have frontal, urogenital and sternal scent glands. Females have a ventral abdominal pouch that opens cranially. Unlike other marsupials, they have no eupubic bones, which support the pouch. They have urogenital scent glands.

Diet

Sugar gliders should be given a daily diet that totals 15–20% of the bodyweight.

The diet of a sugar glider should consist of:

- A variety of fruit, e.g. pears, oranges, kiwi, bananas, grapes, melons, mangos, berries (70% of the diet should be made up of fruit)
- Invertebrates, e.g. mealworms, grasshoppers, crickets, moths
- Nectar (commercially prepared nectar mixes are available)
- Vitamin and mineral supplement
- Fresh water.

Housing

Sugar gliders should ideally be housed in pairs. A fairly large enclosure is required; 2 m x 2 m x 2 m will house up to six animals. They are arboreal and require lots of branches for climbing. A nest box and hide area should also be available and the enclosure should ideally be lined with shredded bark and dried leaves. The enclosure temperature should be maintained between 18 and 24°C, as exposure to temperatures higher than 26.6°C can predispose sugar gliders to hyperthermia.

Wallabies

Species

Wallabies are macropods belonging to the Macropodidae family, along with kangaroos. There are over 30 species of wallaby with several species being kept in captivity, including the tammar (or dama) wallaby, Parma wallaby, red-necked wallaby and Bennett's wallaby, a Tasmanian subspecies of the red-necked wallaby (Figure 2.44).

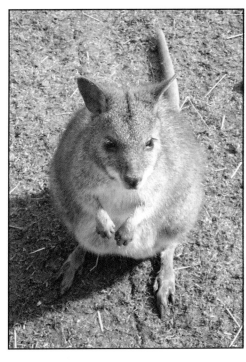

2.44   A Bennett's wallaby.

Anatomy and physiology

Biological data for wallabies are given in Figure 2.45.

- Wallabies possess one pair of lower incisors and one to three pairs of upper incisors. The molar teeth are curved so that only the first two molars are in occlusion. These are shed once they become worn and the more caudal molars move forwards; this is known as molar progression and is also seen in elephants and manatees.
- Wallabies are foregut fermenters, possessing a large sacculated stomach.
- Wallabies have a backward-facing pouch. They can have joeys (young) of different ages nursing at the same time, as they have four teats within the pouch. The older joey will be expelled from the pouch when the new embryonic joey arrives. Reproductive data for wallabies are given in Figure 2.46.
- The hindlimbs are large; the fourth toe is longer than the others, while the first toe is the smallest and the second and third toes are fused. Wallabies have eupubic or marsupial bones, which are boot-shaped, flattened and can vary in size. These bones are found in both males and females and serve as attachment surfaces for several of the abdominal muscles that rest on and articulate with the pubic and pelvic bones.

	Tammar wallaby	Bennett's wallaby
Average life expectancy (years)	10–15	12–15
Bodyweight (kg)	3.5–5.5	Male: 15–26.8 Female: 11–15.5
Body temperature (°C)	35–36	35–36
Heart rate (beats/min)	125–150	120–150

2.45   Biological data for wallabies.

	Tammar wallaby	Bennett's wallaby
Age at sexual maturity (months)	Male: >14 Female: 11–16	Male: 19 Female: 14
Oestrous cycle	30 days	Seasonal
Gestation period (days)	25–28	30
Birth weight (g)	<1	<1
Age at weaning	Joey leaves pouch at approximately 250 days. Weaned at 10–11 months	Joey leaves pouch at approximately 7–8 months. Weaned at 12–17 months

2.46   Reproductive data for wallabies.

Natural history and normal behaviour

The tammar (or dama) wallaby is found in the south-west coastal area of Western Australia. Bennett's wallaby is found in Tasmania.

Wallabies are social animals that can live alongside rabbits and other herbivores quite happily.

Sexing

In males, the scrotum hangs ventrally from the abdomen. Females have pouches.

Diet

The diet of a wallaby should consist of:

- Fresh grazing
- Timothy or other grass hay
- Small amount of dark green leaves
- Small amount of commercial pelleted diet, e.g. Mazuri Kangaroo/Wallaby Diet.

Starches, processed fruits and carbohydrates should be avoided as these can have a harmful effect on the gastrointestinal flora and can lead to dental disease and tooth root infection.

Housing

Wallabies need as large an enclosure as possible to allow the animal plenty of space to hop around. The smallest enclosure acceptable would be 900 cm × 900 cm. The enclosure should be fenced; remembering that wallabies may try and jump over the fence, it should be at least 2.4 m high. Wallabies are also good diggers; the enclosure should therefore extend more than 60 cm below ground. They should be provided with a shaded area. Enclosure

temperatures for the tammar wallaby should be above 16°C; Bennett's wallabies are more tolerant of lower temperatures. If the temperature drops below freezing at night, additional heat should be supplied to keep the enclosure between 15 and 16°C.

Primates

Common marmosets

Species

The common marmoset (Figure 2.47) belongs to the Callitrichidae family of primates.

Natural history and normal behaviour

Common marmosets originate from Central and South America (primarily tropical rainforests of northeast Brazil). They are arboreal and live in groups of eight to ten.

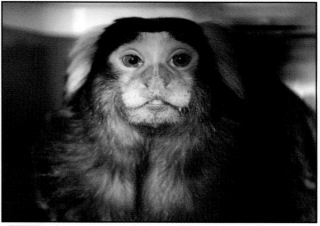

2.47   A common marmoset. (Courtesy of Alistair Lawrie)

Anatomy and physiology

Biological data for the common marmoset are given in Figure 2.48.

- Marmosets have high brain development with stereoscopic vision.
- Deciduous dentition is I2/2 C1/1 M3/3; permanent dentition is I2/2 C1/1 PM3/3 M2/2. The lower incisors are elongated and have a similar crown length to the canines. This enables them to gouge holes when feeding, to access gum, resin and sap.
- Marmosets have five digits on both hands and feet. Nails have been replaced by claws on all except the first digit on the feet.
- The tail is not prehensile.
- Reproductive data for common marmosets are given in Figure 2.49.

Average life expectancy (years)	15
Bodyweight (g)	Male: up to 350 Female: up to 300
Body temperature (°C)	39–40
Heart rate (beats/min)	200–350
Respiratory rate (breaths/min)	30–70

2.48 Biological data for the common marmoset.

Age at sexual maturity (months)	Male: 16 Female: 12 (first reproduction at 20 months)
Oestrous cycle (days)	16–30
Gestation period (days)	148
Litters per year	2
Average litter size	2 (1–4)
Birth weight (g)	35–40
Age at weaning (months)	2–4

2.49 Reproductive data for the common marmoset.

Sexing

The genitalia of females closely resemble those of males; sex determination is therefore difficult in this species. Accurate sex determination is easier in adult animals and is based on shape of the genital opening, eversion of the penis from the prepuce, and palpation of the testes in the scrotum or inguinal region.

Diet

Wild callitrichids are omnivorous, consuming fruit, insects, small birds, reptiles, amphibians, small rodents, birds' eggs, nectar, flowers and gum. In captivity, adult callitrichids should consume 20% of their bodyweight on a daily basis and should be fed twice daily. Pelleted food should be offered first thing in the morning when the animals are most hungry. Produce should then be offered in the afternoon and should represent no more than 30% of the energy intake. In practice, a feeding regime of 70% produce and 30% dry food (by weight) should provide proper energy intake.

The diet of a common marmoset should consist of:

- Complete feed, e.g. pellets (e.g. Mazuri NW Primate), canned marmoset diet (Zupreem) or marmoset jelly (Mazuri)
- Fruit, e.g. apples, pears, bananas, grapes, kiwi, mangos
- Vegetables, e.g. tomatoes, carrots, peas, sweet potatoes, boiled potatoes
- Grated cheddar cheese
- Hardboiled eggs
- Live insects, e.g. mealworms, crickets, locusts. The insects themselves should be fed on an 8% calcium diet 48 hours prior to being used as food
- Vitamin D3 supplement – callitrichids are unable to utilize vitamin D2 from plants efficiently; supplementation with D3 is essential (250–400 IU daily requirement). They also have a higher calcium requirement than other mammals. The calcium to phosphorus (Ca:P) ratio of the diet should be between 1:1 and 2:1
- Gum arabic provided daily as a treat and dietary enrichment.

Further husbandry guidelines for callitrichids can be obtained from The European Association of Zoos and Aquaria (EAZA) at www.eaza.net.

Housing

Callitrichids should be housed in an enclosure with indoor and outdoor areas; a double door for entry to the enclosure is advisable. The indoor enclosure should ideally be constructed of brick or concrete, with wood shavings or bark used as substrate. There should be adequate ventilation, and an active air circulation system should also be considered. The floor area should be no less than 3 m², with a minimum height of 2.5 m. Doors or tunnels in the enclosure should be controllable from outside the enclosure and should be situated at least 1.5 m above the substrate; marmosets are arboreal and so it is unnatural for them to travel close to the ground. There should be two routes of entry/exit between enclosure areas; this will ensure that dominant animals cannot prevent subordinates from entering or leaving certain areas.

The outdoor enclosure should be constructed of wire mesh or glass. If glass is used it should be made temporarily opaque for a short period of time to prevent the animals from running into the glass and injuring themselves. Grass or soil can be used as the substrate. Enclosure furniture should consist of a nest box (25 cm × 25 cm × 25 cm, with a door no smaller than 10 cm²), tree branches, ropes and ladders.

Callitrichids should have access to natural sunlight for ultraviolet exposure and should have a photoperiod of 12 hours. The temperature of the indoor enclosure should be between 18 and 24°C, with 60% humidity. When the outside temperature drops below 5°C, access to the outdoor enclosure should be limited.

Native UK wild mammals

Foxes

Species

In the UK the only species of fox is the red fox, sometimes also referred to as the European fox (Figure 2.50). It belongs to the family Canidae.

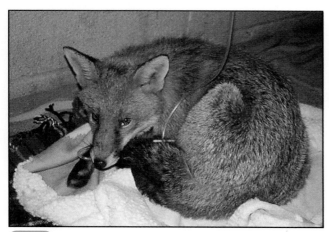

2.50   A red fox.

Natural history and normal behaviour

Foxes are ubiquitous in the UK, although they are absent from many coastal islands. They are often found in urban environments, and encounters with humans are common. They live in small family groups, consisting of an adult pair and cubs. The family disperses in the autumn when the cubs are able to fend for themselves. Adults are solitary during the autumn and winter months, meeting only for mating.

Foxes, unless very debilitated, will attempt to bite anyone handling them. It should be kept in mind that they are extremely strong and surprisingly agile.

Anatomy and physiology

Biological data for the red fox are given in Figure 2.51.

- Hearing is acute and is used to detect prey.
- Foxes are similar anatomically to domestic dogs.
- Coat colour may vary, but is usually reddish brown with a white underside. Albino foxes can also occur. Pups are brown-black in colour. Foxes moult once a year in the spring, which can sometimes be confused with mange infection.

Average life expectancy (years)	Captivity: 14 Wild: 1.5–2
Bodyweight (kg)	Adult male (dog): 6.5 Adult female (vixen): 5.5
Body temperature (°C)	38–39
Heart rate (beats/min)	75–185
Respiratory rate (breaths/min)	11–20

2.51   Biological data for the red fox.

- Pups are born in March or April, with average litter sizes of three to six. Orphan cubs are commonly picked up by well meaning members of the public and may be mistaken for kittens. They should be kept warm and are easy to rear using a canine milk replacer offered every 3 hours. Stimulation of the perineal area for toileting is required after feeding. Reproductive data for the red fox are given in Figure 2.52.

Age at sexual maturity (months)	9–10
Gestation period (days)	49–58 (average 53)
Average litter size	3–6
Age at weaning (weeks)	6
Comments	Pseudopregnancy can occur. Pups born blind and deaf and are unable to thermoregulate for first 2 weeks. Eyes open 11–14 days. Start picking at solid food at 21–28 days

2.52   Reproductive data for the red fox.

Sexing

Sexing is as for domestic dogs. Males have a small scrotum and ventral midline prepuce and penis.

Diet

In the wild, foxes eat small mammals, birds, insects and scraps from bins. In captivity, foxes can be given tinned dog food mixed with dry biscuits for a short period of time. Whole chicks, rabbit pieces or small rodents may also be offered to provide a more varied diet.

Housing

Foxes should be housed in well built, secure cubicles or in portable kennels. Foxes are extremely agile and can escape easily. They can be temporarily housed in large dog kennels, although they should be moved to more secure housing once stabilized. Sawdust or paper makes a good substrate, and a hide area such as a cardboard box, an upturned dog basket, a pile of blankets or shredded paper should be provided. Foxes rely heavily on their sense of smell; an item that contains the animal's smell should therefore be left when cleaning out bedding so that the fox is less stressed by the change.

Badgers

Species

The Eurasian or European badger (Figure 2.53) is found throughout Europe. Badgers are mustelids, related to ferrets and otters.

Natural history and normal behaviour

Badgers are strongly territorial, with a complex family hierarchy. They live in underground setts in groups

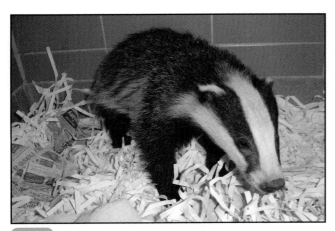

2.53   A badger cub.

Age at sexual maturity (months)	12–15
Gestation period (weeks)	7
Average litter size	3
Age at weaning (weeks)	15
Comments	Delayed implantation common, ranging from 2–10 months. Cubs born mid-January to mid-March in UK, blind and without fur. Eyes open at 5 weeks

2.55   Reproductive data for the Eurasian badger.

of around five animals of mixed sexes. They are nocturnal and, although they do not undergo a true hibernation, their activity is reduced over the winter months. Badgers bite when cornered or stressed; care must therefore be taken with this species. They are clean animals and toilet in one area, known as a latrine. Badgers groom each other and are highly sociable. When excited or threatened, badgers will raise their tails and fluff up their coat to look bigger. They may vocalize using a growl, bark or 'whicker'.

Anatomy and physiology

Biological data for the Eurasian badger are given in Figure 2.54.

Average life expectancy (years)	Captivity: 19 Wild: 10
Bodyweight (kg)	Adult male (boar): 9–16 Adult female (sow): 6–14
Body temperature (°C)	37
Heart rate (beats/min)	70–120
Respiratory rate (breaths/min)	18–30

2.54   Biological data for the Eurasian badger.

- Badgers have good night vision, as they are nocturnal, but may be blinded by bright lights.
- Badgers have an acute sense of smell, which is used for communication with other badgers.
- Females are induced ovulators and show delayed implantation, with cubs born in February. Orphans are common in areas with high population density. Reproductive data for the Eurasian badger are given in Figure 2.55.
- Badgers have very tough skin with dense fur, particularly around the neck area. Coat colour may vary; albino animals have been recorded.
- A large sub-caudal scent gland is situated at the base of the tail, dorsal to the anus, and this excretes a musk-like substance.

Sexing

Sexing is as for the domestic dog. Testes are more prominent during the breeding season.

Diet

Badgers are in the order Carnivora but are actually omnivores, feeding in the wild on worms, insects, mammals, birds, cereals and fruit. In captivity they should be fed as for the red fox (see earlier). Mealworms and peanuts can also be scattered for environmental enrichment. Water should be provided in a bowl.

Housing

Badgers are extremely strong and will chew, bite or dig their way out of any enclosure that is not metal or concrete. Bedding should be provided, such as shredded paper, blankets or straw. Noise should be limited as they are nocturnal. Long-term care requires specialist facilities.

 WARNING
Badgers should be isolated from other animals as there is a risk of them carrying tuberculosis (TB). Gloves and masks should be worn when handling this species and contact surfaces should be thoroughly disinfected. A risk assessment for handling badgers should be put in place for staff.

Otters

Species

The only native UK species is the Eurasian or European otter (Figure 2.56). Asian small-clawed otters are commonly kept in zoos and wildlife parks but are non-indigenous. They are smaller, with rounder faces. Otters belong to the family Mustelidae.

Natural history and normal behaviour

Otters are occasionally encountered at veterinary practices in areas where they are prevalent, such as Scotland, Wales, East Anglia and the West Country. Otters are solitary animals with distinct territories. Their habitat is primarily river or seacoast. Otters are secretive, nocturnal animals and if found are likely to be injured or in a severely debilitated state; with the exception of 'orphans' it is unusual for a healthy otter to be presented to the veterinary practice. Otters are highly vocal and use noises to communicate.

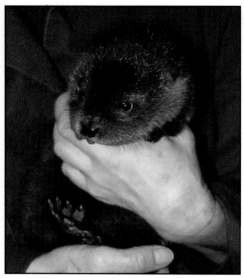

2.56
A Eurasian otter cub.

Anatomy and physiology

Biological data for the Eurasian otter are given in Figure 2.57.

- Sensory whiskers called vibrissae are present on the face and are important for tactile navigation in low water visibility.
- Cubs may be born at any time of the year. They are reared solely by the mother and remain dependent on her for almost a year. Reproductive data for the Eurasian otter are given in Figure 2.58.
- The coat is dense and traps air for buoyancy when diving.
- Large scent glands are associated with the anus; these deposit a musky smell on their spraint (faeces) and are typical of mustelids.
- Otters have webbing between the toes to aid propulsion through the water.

Average life expectancy (years)	Captivity: 10 Wild: 2
Bodyweight (kg)	Adult male (dog): 7.5–10 Adult female (bitch): 5–7
Body temperature (°C)	38
Heart rate (beats/min)	60–170
Respiratory rate (breaths/min)	20–40

2.57   Biological data for the Eurasian otter.

Age at sexual maturity (months)	18–24
Gestation period (days)	60–64
Average litter size	2–3
Age at weaning (months)	10–12
Comments	Cubs born blind and without hair. Eyes open at 30–35 days

2.58   Reproductive data for the Eurasian otter.

Sexing

Males have a larger anogenital distance than females, with a palpable os penis and a midline ventral prepuce. Males are larger and have a stronger musky smell.

Diet

In the wild otters eat fish, eels, frogs, insects, crustaceans and water birds. In captivity, otters should be fed fresh fish, such as trout. If a diet of frozen fish is given, this should be supplemented, e.g. with Fish Eater Tablets (Mazuri Zoo Foods).

Housing

Housing for otters should be as for badgers in the short term (see above). Longer periods in captivity require specialist facilities, as otters require access to water for swimming.

Hedgehogs

Species

The only wild species of hedgehog found in the UK is the European hedgehog (Figure 2.59); it belongs to the order Erinaceomorpha. African pygmy hedgehogs are often kept as pets and are discussed earlier.

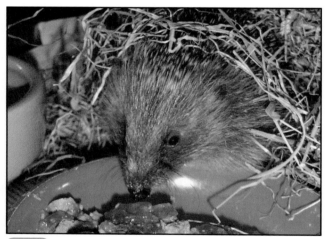

2.59   A European hedgehog.

Natural history and normal behaviour

Hedgehogs are widespread in the UK, with only a few Scottish islands free from this species. They are nocturnal and build nests from vegetation in sheltered places during the day. Hedgehogs hibernate over winter, when temperatures drop below 8°C. They are solitary and rarely fight. They can run fast and may reach speeds of up to 150 m/min. They are good climbers and can also dig well. It is unusual to see a healthy hedgehog out during the daytime. Hedgehogs are fairly vocal and communicate through a combination of grunts, snuffles and/or squeals, depending on species. A normal behaviour exhibited by hedgehogs is 'self-anointing'. This is usually in response to a new scent. Excessive saliva is produced, which is licked over the spines. The purpose of this behaviour is not known.

Anatomy and physiology

Biological data for the European hedgehog are given in Figure 2.60.

- Hedgehogs have a keen sense of smell and acute hearing to locate food.
- Spines cover the dorsal body surface and are replaced throughout the year.
- The orbicularis muscle is well developed over the dorsum, enabling the hedgehog to roll into a ball as a defence mechanism.
- The breeding season lasts from mid-May through to September/October. Females are seasonally polyoestrous and late litters are common in the UK. These offspring have little chance of surviving the winter and will either die or be picked up by members of the public and brought in to the surgery or to a local rehabilitator to over-winter. Hedgehogs weighing less than 550 g should not be released over winter as they will not have enough body reserves to survive. Reproductive data for the European hedgehog are given in Figure 2.61.

Average life expectancy (years)	Captivity: 10 Wild: 2
Bodyweight (g)	800–1200
Body temperature (°C)	35
Heart rate (beats/min)	200–280
Respiratory rate (breaths/min)	20–25

2.60   Biological data for the European hedgehog.

Age at sexual maturity (months)	8–10
Gestation period (days)	35
Average litter size	3–5
Age at weaning (weeks)	5–6
Comments	Hoglets are born with their eyes closed, without spines. These develop after 24 hours. The eyes open at 17 days

2.61   Reproductive data for the European hedgehog.

Sexing

Males have a midline ventral preputial opening. Females have a short anogenital distance and obvious vulval opening below the anus.

Diet

Hedgehogs are insectivorous and in the wild they primarily eat beetles, earthworms, slugs, caterpillars, snails and occasionally carrion and birds' eggs. In captivity, fresh water as well as cat food, minced meat and insectivorous commercial diet should be offered. For long periods in captivity, whole day-old chicks and mealworms may also be offered, as well as cat biscuits to help prevent build-up of dental plaque.

Housing

Hedgehogs can be housed in cat kennels. They are good at climbing so must be housed securely. They should be provided with a towel or shredded paper to hide in.

WARNING
When handling hedgehogs, gloves should always be worn due to the risk of direct contact zoonoses.

Red squirrels

Species

The red squirrel (sometimes called the Eurasian red squirrel), is a sciuromorph rodent that is common across Eurasia. It has become less common in Britain and Ireland due to the introduction of the Eastern grey squirrel and also habitat fragmentation. The red squirrel is protected across most of Europe and it is listed as 'least concern' on the IUCN Red List.

Natural history and normal behaviour

Red squirrels are arboreal mammals, found in both coniferous and broadleaf woodland. They are solitary and make nests (dreys) in the branches of trees. They have complex social hierarchies but do not maintain territories and the feeding areas of local individuals may overlap significantly.

Anatomy and physiology

Biological data for the red squirrel are given in Figure 2.62.

Average life expectancy (years)	Captivity: up to 10 Wild: 3
Bodyweight (kg)	250–340
Body temperature (°C)	38
Heart rate (beats/min)	105–280
Respiratory rate (breaths/min)	No reliable reference found. Squirrels tend to breath-hold when handled

2.62   Biological data for the red squirrel.

- Body length is 19–23 cm (not including the tail, which can be 15–20 cm).
- Coat colour can be variable depending on the geographical region of origin but is always pale cream ventrally.
- The coat is shed twice yearly and the winter coat is much thicker and darker.
- Reproductive data for the red squirrel are given in Figure 2.63.

Age at sexual maturity (months)	Dependent on bodyweight, usually spring of second year
Oestrous cycle	Seasonally polyoestrous
Gestation period (days)	38–39
Litters per year	2
Average litter size	3–4
Post-partum oestrus	Possible, dependent on food availability and bodyweight
Birth weight (g)	10–15 g
Birth characteristics	Altricial, born hairless with eyes closed
Age at weaning (days)	56–70

2.63   Reproductive data for the red squirrel.

Sexing

The anogenital distance is greater in males than females.

Diet

Red squirrels are omnivorous but the greatest part of the diet comprises seeds and nuts from trees. They will also eat fungi, berries, shoots and occasionally birds' eggs.

Housing

Squirrels are able to chew through many materials; stainless steel or galvanized wire cages are suitable. A nest box should be provided with paper for bedding. Tree branches for gnawing are appreciated.

WARNING
- **Squirrels have very sharp incisors and a strong bite that can penetrate leather gauntlets.**
- **Red squirrels often 'breath-hold' during handling, developing a fixed stare. This leads to hypoxia, hypercapnia and bradycardia. This can be fatal if handling is prolonged.**

Bats

Species

Bats belong to the order Chiroptera. There are 18 species of bat in the UK, ranging from 4 g pipistrelles to 40 g noctules. The most commonly encountered species throughout the UK is the pipistrelle. Further information on species identification is provided by the Bat Conservation Trust (www.bats.org.uk).

Natural history and normal behaviour

Bats can live for up to 30 years and all British bats are insectivorous. During the day, body temperature drops and bats go into a state of torpor. They are nocturnal, coming out at dusk to seek food. Bats hibernate over winter in roosts. Male bats roost singly or in small groups over the summer. Both bats

and their roosts are protected under the Wildlife and Countryside Act 1981 (as amended). It is illegal to disturb a bat at roost, except with a special licence. It is also illegal to damage a roost site or obstruct the entrance. For up-to-date legislation on bats, visit www.bats.org.uk.

Anatomy and physiology

Biological data for the pipistrelle bat are given in Figure 2.64.

Average life expectancy (years)	Male: 5 Female: 11
Bodyweight (g)	3–8
Body temperature, respiratory rate and heart rate	Variable in bats depending on ambient temperature, seasonal fluctuations, level of activity and reproductive stage. Torpor is common

2.64   Biological data for the pipistrelle bat.

- Bats are adapted for flight, with a patagium stretched between the digits of the forelimbs to form the wings. Ultrasonic echolocation is used to locate prey and to manoeuvre around objects.
- Mating takes place from July to early September, with males attracting females by making repeated flights around their roost and singing social calls. Reproductive data for the pipistrelle bat are given in Figure 2.65.

Age at sexual maturity (months)	Male: 12–24 Female: 12
Gestation period (days)	44
Average litter size	1–2
Age at weaning (weeks)	6
Comments	Mating may occur in the autumn, with sperm stored by the female until the following spring. Females congregate in maternity roosts in the summer, giving birth from June to July. Young start flying at around 4 weeks old

2.65   Reproductive data for the pipistrelle bat.

Sexing

Bats are easily sexed: males have a longer anogenital distance than females and an obvious ventral midline prepuce.

Diet

In the wild a pipistrelle bat can eat over 3000 insects in one night. Their diet consists of small flies, midges and mosquitos. In captivity, a jam jar lid may be filled with water or soaked cotton wool as a source of water. Bats may be fed jelly from cat food, or, ideally, mealworms dusted in a vitamin/mineral supplement (e.g. Nutrobal, Vetark) should be offered. A cotton bud or small brush may be soaked in electrolyte solution and offered to dehydrated animals. A catheter sleeve attached to a 1 ml syringe may also be used to drop fluid into the mouth.

Housing

Bats can be kept in small boxes or plastic containers with a heat mat against the side set to a maximum of 32°C. Paper towels should be draped over the sides to enable the animal to hang as if roosting.

> **WARNING**
> **Gloves should always be worn when handling bats due to the risk of rabies (European bat lyssavirus (EBLV) 1 and EBLV–2) following a bite or scratch. Staff handling bats should be vaccinated against rabies and, if bitten, post-exposure vaccination is recommended. To date, live rabies virus (EBLV–2) has only been identified in Daubenton's bats in the UK.**

References and further reading

Denver M (2003) Procyonidae and Viverridae. In: *Zoo and Wildlife Medicine, 5th edn*, ed. ME Fowler and RE Miller, pp. 516–523. WB Saunders, St Louis

Keeble E and Meredith A (2009) *BSAVA Manual of Rodents and Ferrets*. BSAVA Publications, Gloucester

Long C (2007) Degu cardiopulmonary values. In: *Exotic Animal Care and Management*, ed. V Judah and K Nuttall, p. 85. Thomson Delmar Learning, New York

Meredith A and Flecknell P (2006) *BSAVA Manual of Rabbit Medicine and Surgery, 2nd edn*. BSAVA Publications, Gloucester

Meredith A and Johnson-Delaney C (2010) *BSAVA Manual of Exotic Pets, 5th edn*. BSAVA Publications, Gloucester

Müller EF and Lojewski U (1986) Thermoregulation in the meerkat (*Suricata suricatta* schreber, 1776). *Comparative Biochemistry and Physiology A: Comparative Physiology* **83**(2), 217–224

Mullineaux E, Best D and Cooper JE (2003) *BSAVA Manual of Wildlife Casualties*. BSAVA Publications, Gloucester

O'Malley B (2005) *Clinical Anatomy and Physiology of Exotic Species: Structure and Function of Mammals, Birds, Reptiles and Amphibians*, pp. 173–195. WB Saunders, St. Louis

Quesenberry and Carpenter (2012) *Ferrets, Rabbits and Rodents: Clinical Medicine and Surgery, 3rd edn*. Elsevier, St. Louis

Rivera S (2003) *Exotic Animal Medicine for the Veterinary Technician*, ed. B Ballard and R Cheek, pp. 269–270. Iowa State Press, Ames

Stein FJ (1978) Sex determination in the common marmoset (*Callithrix jacchus*). *Laboratory Animal Science* **28**(1), 75–80

Vogler BR, Elias K and Steiner-Valentin KHS (2010) Anaesthesia in captive raccoons (*Procyon lotor*) during seasonal obesity. In: *Proceedings of the International Conference on Diseases of Zoo and Wild Animals, Madrid, 12 May 2010–15 May 2010*, pp. 6–9

Self-assessment questions

1. What is the dental formula of a rabbit? How do rabbit's teeth differ anatomically from those of cats and dogs?
2. Why is it recommended to breed female guinea pigs before they are 12 months old?
3. How is persistent oestrus identified in the ferret? What are the potential complications associated with this condition in female ferrets and how may these be avoided?
4. What husbandry-associated problem is common in pet skunks and raccoons?
5. What temperature should African pygmy hedgehogs be kept at?
6. Briefly describe what to feed a pet sugar glider.
7. Describe the dental anatomy and tooth wear pattern in a pet wallaby. What other species show this pattern of wear?
8. Describe how to sex a pet marmoset.
9. What bodyweight should hedgehogs be prior to release in order to be able to survive the winter in the wild?
10. What is the zoonotic risk when handling wild bats and what precautions should be taken?

3

Birds: biology and husbandry

Richard Jones and Carli Dodd

This chapter is designed to give information on:

- Common species seen in practice
- The anatomy and physiology of birds
- Dietary and housing requirements
- Some common behavioural issues

Common species seen in practice

Examples of bird species commonly encountered in small animal practice are given in Figure 3.1.

Psittaciformes (see Figure 3.2)

Characterized by a powerful hooked beak that is designed to facilitate foraging behaviour, including cracking into nuts and stripping bark from trees. Their popularity as pet birds stems from their ability to mimic noises and speech. They are gregarious by nature and highly intelligent. Examples:

- African grey
- Timneh grey
- Blue-front Amazon
- Double yellow-headed Amazon
- Budgerigar
- Yellow-sided caique
- Cockatiel
- Galah/roseate cockatoo
- Lesser sulphur-crested cockatoo
- Maroon-bellied conure
- Sun conure
- Grande eclectus
- Lovebird
- Blue and gold macaw
- Greenwing macaw
- Quaker/monk parakeet
- Blue-headed pionus
- White-capped pionus

▶

Passeriformes (see Figure 3.3)

Contains over 5000 identified species (more than half of all known bird species), many of which are encountered in practice. Wild passeriformes include a wide variety of songbirds and corvids; having a British bird book in the practice can be helpful. Examples:

- Canary
- Finches: zebra, Gouldian and society (Bengalese)

Falconiformes (see Figure 3.4)

Falcons: All have relatively long, pointed wings, a dark brown iris and a 'tooth' on the upper beak used for dislocating the cervical vertebrae of prey. They have a 'malar stripe' (a moustachial strip of dark coloured feathers below the eyes to reduce the sun's glare) and have an elongated centre toe to aid in capture of prey in mid air. The species of falcon encountered in practice range in size from the tiny male American kestrels, weighing only 110 g, through to the female gyr falcon, coming in at 2 kg. Examples:

- Gyr falcon
- Kestrel
- Peregrine falcon
- Lanner falcon
- Saker falcon

Shortwing hawks: The sprinters of the raptor world. They have relatively short, rounded wings, long tails (to increase manoeuvrability through woodland), a yellow/orange iris and a prominent orbital ridge to protect their eyes. They are generally

▶

3.1 Bird species commonly encountered in practice. (continues)

Falconiformes (continued)

highly strung species and so are often hand-reared and 'imprinted' to accustom them to human contact. Examples:

- Goshawk
- Sparrowhawk

Broadwing hawks: Soaring birds. The common buzzard, the only indigenous bird in this group, is essentially a scavenger but the North American red-tailed and Harris' hawks can become proficient hunters. They are robust and are highly recommended as a beginner's bird. The Harris' hawk, one of the few truly social raptors, adapts very well to its falconry role and as such has become the most popular falconry bird in the UK. They are highly intelligent birds and need constant stimulation in the form of regular flying/hunting. They are one of the few raptor species that can demonstrate psychological feather plucking. Examples:

- Common buzzard
- Harris' hawk
- Red-tailed hawk

Eagles: Generally large, broad-winged raptors. They have extremely powerful feet and beaks and any handling should be performed by experienced personnel only. Apart from specialist centres they are rarely kept in captivity due to the fact that the majority of the UK (apart from the extremely remote areas of Scotland) is unsuitable for hunting such a large and potentially wide-ranging raptor. Examples:

- Golden eagle
- Bald eagle
- Steppe eagle
- Tawny eagle

Strigiformes (see Figure 3.5)

Owls vary greatly in size and nature and, although generally not used for falconry, appear to cope very well in captivity and breed quite readily in an aviary situation. Some of the larger owls (e.g. European eagle owls) have extremely powerful beaks and feet and so must be handled with care. This is especially important in the case of hand-reared/imprinted owls, which can become quite aggressive to anyone other than their handler. Examples:

- Barn owl
- African spotted eagle owl
- Bengal eagle owl
- European eagle owl
- Little owl
- Tawny owl

Struthioniformes

Ratites are large, long-legged flightless birds, with long necks, underdeveloped pectoral musculature and no keel bone. Example: Rhea

Anseriformes (see Figure 3.6)

Anseriformes are characterized by their bill, dense feathering, elongated neck and webbed feet. All domestic ducks are derived from the mallard, with the exception of the Muscovy. Domesticated geese (i.e. those kept for eggs/meat production) are derived from the greylag goose. Examples:

- Ducks: Aylesbury, Call, Campbell, crested, Indian runner, mallard, Muscovy
- Geese: Brecon buff, Canada, Embden, Hawaiian/nene, Toulouse
- Swans: black, mute ▶

3.1 (continued) Bird species commonly encountered in practice. (continues)

Columbiformes

Pigeons and doves vary in size depending on species. They are generally characterized by 'stocky' body, slender beak and fleshy cere. Examples:

- Collared dove
- Diamond dove
- Racing pigeon
- Wood pigeon

Galliformes (see Figure 3.7)

Examples:

- Chickens: Ancona, Araucana, Barnevelder, Dutch bantam, Frizzle, Buff laced frizzle, Frizzle bantam, Leghorn, Marans, Orpington, Plymouth Rock, Rhode Island red, Sebright bantam, Silkie, Blue silkie bantam, Buff silkie, Sussex, Buff Sussex bantam, Speckled Sussex, Wyandotte, Blue laced Wyandotte, Golden laced Wyandotte
- Hybrid chickens: Bovans goldline (Rhode Island red/light Sussex), Bovans near (Rhode Island red/barred Plymouth Rock), Legbar (Leghorn/Araucana/barred Plymouth Rock), Marans cuivre (Rhode Island red/marans), Speckledy (Rhode Island red/Marans)
- Turkeys: Bourbon red, Bronze, Norfolk black

3.1 (continued) Bird species commonly encountered in practice.

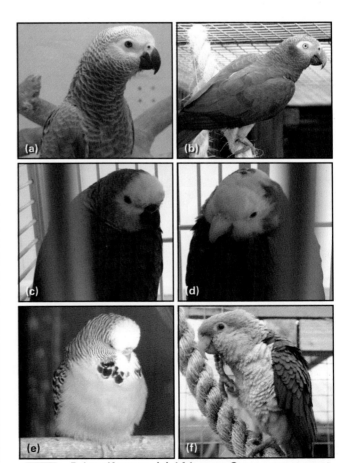

3.2 Psittaciformes. **(a)** African or Congo grey parrot. **(b)** Timneh grey. **(c)** Blue-fronted Amazon. **(d)** Double yellow-headed Amazon. **(e)** Budgerigar. **(f)** Yellow-sided caique. (continues) ▶

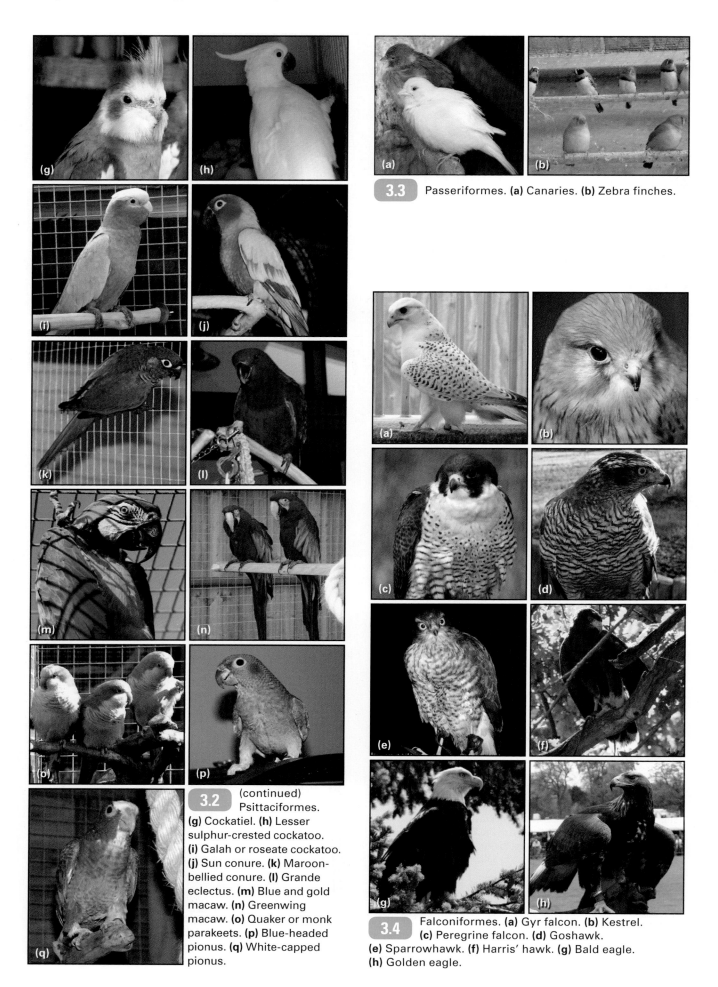

3.3 Passeriformes. **(a)** Canaries. **(b)** Zebra finches.

3.2 (continued) Psittaciformes. **(g)** Cockatiel. **(h)** Lesser sulphur-crested cockatoo. **(i)** Galah or roseate cockatoo. **(j)** Sun conure. **(k)** Maroon-bellied conure. **(l)** Grande eclectus. **(m)** Blue and gold macaw. **(n)** Greenwing macaw. **(o)** Quaker or monk parakeets. **(p)** Blue-headed pionus. **(q)** White-capped pionus.

3.4 Falconiformes. **(a)** Gyr falcon. **(b)** Kestrel. **(c)** Peregrine falcon. **(d)** Goshawk. **(e)** Sparrowhawk. **(f)** Harris' hawk. **(g)** Bald eagle. **(h)** Golden eagle.

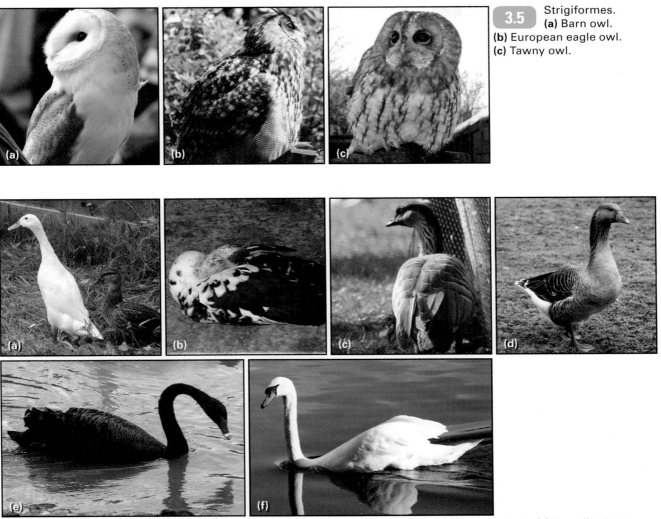

3.5 Strigiformes. **(a)** Barn owl. **(b)** European eagle owl. **(c)** Tawny owl.

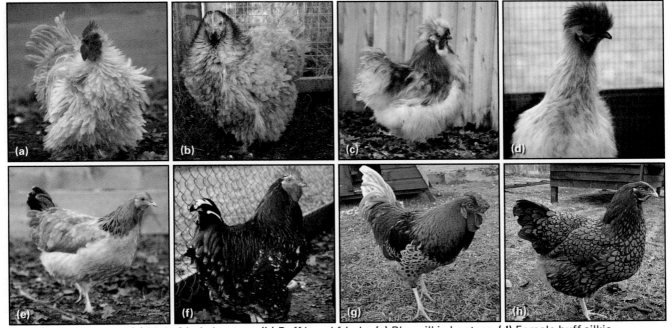

3.6 Anseriformes. **(a)** Indian runner duck (left) and female mallard (right). **(b)** Muscovy duck. **(c)** Hawaiian/nene goose. **(d)** Toulouse goose. **(e)** Black swan. **(f)** Mute swan.

3.7 Galliformes. **(a)** Male frizzle bantam. **(b)** Buff laced frizzle. **(c)** Blue silkie bantam. **(d)** Female buff silkie. **(e)** Female buff Sussex bantam. **(f)** Male speckled Sussex. **(g)** Male blue laced Wyandotte. **(h)** Female golden laced Wyandotte.

Anatomy and physiology

Biological and reproductive data for selected species are given in Figure 3.8. Average heart and respiratory rates are given in Figure 3.9.

Nervous system

The avian nervous system is similar to that of mammals, although the brain is proportionately smaller in comparison, with a much larger percentage of its mass dedicated to the optic lobe.

Structural features of the avian spinal cord are comparable to those in mammals, although they lack a cauda equina; thus the length of the spinal cord equals that of the vertebral column. Both brain and spinal cord are ensheathed in the meninges, although the epidural space is filled with a gelatinous rather than a liquid substance.

Cervicothoracic and lumbosacral swellings of the cord represent the origins of the brachial and lumbosacral plexus for the spinal nerves supplying the wing and leg. The nerves arising from the lumbosacral plexus pass between the pelvis and kidneys/gonads before reaching the leg; thus any inflammation involving the latter can result in hindlimb paresis.

The autonomic nervous system is comparable to that of mammals.

The eye and vision

Special adaptations of the avian eye include bony plates (the scleral ossicles) within the eye that stabilize the large globe to prevent its collapse. Unlike mammals, the pupil is under voluntary control. The lens is softer, allowing rapid change in focus, and is transparent to ultraviolet rays; birds can therefore see within the UV spectrum. The retina, unlike that of mammals, is devoid of blood vessels in order to

Common name	Adult bodyweight [a] (kg)	Lifespan [b] (years)	Incubation period (days)	Clutch size
Psittaciformes				
African grey	0.39–0.6	50–70	28	2–3
Timneh grey	0.3–0.36	50–60	26	2–3
Green-cheeked (red-crowned), blue-fronted and orange-wing Amazons	0.27–0.5	50–60	25–26	3-4
Yellow-naped, yellow-faced, yellow-crowned and double yellow-headed Amazons	0.375–0.58	50–60	28–29	3–4
Australian king parrot	0.20–0.24	25	20–21	3–6
Budgerigar	0.3–0.8	15	16–18	4–8
Cockatiel	0.8–0.11	20	18–20	1–7
Citron cockatoo	0.33–0.4	40–60	25–26	2–3
Galah cockatoo	0.27–0.39	25–40	22–24	3–6
Greater sulphur-crested cockatoo	0.8–0.95	57	27–28	2–3
Leadbeater's cockatoo	0.34–0.41	40–60	25–26	2–4
Lesser sulphur-crested cockatoo	0.32–0.4	40–60	24–25	2–3
Mollucan cockatoo	0.78–0.95	25–55	28–29	2
Umbrella cockatoo	0.55–0.6	40–60	28	2
Maroon-bellied/green-cheeked conure	0.6–0.95	25–30	23	4–6
Nanday conure	0.125–0.14	25	21–23	3–5
Patagonian conure	0.25–0.29	35	24–25	2–5
Sun conure	0.12–0.14	30	27–28	3–4
Eclectus	0.375–0.55	30	26–28	2
Rainbow lorikeet	0.1–0.16	16	23–25	2–3
Chattering lory	0.14–0.22	20–26	26	2
Lovebird	0.4–0.7	10–20	18–24	4–6
Blue and gold macaw	0.9–1.2	40–60	22–26	2–4
Greenwing macaw	1.0–1.35	30–60	24–28	2–3
Hahn's macaw	0.14–0.17	23	23–26	2–5
Ringneck parakeet	0.115–0.15	25–30	22–23	4–6
Blue-headed pionus	0.23–0.26	15–20	24–26	3–4

3.8 Biological and reproductive data for selected species. [a] Guideline only – large variation within species; must use in conjunction with body condition scoring. [b] Maximum lifespan collated data – may be considerably lower for captive species. (continues) ▶

Common name	Adult bodyweight [a] (kg)	Lifespan [b] (years)	Incubation period (days)	Clutch size
Passeriformes				
Canary	0.1–0.4	24	12–14	3–5
Zebra finch	0.1–0.2	14	12–16	4–7
Common hill mynah	0.175–0.25	8	14–15	1–3
Falconiformes				
Gyr falcon	0.8–2.1	16	32–33	3–5
Kestrel	0.15–0.3	16	29	4–5
Lanner falcon	0.5–0.8	14	31–33	3–5
Merlin	0.15–0.3	12.5	28–30	3–4
Peregrine falcon	0.5–1.0	18–20	31–33	3–5
Saker falcon	0.7–1.3	15	31–33	3–5
Northern goshawk	0.6–1.3	19	32–34	3–5
Eurasian sparrowhawk	0.1–0.3	15	32–34	3–6
Common buzzard	0.6–1.0	25	33–38	3–5
Harris' hawk	0.6–1.2	25	32–34	3–6
Black kite	0.7–1.0	24	31–32	3–5
Red kite	0.7–1.0	28	31–32	3–5
Bald eagle	4.0–5.5	45	35–36	2
Golden eagle	3.0–5.0	40	43–45	2
White-tailed sea eagle	4.0–5.5	42	34–42	2
Griffon vulture	6.0–8.0	40	48–54	2
Strigiformes				
Barn owl	0.3–0.4	20	32–34	4–7
Snowy owl	1.5–2.0	25	33–36	5–7
Tawny owl	0.35–0.45	18	28–30	3–5
Struthioniformes				
Emu	20.0–48.0	20	50–57	7–12
Ostrich	63.0–120.0	50	41–43	15–20
Rhea	18.0–40.0	15–20	36–40	10–12
Anseriformes				
Mallard	1.0–1.5	20–30	23–29	8–12
Muscovy duck	2.0–4.0	8–18	35	8–15
Canada goose	3.0–4.0	22–24	28	4–6
Hawaiian goose	2.0–3.0	18–19	29	3–5
Black swan	4.0–7.0	10–18	35–40	4–10
Mute swan	8.0–10.0	13–27	35–40	4–8
Columbiformes				
Pigeon	0.35–0.55	30	17–18	2
Galliformes				
Chicken	0.5–3.0	7–9	19–21	5–8
Turkey	5.0–8.0	12–13	28	8–5
Common pheasant	0.9–1.2	18–27	22–24	8–12
Grey partridge	0.4–0.5	5	24–25	8–20
Helmeted guinea fowl	1.0–2.0	10–15	27	8–12
Indian peafowl	4.0–5.0	18–24	28–30	3–5

3.8 (continued) Biological and reproductive data for selected species. [a] Guideline only – large variation within species; must use in conjunction with body condition scoring. [b] Maximum lifespan collated data – may be considerably lower for captive species.

Bodyweight	Heart rate at rest (beats/min)	Respiratory rate at rest (breaths/min)
25 g	274	60–70
100 g	206	40–52
200 g	178	35–50
300 g	163	30–45
500 g	147	20–30
1 kg	127	18–30
2 kg	110	19–28
5 kg	91	18–25
10 kg	79	17–25
100 kg	49	15–20
150 kg	45	6–10

3.9 Average heart and respiratory rates in relation to the weight of a bird. Restraint can cause a 1.5–2-fold increase in the rates given.

accommodate an increased density of sensory receptors. The fovea is the retinal area with the greatest density of receptors and represents the centre of maximum optical resolution. Birds possess a pecten oculi, which is a network of blood vessels that supply nutrition and oxygen to the vitreous, which then diffuse into the retina.

The ear

The external ear is a relatively short canal, extending ventrally and caudally from the external acoustic meatus to the tympanic membrane. The external acoustic meatus is a small aperture, nearly always circular, which opens externally on the side of the head and is protected by specialized contour feathers, which diminish the masking of sound from air turbulence generated by flight. The middle ear is the air-filled cavity between the tympanic membrane and the inner ear. The tympanic membrane projects outwards, unlike in mammals. Vibrations of the tympanic membrane are carried to the perilymph of the inner ear by the extracolumella cartilage and rod-like bony columella (homologous to the mammalian stapes), which is implanted medially in the vestibular window. The inner ear consists of bony and membranous labyrinths. The bony labyrinth, comprising the vestibule, semicircular canals and the cochlea, encloses the membranous labyrinth. Of the membranous labyrinth, the utricle, saccule and semicircular ducts are concerned with the position and movement of the head in space, whereas the cochlear duct is involved in hearing. The actual auditory performance of birds differs from that of mammals in several characteristics. The capacity to discriminate pitch is similar to that of humans; however, the temporal resolution is about ten times faster. Thus, the song of a chaffinch, for example, would have to be slowed down ten times before the human ear could resolve all of the detail that is learned by the chaffinch chick. As far as directional analysis of sound, that of diurnal birds once again appears similar to that of humans, although studies on the barn owl demonstrate that it has an acuity of localization surpassing all terrestrial animals so far tested, which enable it to hunt moving prey in total darkness.

Olfaction and taste

The visual lifestyle of the great majority of birds, coupled with the fact that odours are quickly dispersed high above the surface of the land and water, probably accounts for the popular assumption that birds have very little sense of smell. There is, however, abundant anatomical, physiological and behavioural evidence that birds do perceive olfactory stimuli. Vultures, for example, have been shown to congregate over odiferous up-draughts of hidden food items. Anatomically, the olfactory region of the nasal cavity lies in the region of the dome-like caudal nasal concha, which is lined with the olfactory epithelium.

In the past it has been widely believed that the sense of taste is poorly developed in birds. However, recent work has shown that taste buds are much more numerous than previously supposed. In most species the taste buds lie at the base of the tongue; however, in waterfowl they occur within the bill and in parrots they occur on the roof of the oral cavity.

Respiratory system

Nares

The position of the nares varies between species. Most commonly they are sited at the base of the beak. In some species they are surrounded by a waxy layer of skin (the cere) and in others they are surrounded by feathers. In some species the nostrils are found on the beak. Many species have a protuberance within each naris, known as the operculum. In falcons this is specially modified to act as a baffle, which regulates the amount of air entering the nasal cavity during high speed flight and may act as an indicator of air speed by detecting changes in pressure and temperature.

Nasal cavity

The nasal cavity contains a series of conchae, which increase the surface area over which inspired air must pass. The conchae have an epithelial lining, which secretes mucus. They cause the air to become turbulent and act to filter, warm and moisten it. In species that have a sense of smell, the olfactory region is found in the caudal nasal concha.

The nasal cavity also communicates with the infraorbital sinus, which surrounds and cushions the structures of the skull and helps to decrease the weight of the head.

Birds have a nasal gland, which, in marine species, enables the intake of salt water by secreting a hypertonic solution of sodium chloride. In some desert-dwelling species it is involved in osmoregulation. In other species it does not produce salt.

The inspired air passes through the nasal cavity and exits via the choana, which lies in close proximity to the larynx and glottis when the beak is closed.

Larynx

The larynx consists of four partially ossified cartilages, a dilator and a constrictor muscle. It has a mucus-secreting epithelial lining. The slit-like opening to the trachea created by the larynx is known as the glottis and is sited at the base of the tongue. The larynx is not involved in sound generation.

Trachea

The trachea is formed by complete cartilaginous rings that progressively decrease in diameter caudally. It has a mucus-secreting epithelial lining similar to that in the larynx. In some species the trachea is elongated and convoluted. In swans the sternum is modified to accommodate the trachea.

Syrinx

The trachea bifurcates to form the right and left primary bronchi. This is the site of the syrinx (Figure 3.10). The syrinx comprises ossified cartilaginous rings and soft tissue membranes of the caudal trachea and of the cranial bronchi and the syringeal muscles. It is the site of voice production.

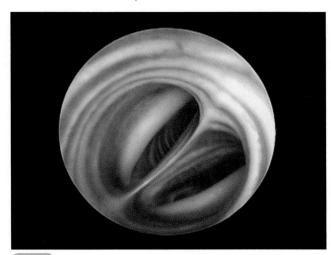

3.10 Endoscopic view of the syrinx.

Bronchi and lungs

The primary bronchi pass through the rigid lungs and terminate at the ostia, where they open to the air sacs (Figure 3.11). The lungs are fixed structures; they attach to the body wall dorsally and embed the ribs.

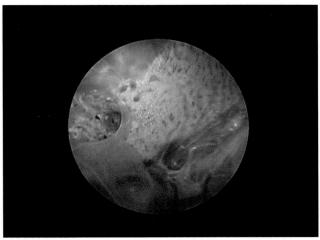

3.11 Endoscopic view of the lung and ostia.

Secondary bronchi branch off the intrapulmonary primary bronchi; and parabronchi branch off the secondary bronchi. The parabronchi contain atria and exchange tissue. Air capillaries branch off from the parabronchi; these air capillaries are tiny in diameter and anastomose with each other to form an extensive network. The air capillaries are interlaced by blood capillaries and are the site of gaseous exchange. The highly efficient gaseous exchange is facilitated by the cross-current flow of the air and blood capillaries.

The lung is 'divided' into the paleopulmonic and neopulmonic regions. The craniodorsally sited paleopulmonic parabronchi demonstrate parallel alignment, providing a platform for a unidirectional constant air flow. The neopulmonic parabronchi anastomose freely with other parabronchi to form a complex meshwork through which the airflow is tidal. The neopulmonic region constitutes no more than 25% of the whole lung and is absent in 'primitive' birds, e.g. some species of penguin and the kiwi.

Air sacs

Birds possess a system of air sacs, which are thin, poorly vascularized membranes that are not involved in gaseous exchange but act as bellows, ventilating the lung. The number of air sacs varies, as the cervical and clavicular air sacs are paired in some species and not in others. The cranial thoracic, caudal thoracic and abdominal air sacs are always paired.

The cranial air sacs

The cervical air sac(s) lies between the lungs, dorsal to the oesophagus. It diverticulates bilaterally and communicates with the vertebral canal. The clavicular air sac(s) occupies the thoracic inlet and diverticulates to communicate with the sternum, heart, thoracic girdle and humerus. The cranial thoracic air sacs are situated dorsolaterally within the thoracic region and communicate with the paleopulmonic secondary bronchi.

The caudal air sacs

The caudal thoracic air sacs communicate with the neopulmonic or caudal paleopulmonic secondary bronchi. The abdominal air sacs communicate directly with the primary bronchi. They diverticulate and are associated with the kidney, pelvis and synsacrum and, in some species, the muscles and bones of the pelvic limb.

During inspiration, the caudal air sacs receive half of the 'fresh air', while the other half passes into the parabronchi and air capillaries. Thus during expiration the 'fresh air' received by the caudal air sacs is passed back through the lung, allowing for gaseous exchange on both inspiration and expiration. This means that the volume of air in the lungs remains constant, which makes for an extremely efficient system.

Cardiovascular system

The heart is located in the middle of the thoracic region (Figure 3.12). It lies in an indentation of the sternum and is covered caudoventrally by the liver. Anatomically it is similar in structure to the

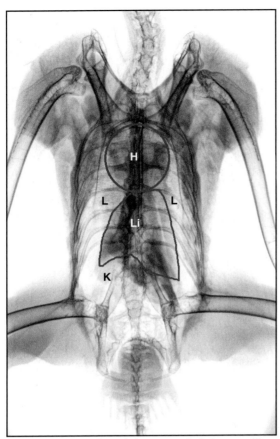

3.12 Ventrodorsal thorax and abdomen, illustrating the position of organs. H, heart; Li, liver; L, lung; K, kidney.

mammalian heart but is relatively larger. The right atrioventricular valve is devoid of chordae tendineae and the left bicuspid valve is a thin membrane. Pulse rate and blood pressure are increased when compared with mammals, and the ascending aorta curves to the right, in contrast with mammals.

Blood cells

- Erythrocytes are ovoid in shape with an ovoid nucleus. They are larger than mammalian erythrocytes.
- Thrombocytes are haemostatic cells, analogous to mammalian platelets. They are small cells with an ovoid nucleus.
- Heterophils are the equivalent of the mammalian neutrophils, as they are phagocytic. They are round cells with a bi- or trilobed nucleus and red-staining fusiform cytoplasmic granules. These granules are noted when blood films are stained with Romanowski type stains.
- Eosinophils are irregularly round cells with a bilobed nucleus and red-staining cytoplasmic granules.
- Basophils are round cells with an indented, single-lobed nucleus and densely packed blue-staining cytoplasmic granules. They are involved in the inflammatory process.
- Lymphocytes are round mononuclear cells and are found in three distinct sizes: large, medium

and small. T-lymphocytes (derived from the thymus) are concerned with the development of cellular immunity. B-lymphocytes (derived from the cloacal bursa) are concerned with humoral immune responses.
- Monocytes are large, round, pleomorphic cells. The nucleus can be round, horseshoe-shaped, indented or ovoid. Monocytes circulate for a short period before passing into tissues and becoming macrophages.

Digestive system

Oral cavity and pharynx

Birds lack a soft palate and thus have a single cavity known as the oropharynx. The choana is the fissure in the palate that connects the nasal cavity and the oropharynx. The palate is ridged both laterally and caudally to the choana. Another slit-like opening immediately caudal to the choana is the infundibular cleft; this is the common termination of the right and left Eustachian tubes. Caudally directed papillae are distributed on the edges of the choana and infundibular cleft.

The shape and structure of the tongue varies greatly and is directly related to the types of food eaten:

- Protrusible tongues are adapted for collecting food (nectar, insects, sap, etc.). They are generally long and narrow and can function as a spear, probe, brush or capillary tube
- Non-protrusible tongues are adapted for manipulation of food and swallowing
- Seed-eaters tend to have a stout, fleshy tongue
- Most birds of prey have a hard, roughened rostral portion to their tongue; some eagles and vultures have a trough-like curl to the tongue
- Piscivorous birds often have stiff papillae to facilitate holding slippery prey
- Many water-based birds have processes that interdigitate with the lamellae of the beak and a scoop-like portion to allow for collection of water and the filtering of foodstuffs
- Many species have a simple tongue structure with caudally directed papillae to facilitate swallowing.

The tongue is supported by the hyobranchial apparatus and, with the exception of psittacine birds, has no intrinsic musculature.

Oesophagus and crop

Situated on the right side of the neck, the oesophagus is a thin-walled distensible tube. It contains mucous glands but, in almost all cases, is not actively involved in digestion.

In many species there is a diverticulum of the oesophagus known as the crop (or ingluvies), which is found immediately cranial to the thoracic inlet. This is essentially a storage space to allow for the rapid collection/consumption of food. Pigeons and doves produce a 'crop-milk' for their chicks. This is generated by the crop lining in both sexes and has a high fat and protein content. Prolactin is the pituitary hormone that stimulates the proliferation of the epithelial lining, which secretes the 'milk'.

Proventriculus/glandular stomach

The oesophagus empties into the first stomach, the proventriculus. The lining of the proventriculus has two types of gland: one that secretes mucus and one that secretes hydrochloric acid and pepsin.

Ventriculus/gizzard

The proventriculus empties into the ventriculus (or gizzard) via the intermediate zone. In birds that consume relatively soft food (e.g. carnivores) the gizzard is less developed, is uniform in thickness and acts as a storage area in which the gastric juices can work. It is also responsible for the production of the pellet (or casting) in birds of prey (see later). In species that consume food items that are more difficult to digest (e.g. granivores) the gizzard is highly developed and well muscled to enable mechanical digestion, i.e. grinding the consumed food into smaller pieces that can be broken down by the gastric juices. The lining of the gizzard is known as the cuticle or koilin layer and is a carbohydrate–protein complex that varies in thickness and has a distinct coloration, caused by bile pigments regurgitated from the duodenum.

Intestine

The duodenum is the first portion of the intestine. In most species it is a U-shaped loop. It secretes mucus, and the bile and pancreatic ducts empty into it. The jejunum and ileum follow the duodenum. In neonates the yolk sac empties into the intestine at the junction of the jejunum and ileum. This is resorbed and the yolk sac is converted to scar tissue; depending on the species this occurs by 4–9 days of age. The large intestine comprises, where present, the caecum and the rectum. The caecum is sometimes paired (caeca) and occasionally sacculated. It is vestigial in psittacine birds. The ileum continues into the rectum, which is usually straight and relatively short and terminates at the coprodeal portion of the cloaca.

Pancreas

The pancreas is a trilobed organ closely associated with the duodenal loop. It is pale red or yellow in colour. It has both endocrine and exocrine functions, producing amylase, lipases and proteases including trypsin.

Liver

The liver is a bilobed organ (Figure 3.13). The right and left lobes are each drained by their own bile duct. In most species the right bile duct diverticulates to form the gall bladder, which is found on the visceral aspect of the right liver lobe.

Urinary system

The kidneys (Figure 3.14) are paired and are located on the dorsal aspect of the abdominal wall in the renal fossae of the synsacrum. They each have three lobes, or poles: the cranial, middle and caudal. The

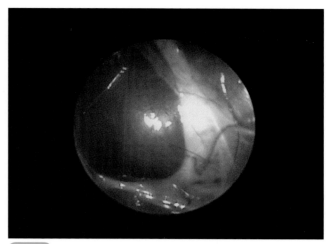

3.13 Endoscopic view of the liver.

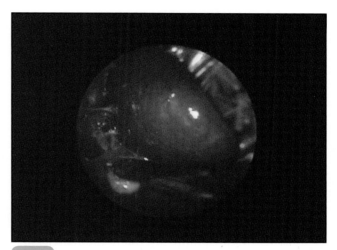

3.14 Endoscopic view of the kidney.

kidneys comprise a cortex and medulla, although there is not a clear demarcation as is seen in mammals. The kidney contains two types of nephron: those with a loop of Henle (mammalian type), which produce the urine, and those without (reptilian type), which excrete uric acid. The nephrons empty into a collecting tubule that serves the lobule; this joins a collecting duct, which in turn joins other ducts that combine to form a secondary branch of the ureter. Five to six secondary branches join to form a primary branch, which empties into the ureter. The pelvic ureter has mucous glands in its lining, thought to facilitate the transportation of uric acid and its salts. The ureters empty into the urodeal portion of the cloaca. Urine is then moved from the urodeum into the rectum via the coprodeum, by retroperistalsis, for storage until defecation. This affords the opportunity for resorption of water and salts, should it be required.

Renal portal system

The development of the renal portal system is another distinct feature of the avian kidney. One-half to two-thirds of the blood supply to the kidney comes from the hindlimbs via veins comprising a 'portal ring' and terminating in the counterflow peritubular capillary plexus, where it is mixed with arteriolar blood from the glomeruli. A valve within the portal ring is able to shunt the venous blood either away from or through the whole kidney or parts of the kidney. The smooth muscles within the shunt are innervated by adrenergic (relaxation) and cholinergic (contraction) nerve fibres, and it has been suggested that in times of exertion, such as during flight, the valve is open and blood from the hindlimbs is directed to the central circulation. A clinical implication of this renal shunt system is that injections of medication into the legs may lead to toxic levels within renal tissue, or even direct excretion of the drug without achieving therapeutic dosage in other parts of the body.

Cloaca

The cloaca is the common collecting chamber for the urogenital and digestive tracts, which opens to the outside at the vent. It is separated by two mucosal folds into three areas: craniocaudally the coprodeum, urodeum and proctodeum.

The proctodeum is the site of the phallus and the proctodeal glands and, in young birds, communicates with the cloacal bursa (bursa of Fabricius). The cloacal bursa is most prominent between 4 and 12 weeks of age. It contains lymphoid tissue and is an important site of B-lymphocyte maturation. This bursa regresses as the bird matures.

Lymphatic system

Lymphatic vessels are present as in mammals but are relatively less numerous. With very few exceptions, they closely follow the blood vessels, usually accompanying the arteries within the trunk. The central lymphatic organs of birds are the bone marrow and the thymus, and also the cloacal bursa. Both thymus and cloacal bursa, however, undergo fatty involution with the onset of sexual maturity. The spleen lies within the dorsal mesentery, between the proventriculus and ventriculus. As well as its lymphatic function, the spleen is also responsible for the recycling of aged erythrocytes, although this is primarily undertaken by the liver in birds. Peripheral lymphatic tissue can be found within the spleen and within the walls of the respiratory and gastrointestinal tracts. True lymph nodes occur only in certain aquatic birds, including ducks and geese, in the region of the thyroid gland and kidneys.

Endocrine system

The pineal gland is located between the cerebral hemispheres and the cerebellum. It is thought to be involved in photoreception, circadian rhythms and the control of reproduction.

The hypophysis or pituitary gland and the neurohypophysis (a direct extension of the hypothalamus) are located in the brainstem. The hypophysis produces follicle-stimulating hormone (FSH), thyroid-stimulating hormone (TSH), luteinizing hormone (LH), adrenocorticotropic hormone (ACTH) and melanotropic hormone (MSH). The neurohypophysis produces the hormones vasotocin and mesotocin, and controls part of the hypophysis.

Glands of the thoracic inlet

- The paired thyroid glands are the most cranial glands, located medial to the jugular vein. They secrete thyroxine and triiodothyronine. Both hormones have a similar activity, controlling moulting, stimulating metabolism, and regulating heat production and body growth, particularly reproductive tissues.
- Caudal to the thyroids are the paired parathyroid glands, which secrete parathyroid hormone (PTH). This initiates the resorption of bone to increase blood calcium levels, and increases the renal excretion of phosphate.
- Caudal to the parathyroids are the ultimobranchial glands. They comprise four distinct components: C-cells, which produce calcitonin; the parathyroid nodules; the vesicles; and lymphoid tissue.
- The carotid bodies are found in the thoracic inlet. Functionally they are associated with the APUD (amine precursor uptake decarboxylation and storage) system of cells, discussed below.

Adrenal glands

The paired adrenal glands are located at the cranial aspect of the kidney, in close proximity to the gonad. They have medullary and cortical cells that are interwoven. The medullary cells secrete adrenaline and noradrenaline. The cortical cells secrete corticosterone and aldosterone.

Gastroentero-pancreatic system

The APUD system of cells is a diffuse complex scattered throughout the gastrointestinal tract, pancreas and carotid bodies. It takes up amino acid precursors, decarboxylates them and stores the amines.

Pancreatic islets

Pancreatic islets secrete glucagon, insulin and somatostatin, involved in carbohydrate and lipid metabolism.

Reproductive system

Male

Testes

The testes (Figure 3.15) are paired and are located near to the cranial aspect of the kidney. They are bean-shaped and are commonly pale yellow or white, although in some species (e.g. some cockatoos) they are black due to the presence of melanocytes. Their function is the same as in mammals, i.e. spermatogenesis and testosterone production. During the breeding season the testes increase in size and weight; in some species this is dramatic, with up to a 500-fold increase.

Mature spermatozoa pass from the testis into the ductus deferens via the rete testis (if present) and the epididymus. Each ductus deferens runs along the medial aspect of the kidney in close proximity to the ureter. Each ductus deferens penetrates the urodeal portion of the cloaca to form a papilla that, in some

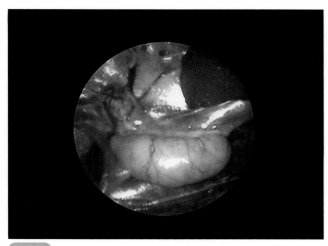

3.15 Endoscopic view of the testes.

species, swells during the breeding season to facilitate the storage of sperm. Some species, including ratites and waterfowl, have 'phalli' that are introduced into the cloaca of the female during copulation to facilitate the transport of semen. The 'phallus', if present, is located ventrally in the proctodeum, and dysfunction or disease of this organ may result in reproductive failure.

Female

In most species only the left ovary and oviduct are functional.

Ovary

The ovary (Figure 3.16) is located near to the cranial aspect of the kidney. It is suspended from the body wall by the mesovarian ligament. In immature birds the ovary is flattened. As the bird matures the ovary takes on a more cobble-stoned appearance. Under the influence of gonadotrophins the ovary produces follicles; this gives the classic 'bunch of grapes' look to the ovary. As the breeding season approaches, yolk, lipids and proteins made by the liver are deposited into these follicles, which increase in size and become suspended by stalks. Oestrogen, luteinizing

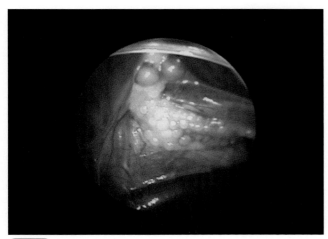

3.16 Endoscopic view of the ovary.

hormone and prolactin stimulate rupture of the follicle wall and ovulation. At this time the follicle is a thin sac, which is thought to secrete hormones including progesterone, associated with oviposition and incubation/nesting behaviours. During non-breeding times the follicles collapse and are resorbed.

Oviduct

During the breeding season the oviduct occupies the majority of the left caudal abdominal region; it reduces considerably in size when the bird is not breeding. It is suspended from the body wall by lateral and ventral ligaments.

There are five regions of the oviduct, with distinct functions: the infundibulum, magnum, isthmus, uterus and vagina.

Cranially, the infundibulum has a relatively thin-walled finger-like projection that 'catches' the ovulated follicle. This is then passed to the thicker-walled caudal tube-like progression, where fertilization occurs. The sperm is held in the grooves of the lining until required. The chalaziferous layer of albumen and the paired chalazae (twisted strands of albumen) are produced by the infundibulum. This process takes less than an hour. The ovum progresses to the magnum, which is the largest region of the oviduct. It is highly glandular and is responsible for the deposition of the majority of the 'egg-white': albumen, sodium, magnesium and calcium. This process takes approximately 3 hours. The isthmus, which is the next region, is much reduced in comparison with the magnum; it is short and less glandular. It produces the inner and outer shell membranes, taking between 1 and 2 hours. The uterus or shell gland 'holds' the egg for 20–26 hours. It is ovoid in shape and highly vascularized, with numerous longitudinal folds and glands. It produces salts, water, the shell and shell pigments. The final region of the oviduct is the vagina; while it is not involved in egg production, it contributes to the muscular expulsion of the egg and serves to store sperm. If positioned correctly, the egg will pass through the vagina in a matter of seconds.

Musculoskeletal system

The skeletal system of birds is characterized by weight reduction in order to facilitate flight. For example, the medullary cavities of certain bones (e.g. the humerus, femur and some vertebrae) are replaced by air-filled projections of the air sacs; strength is compensated for by increased mineral content of cortices and a series of bony 'cross beams' traversing the medullary cavity.

In female birds the medullary cavities, under the influence of reproductive hormones, can become filled with labile or medullary bone. This serves as a repository for egg-shell production and phases of its formation and destruction alternate during the laying cycle.

Skull

The structure of the skull (Figure 3.17) is modified to accommodate the beak, enormous eyes and a relatively large brain; it contains a large air-filled sinus to reduce the overall weight.

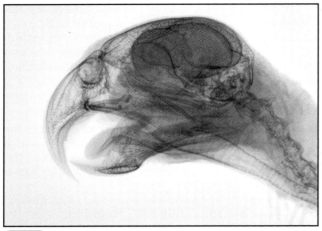

3.17 Positive radiographic image of the lateral skull.

In many species the nasal, premaxillary and maxillary bones form a rigid triangular block that constitutes the upper jaw, which can move independently of the rest of the skull due to the craniofacial elastic zone. In parrots this elastic zone has further evolved into a synovial articulation (hinge joint).

The quadrate bone forms the link between the mandible (lower jaw) and the cranium. A series of small bones, ligaments and seven paired muscles are involved with the kinetic movement of the beak.

The bones of the cranium are infiltrated by a system of pneumatic diverticula, presumably to decrease weight.

Neck

Birds have an increased number of cervical vertebrae when compared to mammals. They vary in number from 14 to 25 and, combined with the highly mobile atlanto-occipital joint, result in an extremely manoeuvrable neck, which compensates for the total commitment of the thoracic limb.

Thoracic vertebrae

In many species the thoracic vertebrae are fused, forming a bony plate known as the notarium. This provides a more stable structure to accommodate for the forces acting on the ribcage during flight. In other species there are distinct thoracic vertebrae with limited mobility.

Ribs

The 'true ribs' vary in number from three to nine. They articulate dorsally with the thoracic vertebrae and ventrally with the sternum, where they are ossified cartilages. In some species the last few ribs do not articulate with the sternum but with the rib cranial to it. There are a varying number of 'floating ribs', which comprise the bony ventral portion that articulates with the cranial aspect of the ilium.

Sternum

The sternum is highly developed in birds and has a prominent ventral median keel, which strengthens the sternum and provides attachment for the flight muscles.

Synsacrum

The last few thoracic vertebrae, all of the lumbar and sacral vertebrae and the first few caudal vertebrae are fused to form a bony plate known as the synsacrum. This provides protection to the viscera and a rigid framework to support the pelvic limbs.

Free caudal vertebrae

Varying from five to eight in number, the free caudal vertebrae provide attachment for the tail muscles.

Pygostyle

In many species the last of the caudal/coccygeal vertebrae are fused to form the pygostyle. This is usually slightly upturned and provides attachment for the retrices (tail feathers).

Thoracic girdle

The thoracic girdle comprises the scapula, clavicle and coracoid bones, which form a pyramid strut that maintains the position of the wing and provides support and attachment for flight muscles.

The scapula is a blade-like bone that is attached to the ribs. The clavicles are fused in most species to form the furcula (wishbone), which is attached to the keel. The coracoid articulates with the sternum and acts as a strut, holding the wing away from the sternum and preventing the ribs from collapsing during the downstroke of the wing. At the point where these three bones meet is the triosseal canal, through which the tendon of the supracoracoid muscle passes. This enables attachment of this tendon on the dorsal aspect of the humerus and results in the upstroke of the wing. The 'tip of the pyramid' articulates with the humerus.

Thoracic limb/wing

The bones of the wing are shown in Figure 3.18.

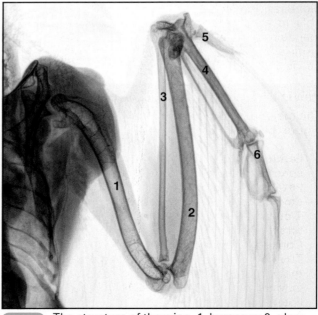

3.18 The structure of the wing. 1, humerus; 2, ulna; 3, radius; 4, major metacarpal; 5, alula; 6, digits.

Humerus

In most species the humerus is relatively short and broad, with the proximal end being expanded with a highly developed pectoral crest for attachment of the pectoral musculature. The humerus is pneumatized via a large foramen and a lateral diverticulum of the clavicular air sac.

Radius and ulna

In birds the ulna is the dominant bone of the forearm. The radius and ulna are reasonably widely separated, and both are bowed slightly to produce a unit that is resistant to the bending forces applied during the wing beats. The ulna provides attachment for the secondary remiges (flight feathers).

Manus

The radial and ulnar carpal bones articulate with the radius and ulna proximally and the metacarpals distally. The major and minor metacarpals are fused and provide attachment for the primary remiges. The digits are reduced in number to three: the alular digit, the major digit and the minor digit. The alular digit has limited independent movement and gives rise to the alula or 'bastard wing'. The major digit has two phalanges and the minor digit has one phalanx.

Flight muscles

The main muscles involved in flight are the supra-coracoideus for the upstroke and the pectoralis for the downstroke. These are highly developed in flighted birds and constitute 15–21% of the bodyweight.

Pelvic girdle

The pelvic girdle comprises the ilium, ischium and pubis, which are partially fused. The pelvis is elongated and arched in shape when compared to that of mammals. The ilium is fused with the synsacrum. In the majority of birds the pelvic girdle is incomplete ventrally to accommodate the passage of eggs. In flightless birds there is a ventral symphysis, presumably to accommodate increased bodyweight and maintain the body cavity when the bird sits. The pelvic girdle allows for attachment of the musculature of the pelvic limb and provides protection for the viscera.

Pelvic limb

The major bones of the pelvic limb (leg) are shown in Figure 3.19.

- **Femur:** The femur is short and broad. In many species it is pneumatized.
- **Patella:** Present in most species and well developed in aquatic birds.
- **Tibiotarsus and fibula:** The tibia and proximal tarsal bones are fused to form the tibiotarsus. Consequently, the hock is an intertarsal joint. The fibula is much reduced (in comparison with that of mammals) to a tapered rod and usually extends two-thirds of the tibiotarsal length with ligamentous attachment.
- **Tarsometatarsus:** The distal tarsal bones and three main metatarsals are fused to form the

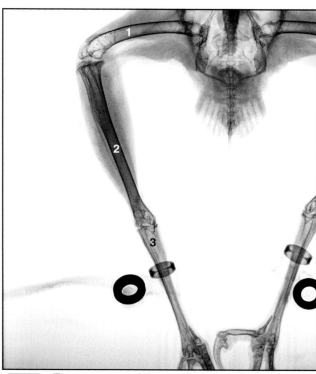

3.19 The structure of the leg. 1, femur; 2, tibiotarsus; 3, tarsometatarsus.

tarsometatarsus. In most species it is shorter than the tibiotarsus; however, in long-legged birds they are of similar length, which results in the centre of gravity remaining above the toes when crouching. Distally there are three trochleae for articulation with digits II, III and IV. Between the trochleae for digits III and IV there is a canal for the extensor tendon. There is a fossa medially for the first metatarsal.

- **Digits:** Digit I, the hallux, has two phalanges, digit II has three, digit III has four and digit IV has five phalanges. The distal phalanx of each digit is claw-shaped. The direction of the digits varies depending on the species. The majority of birds are termed anisodactyl, whereby digit I is directed caudally and digits II, III and IV are directed cranially. Zygodactyl birds have two digits directed caudally (I and IV) and two cranially (II and III). Owls, turacos and ospreys have a basic zygodactyl foot, but can move digit IV to direct it cranially. In most swift species all four digits are directed cranially to facilitate climbing. In terrestrial birds digit I is often greatly reduced so that it does not contact the ground.
- **Muscle:** The main muscle mass of the leg is positioned close to the body and therefore the centre of gravity; thus many muscles have long tendons of insertion. In some species (including raptors) many leg tendons become ossified, especially those involved in flexion of the leg and toes. It is suggested that this is an adaptation to prevent overstretching of such tendons in those species that feature heavy or prolonged loading (e.g. during climbing in tree creepers or capture and transport of heavy prey items in raptors).

Integument

Feathers

Feathers are unique to the class Aves. They provide insulation and protection, enable flight and are vital to behavioural and communicative function. Feathers are divided into three categories:

- Pennaceous, contour or vaned feathers
- Down feathers
- Filoplumes.

Pennaceous feathers are further sub-divided:

- Tetrices – Contour or cover feathers
- Remiges – Flight feathers
- Retrices – Tail feathers
- Ornamentrices – Ornamental feathers.

All feathers arise from feather follicles. The calamus is the 'end' of the feather, which is embedded in the follicle. The calamus extends into the rachis, which is the feather shaft. On either side of the rachis, at a 45-degree angle, are the barbs, each of which has two series of barbules at 45-degree angles, extending distally and proximally. The distal barbules have tiny hooks (barbicles), which interlock with the proximal barbules of the adjacent barb. This creates an almost airtight seal to each vane of the feather.

Down feathers provide thermal insulation and increase buoyancy in aquatic species. Down feathers are further sub-divided.

- Semiplumes – The feather shaft is longer than the barbs, and the vanes are 'fluffy' at the proximal end of the shaft.
- Down feathers – The shaft is shorter than the barbs or absent, and vanes are wholly 'fluffy'.
- Powder down feathers – These are continually growing feathers that shed minute particles of keratin (feather dust/wax). They are present in herons, pigeons, parrots, bowerbirds and toucans.

Filoplumes are specialized feathers and can be further subdivided.

- Filoplumes – The shaft is long and fine, with a tuft of barbs distally. Filoplumes are thought to be sensory detectors as they are closely associated with Herbst corpuscles (see later). Their close proximity to contour feathers suggests that they maintain normal feather position.
- Bristle feathers – The shaft is long and fine, with a few barbs proximally. Again, these feathers are closely associated with nerve endings. They are found around the nares, eyes and mouth.

Feather colour

Feather colour is generated by pigments, structural adaptations or a combination of the two.

Pigmentary colours

- **Melanin** pigments produce dull yellow, red-brown, brown and black colours. They are found in the epidermal cells of skin and feathers.
- **Carotenoid** pigments are dissolved in the fat globules of the feather and produce yellow, orange and red colours. They are synthesized from dietary carotenoids.
- **Porphyrins** produce pink, brown, red and green colours. They are nitrogenous pigments.

Structural colours

- Iridescent colours are achieved in a variety of ways:
  - The barbules of a feather can be twisted to cause interference in the reflected light (e.g. hummingbirds, starlings)
  - Barbules can have very thin layers of keratin to reflect colours (e.g. peacocks).
- Non-iridescent colours are produced by the scattering of light by minute particles. Most blue colours are achieved by this mechanism. The keratin in the barbs contains tiny air-filled pockets. The colour of white feathers is due to the refraction and reflection of all wavelengths of white light.

Moulting

Feathers are essentially dead structures so have no ability to heal if they become damaged; they are therefore regularly replaced by new feathers. The frequency and pattern of moulting varies between species. Many birds have a full moult once a year, whilst some have a full and a partial moult and others two full moults. Most species moult their flight feathers sequentially and symmetrically, enabling them to maintain flight during the moult. Some species with a high wing-load will replace all of their flight feathers at once, meaning that for 2–4 weeks they are flightless; this is most apparent in some species of duck and seabird and will take place in a secluded body of water or far out at sea, where predators are less common.

Skin

- The epidermis is made up of three layers: the basal (germinative) layer; the intermediate layer; and the outer cornified layer, which contains the striated muscle that moves the skin. The epidermis is thin in the feathered areas, with the basal layer only two to four cells thick. It is much thicker in the unfeathered areas of the legs and feet, where it also interlocks with the dermis.
- The dermis consists of the superficial and deep layers. The superficial dermis contains loosely arranged layers of collagen. The deep layer contains fat, smooth muscle, feather follicles, blood vessels and nerves, including Herbst corpuscles.
- The skin is attached to the muscles in very few places, but has extensive attachments to the skeletal structures of the head and extremities.
- Subcutaneous tissue is most abundant in the dorsal cervical, midline, axillary and inguinal regions. Footpads are present in many species, especially terrestrial birds.
- During the breeding season, many species will develop a brood patch: a thickening and

increased vascularization of the skin in the ventral abdominal region.
- The skin is glandless, with the exception of the ear canals, pericloacal gland and the uropygial (preen) gland. The presence of these glands varies between species.
- The uropygial gland is bilobed and is situated dorsally near the tail. It produces a holocrine lipid secretion via a nipple-like papilla, which commonly has a tuft of down feathers at the tip. The secretion is spread over the feathers during preening and facilitates feather quality maintenance.
- The propatagium is a modified triangular fold of feathered skin on the leading edge of the wing, between the shoulder and carpal joints. In its cranial-free edge is the elastic propatagial ligament. These structures maintain the leading edge of the aerofoil structure of the wing and their integrity is essential for flight.

Modifications of the skin

- **Comb:** Found in species of fowl, cassowaries and male Andean condors, the comb is an ornamental outgrowth of skin on the head (Figure 3.20). It is thickened and highly vascular; the colour of the comb can be useful in assessing health status as it will be pale in cases of hypotension and yellow if the bird is jaundiced.
- **Wattles:** In chickens these ornamental folds of skin extend from the ventral surface of the mandible (Figure 3.20). In some species (e.g. wattled starlings) these structures occur in the rictal region. Bantam silkies and domestic turkeys have a median wattle or dewlap.
- **Ear lobes:** Found in Galliformes, these skin folds hang down from the external ear openings and are either red or white in colour, except in silkies where they are purple.
- **Snood:** Found in turkeys, this is a highly vascularized distensible skin projection that arises from the dorsal surface of the head, between the eyes and nares. The colour and turgidity of the snood varies, depending on the turkey's emotional status.
- **Caruncles:** Found in turkeys, the caruncles are small protuberances similar to the snood, though much less distensible. They are found on the head and upper neck.
- **Scales:** In most species, the distal part of the pelvic limb is covered with scaly skin. Scales are highly keratinized, raised areas of epidermis that are separated by areas of less keratinized skin.
- **Spurs:** In some species (most notably fowl) there is a well developed, pointed keratinized spur on the caudomedial aspect of the tarsometatarsal region (Figure 3.20). It is usually larger in males and after 6 months has a bony attachment. Most commonly there is one spur on each leg; however, they are more numerous in some species (Indian game fowl and peacock-pheasants, for example, have two and four, respectively). In some species there is a spur present in the carpometacarpal region (e.g.

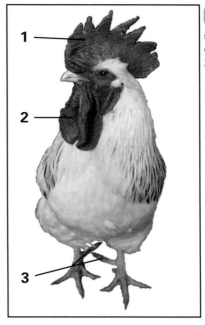

3.20 Chickens exhibit several modifications of the skin. 1, comb; 2, wattle; 3, spurs.

spur-winged plovers, spur-winged geese, sheathbills and jacanas).
- **Claws:** The distal phalanx of each digit is enclosed by a horny claw. The dorsal and lateral aspects of the claw are highly keratinized; the ventral aspect is softer and grows more slowly. This produces the characteristic curve of the claw. In many species a claw on each foot is adapted slightly to facilitate preening and feather maintenance. Foot claws are utilized for perching, climbing, digging, scratching, preening, grasping and as weapons for hunting and fighting. Some nestlings have a claw on the alular digit of the wing. Adult ratites have claws on the wing digits. Ostriches have claws on three of the wing digits. Cassowaries, kiwis and emus have a claw on the alular and major digits.

The beak

The beak is used for feeding, preening, nest building and as a weapon. It is a continually growing structure and is worn down by 'normal use'. Functionally, it replaces the lips and teeth of mammals. The shape and rigidity vary depending on the method of feeding.

The upper and lower jaw bones (maxilla and mandible, respectively) and the horny covering (rhamphotheca) comprise the beak. The dermis is closely associated with the periosteum of the maxilla and mandible and is well vascularized. The epidermis has a very thick stratum corneum, which contains calcium phosphate, hydroxyapatite, calcium, keratin-bound phospholipids and keratin; this gives the required rigidity.

The rhamphotheca is perforated at certain points by tiny pores and contains a dermal core, which communicates with dermal papillae and Herbst corpuscles. These are most commonly situated at the tip of the beak and are collectively termed the beak tip organ. They serve a tactile function, independent of the tongue and eyes. In parrots, they are most numerous in the lower beak tip. In ducks and geese, both the lower and upper bill tips contain these sensory organs. In granivores (grain-eating birds), it is absent.

Most neonates have an egg tooth, which is a small projection on the dorsal aspect of the upper beak that is usually white in colour and facilitates hatching by penetrating the shell.

The nostrils (or nares) are located in the upper beak in some species (notably many Anseriformes) and at the base of the upper beak in other species. In many of these birds they are surrounded by a wax-like area of keratinized skin known as the cere.

Sexing

In some species of bird there are marked differences between the two sexes (sexual dimorphism); in others there are no obvious differences and the only way of sexing them is by DNA polymerase chain reaction (PCR) testing or endoscopic examination.

- **Psittaciformes:** Few species exhibit sexual dimorphism. Males are often very slightly larger, with a broader head than females, but this is only useful if you can make a comparison with a bird of the same species and from the same bloodline. Species that exhibit sexual dimorphism include:
  - Budgerigars: In the 'normal' green coloration adult males have a blue cere and in females it is a fleshy pink/brown. However, this is not applicable to lutino, blue or white mutations.
  - Cockatiels: In the 'normal' grey coloration the cheek patches of males are more vibrant yellow and orange than those of females, which are a duskier yellow/grey. Also, females have bars across the underside of the tail feathers, whereas males do not. These bars are less distinct or absent in the colour mutations.
  - Cockatoos: In many species the iris of adult females will be light brown/red while that of males will be dark brown/black.
  - Australian king parrots: Males have a red head whereas females have a green head (Figure 3.21).
  - Eclectus: Females are red and purple with a black beak whereas males are predominantly green with a yellow/orange beak (Figure 3.22).

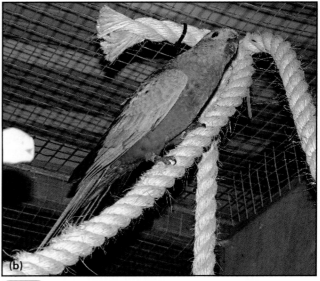

3.21 (continued) **(b)** Female Australian king parrot.

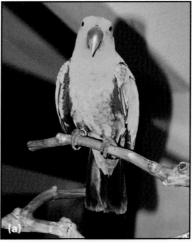

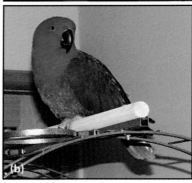

3.22 Male **(a)** and female **(b)** red-sided eclectus.

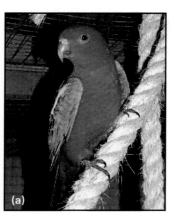

3.21 **(a)** Male Australian king parrot. (continues)

- **Passeriformes:** Many species exhibit sexual dimorphism, with the male being distinctly coloured or patterned. Some males have less obvious characteristics: they are more vocal (e.g. male canaries) and more active during the breeding season (dancing and nest building). Some males have a prominence in the proctodeum that is pronounced during the breeding season. Many passerine birds show no sexual dimorphism.
- **Falconiformes:** Females are larger than males.

- **Strigiformes:** Females are larger than males in many species.
- **Struthioniformes (ratites):** Males have a distinct phallus, which can be visualized by everting the cloaca.
- **Anseriformes:**
  - Ducks: Most species exhibit sexual dimorphism, with the male being more colourful and ornamented. Males also have a phallus that can be visualized by everting the cloaca.
  - Geese: Few species exhibit secondary sexual characteristics (although in Chinese and African geese, head ornamentation is larger in males); however, males have an obvious phallus, which can be visualized by everting the cloaca.
  - Swans: Few species exhibit sexual dimorphism; however, males have a phallus, which can be visualized by everting the cloaca.
- **Columbiformes:** Some species demonstrate chromatic sexual dimorphism. Males possess two conical papillae in the proctodeum, whereas females do not.
- **Galliformes:** Many species exhibit sexual dimorphism. Males tend to be larger in size, distinctly coloured and more highly ornamented. In many species they are more 'vocal' and aggressive.

Diet

Bird nutrition is a complex topic, far beyond the scope of this text. What follows is a general overview with some dietary recommendations for commonly encountered species; this is by no means exhaustive.

Parrots

Parrot diet is an evolving topic. Attempting to replicate a wild diet is very difficult as wild parrots eat a wide variety of foodstuffs depending on location, availability and time of year. Historically, seed diets were fed as standard; however, it is now known that they do not meet the birds' dietary requirements. Current recommendations are to feed an extruded pellet diet and to supplement with vegetables and fruit. This helps to stop 'selective feeding', whereby birds will just eat one type of seed or nut despite being offered a wide choice. There are a variety of pelleted diets available and, while all are better than a seed-based diet, some still require supplementation with certain vitamins and minerals.

If a parrot will not take to a pelleted diet then there are certain foods that can be offered as a better alternative to a complete seed mix. Soaking pulses (e.g. chickpeas, haricot beans, black-eyed beans and mung beans) until they have sprouted, rinsing them thoroughly and regularly throughout soaking, and then mixing them with 'meaty yellow' and 'leafy green' vegetables provides a better source of protein and carbohydrate, as well as a higher vitamin content. Wholewheat pasta and brown rice can be added in moderation to the mix.

Seeds and nuts should make up only 10% of the entire diet, but they do make for a good training aid and occasional treat. Vitamin and mineral supplements made specifically for birds would need to be added. Any food source offered should be fit for human consumption and preferably organic. There have been reported cases of poor quality seeds and nuts being a source of *Aspergillus* spp.

One of the most important dietary minerals for all birds is calcium. To utilize this, birds also require activated vitamin D3. Vitamin D3 is activated by UVB light, which is present in unfiltered sunlight or can be gained from an ultraviolet bird lamp.

Fresh water should always be available. It can be good practice to place this at the opposite end of the cage from the food, to encourage exercise and reduce the risk of contamination.

'Feeding time' for wild parrots is often very social, with large flocks gathering together; this should be acknowledged as a time for 'flock' interaction in the home environment. Indeed, it can be very useful when attempting to convert a bird on to pellets, or when introducing a new food item, to offer it at the time the family is eating.

Many parrot owners share human food with their birds. This is not a problem as long as it is done in a controlled manner. Food should never be passed from mouth to beak as this is part of a mating ritual and can create/reinforce an unnatural bond. Also, the type of food shared needs to be safe for the bird. Dairy produce should be avoided, as birds do not have the ability to digest it. Any high-fat or high-sugar food could be detrimental to a bird's health. Avocado, chocolate, caffeine and alcohol should never be fed to birds. There is regular debate about the feeding of animal protein to parrots. In the wild, parrots have been known to eat invertebrates, carrion and dead fish. In captivity, if they are fed a good quality diet, they do not require the addition of animal protein; however, some owners will utilize sources as occasional treats or for environmental enrichment.

In the wild parrots spend a great deal of their time searching for food. This is one of the reasons they have evolved such a large brain. In captivity they generally have a dish of food placed in front of them, thus eliminating the need to search for it. Good dietary management and environmental enrichment should encourage the bird to forage for food. This can be done in a number of ways, from offering whole foodstuffs (e.g. corn-on-the-cob with the husk still on), to wrapping favoured food items in paper, through to using the most complex purpose-made foraging toys. Allowing the parrot to exhibit this normal behaviour will greatly reduce boredom and will often stimulate the bird to try new foods.

Some parrots are specialist feeders; lories and lorikeets are nectar-feeders and therefore require a specialist diet and lots of fruit.

Passeriformes

This is a very diverse group of birds when considering diet. Attempting to replicate what the bird would eat in the wild is good practice for captive passerine birds and wildlife casualties.

■ Corvids (crows, magpies, etc.) feed on carrion, scraps and insects; jays will forage for acorns during autumn.
■ Blackbirds, robins and thrushes eat insects, worms, fruit and berries.
■ Tits, finches, sparrows and wrens eat seeds and insects.

Historically, seed-only diets have been fed to finches and canaries, and a combination of seed and 'egg-food' is given to other passerine birds. These diets are now known to be lacking in many essential nutrients. Current recommendations are to feed a formulated diet to captive passerine birds, supplemented pre-moult and pre-breeding with limited rations of higher fat content seeds such as linseed and rapeseed.

Fresh water should be made available.

Raptors

Diet is an essential aspect of captive bird of prey management. Raptors are whole-carcass feeders – i.e. they consume fur/feather, skin, muscle, internal organs and bone. The indigestible parts are regurgitated in a pellet, or cast/casting (NB the production of a pellet is also called casting). The time taken between consuming food and casting varies depending on what has been eaten, but should never take longer than 16 hours.

Ideally, food offered should be close to what the bird would eat in the wild. While wild raptors are opportunistic hunters, they do have preferred prey items:

■ Larger falcon species and sparrowhawks feed on birds
■ Kestrels, owls and *Aquila* eagles feed on mammals
■ Goshawks, red-tailed hawks and Harris' hawks feed on a mixture of birds and mammals
■ Smaller falcons, e.g. hobbies and little owls, feed on insects
■ *Haliaeetus* eagles and ospreys feed on fish
■ Kites and buzzards are truly opportunistic, feeding on carrion and a mixture of other feathered, furred, insect and amphibian prey
■ Vultures are specialist carrion feeders.

In captivity, the majority of a raptor's diet consists of day-old chick/turkey poults, quail, rodent and quarry (prey caught while hunting). Day-old chicks, if fed with the yolk-sac, provides a surprisingly adequate level of nutrition for use in combination with adult whole prey. 'Road kill' should never be offered. Even though the majority of water is gained from food, fresh water should always be available for raptors to drink. Appropriate vitamin and mineral supplements should not generally be required in the adult non-breeding bird if fed a balanced whole carcass diet. If supplements are to be used, they should only be those recommended and developed for raptors and should be used precisely according to the manufacturer's instructions. The use of any supplements should be directed towards specific requirements at specific times, e.g. growth, breeding and moulting.

Ratites

Ostrich pellets may provide a better basis for the diet than poultry feeds; however, one should ensure that they come from a reputable source that has proven their diet and ingredients to be of the required standard and is actively involved in nutritional research and development.

Ratites are browsers; however, given the balanced nature of the pelleted diet, access to 'browse' (including new shoots) should be limited so as not to affect the daily nutrient intake. Impaction is an issue with rheas as they have a tendency to eat whatever is available; owners need to be aware of this if they are being kept in a paddock.

Fresh water should be made available.

Waterfowl

All waterfowl should have access to fresh water and to soluble and insoluble grit; this facilitates mineral supplementation and the grinding action of the gizzard, respectively.

Ducks

There are specific duck diets available, but many people will use a chicken/turkey feed (see later). While this is not usually a problem, it can have implications for young birds. Ducklings will eat more quickly than chicks; medicated chick crumbs should therefore be avoided, as overdose of the medication is a real possibility. Using a pellet as a basis and supplementing with vegetable greens, hardboiled egg and invertebrates is standard practice. Ducks will also 'help themselves', eating duckweed and other aquatic plants and invertebrates when available. Bread should not be fed to ducks, due to its poor nutritional value and the fact that selective feeding will inevitably result in dietary deficiencies.

Geese

Geese are grazers and can survive on a diet mainly consisting of grass, supplemented with goose/swan pellets. The grass that they are grazed on should be a maximum of 7.5–10 cm in length; any longer and impaction becomes an issue. Wheat can be offered as an alternative to pellets when grass is in good supply; this should be given in water. When grass is not readily available, a waterfowl pellet should be fed. Access to aquatic plants is also beneficial.

Swans

Aquatic plants, algae, crustaceans, frogs and invertebrates will be readily eaten when available. A waterfowl pellet will provide a good source of nutrition during months where natural food items are scarce. Swans will also graze on grass and vegetation.

Pigeons and doves

For the most part, pigeons are granivores. In captivity their diet constitutes cereal, seed and legumes supplemented with mineral grit. Complete formulated pellet diets are available, which are often geared towards different lifestages (young birds, breeding, racing, moulting, etc.).

Fresh water should be made available. If troughs are used then particular care should be taken with regular replenishment and hygiene, to limit pathogen transfer.

Poultry

A vast amount of research has been done into formulating poultry diets. While they have been developed for the commercial poultry market, they make an ideal basis for the backyard pets seen in practice.

All backyard poultry should have access to fresh water and to soluble and insoluble grit; this facilitates mineral supplementation and the grinding action of the gizzard, respectively.

Chickens

There are different diets for different lifestages, starting with chick crumbs, then grower pellets and progressing to breeder and layer pellets or mash. Feeding a formulated diet ensures that the birds are receiving their basic dietary requirements. Other food items can then be given as treats and for environmental enrichment. Many backyard poultry keepers feed kitchen scraps to their charges. As long as this is done in moderation, and any potentially harmful foods are removed, it should not be a problem. Harmful food items include 'junk-food'; anything processed and high in salt, fat or sugar should be avoided. Avocado, chocolate, caffeine and alcohol must also not be fed. Meat products and meat derivatives should not be offered. Good additions to the diet include fresh cabbage, cauliflower leaves, spinach, grass clods and dandelions. Pasta, hardboiled egg and corn-on-the-cob can be offered, as can invertebrates; chickens will eat worms and other bugs in the garden – mealworms are usually a favourite. All treats should be fed in moderation. Using feed-balls or hiding favoured treats to encourage natural feeding behaviours should be actively encouraged. Some fruits can be given as a treat, such as apples and strawberries, but again this must be very occasionally.

Game birds

Many good quality game bird pellets are available that are specifically formulated for various species. These should make up the major component of the diet. Greens (kale, cabbage, spinach, etc.) and hardboiled egg can be offered, along with invertebrates (such as mealworms) as treats, which can be used for environmental enrichment by encouraging foraging behaviours. These must be given in moderation.

Housing

As for all animals, the five freedoms are paramount when considering husbandry requirements for birds.

Due to the sensitive nature of the respiratory tract, inhaled toxicity is an important consideration when discussing bird husbandry. Aerosols, plug-in air fresheners, smoke, excess dust and paint fumes are potentially toxic, and overheated non-stick pans, new ovens and ironing board covers can release toxic PTFE gases. This list is not exhaustive and, as a general rule, anything that has a 'strong smell' should be avoided.

The five freedoms

- Freedom from thirst and hunger – through ready access to fresh water and a diet to maintain full health and vigour.
- Freedom from discomfort – through provision of an appropriate environment including shelter and a comfortable resting area.
- Freedom from pain, injury, and disease – by prevention or rapid diagnosis and treatment.
- Freedom to express normal behaviour – through provision of sufficient space, good facilities and company of the animal's own kind.
- Freedom from fear and distress – by ensuring conditions and treatment that avoid mental suffering.

Psittaciformes

Aviary design for parrots is similar to that for passerine birds. Two layers of mesh are recommended, and all metalwork must be non-galvanized to prevent zinc toxicity. Natural branches are ideal for indoor and outdoor use but must be thoroughly disinfected prior to use; apple, pear, magnolia, ash and dogwood are appropriate. Ropes and swing perches will be enjoyed, but care must be taken to avoid getting toes caught. The aviary must have a shelter within the covered third, which should be insulated to protect from cold. The base of the aviary should be well drained concrete, which can be top-dressed with pebbles or large non-toxic wood chips. A double-door system should be used.

Cages should be as large as possible, especially if parrots are to be confined to them; the minimum requirement is that the bird is able to open its wings fully in all directions and to turn around easily. Again, all metal should be zinc-free. While toys are highly recommended, the cage should not be overcrowded. It can be useful to rotate toys to maintain interest. Newspaper is the preferred substrate as it is non-toxic, easily replaced and inexpensive. Environmental enrichment should focus on foraging behaviour, as discussed above. Time out of the cage is recommended and should always be monitored. Parrots are intelligent and can be trained. Exercises such as 'step-up' should be regularly practised and a routine established. Access to unfiltered sunlight or artificial full spectrum UV is essential, and daylength should be observed. Parrots require 12–14 hours of sleep; covering the cage or having a 'bedtime cage' in a quiet room is recommended.

Many species are originally from the rainforest so showering or mist spraying should become part of their routine. Some species prefer to bathe in a shallow dish of water, and smaller parrots, e.g. budgerigars, like to bathe in damp foliage; wet lettuce leaves placed on the bottom of the cage usually suffice.

Passeriformes

Husbandry practices will vary depending on the species and the purpose for which the bird is kept. 'Pet' canaries and finches are often housed in cages. The preferred cage substrate is newspaper, for ease of changing, availability and price. Perches should be natural branches (apple or pear tree is ideal), cleaned with a suitable disinfectant. Toys/swings, etc. should be limited in number so as not to crowd the cage; canaries and finches do not enjoy toys as much as psittacine birds. Feed and water containers should be easily cleaned, emptied and filled. Ideally, they should be at opposing ends of the cage to reduce the risk of contamination and to promote exercise. If kept indoors, provision of artificial full spectrum UV light and appropriate daylight lengths is recommended.

Indoor and outdoor aviaries are also utilized for captive passerine birds and wildlife casualties. Substrate in aviaries varies. A concrete base with drainage is required, which can be left bare or top-dressed with gravel or hardwood chips. If a top layer is used then the pieces should be large enough that they cannot be eaten, and care must be taken when selecting the product to avoid potential toxins. The wire on the aviary should be of a suitable gauge to prevent bending and chewing (particularly with corvids), and the gaps between the wire must be small enough that birds cannot poke their heads through. Wire should be square-mesh, to prevent birds from getting their toes and feathers caught. Having non-toxic natural foliage will provide perching and shelter. One-third of the aviary should be solid-sided and have a solid roof to offer protection from the elements. Provision of a nest box is also good practice.

Corvids like to play with toys; foraging toys made for large parrots are suitable and provide a good tool for environmental enrichment.

Food and water receptacles should be easy to access. A double door system should be incorporated in the aviary design.

If breeding, provision of a cup-shaped nest (plastic or clay, with a felt insert) is essential.

Raptors

As a general rule, raptors should be kept in an aviary when not flying. When deciding where to position an aviary, sites with high numbers of potential predators should be avoided, as should sites close to a compost heap or muck/straw piles, due to the risk of *Aspergillus* infection.

Dimensions for aviaries will obviously vary depending on the species and also depending on whether one or two birds are being housed together. The aviary must be big enough to allow for each bird to have its own space, but not too large that it makes catching the birds difficult.

The most common design is three solid sides with a mesh front (square weld mesh rather than chicken wire, as feathers can get caught in the twists). The roof is often one-third solid and two-thirds mesh or a solid roof with skylights of mesh to provide a stronger structure and better protection from the elements. Four solid-sided aviaries with a skylight roof are recommended for breeding pairs and nervous birds as they offer the best security and protection from weather and potential predators. A double door system should be used and the appropriate security devices incorporated.

Within the aviary there should be plenty of perching surfaces in open and secluded areas; these perches should be appropriate for the species. As a general rule, the perches used for falcons are block perches and for most other species (hawks, eagles, etc.) a bow perch is used. This is because in the wild falcons preferentially perch on cliffs (or nowadays rooftops), while other birds prefer branches. Ideally, all perches should be covered with longleaf artificial grass such as Astroturf, as this helps to prevent foot problems by dispersing the pressure on the feet.

The aviary should also have a bath that can be easily cleaned and filled from the outside. There should be a feeding hatch or chute, to allow for remote provision of rations. The floor should be well drained and easy to clean. The provision of natural cover (living shrubs) can be beneficial as long as they do not overcrowd the aviary.

'Flying birds' will usually have a weathering area and separate night quarters. If a permanent weathering is used it should provide protection from extreme conditions. This is usually achieved by having an open-fronted cubicle that allows the bird to be under cover or exposed. The floor of this cubicle should be easy to maintain. A bath should be provided and the area should be predator-proof. When travelling to field meetings the weathering area is often improvised, but one rule must always be adhered to: a tethered bird should be closely monitored. After flying, the bird is put away into its night quarters. This is usually a closed unit with perches in which the bird is either turned loose or kept tethered. The important difference in this area is that the perches are higher off the ground and the bird is kept in darkness. This affords more protection from frostbite and will make the bird feel more secure. Diurnal raptors have poor night vision; it is therefore vital that the night quarters are made rodent-/predator-proof.

During the daytime, most birds are kept tethered (i.e. with their leash attached to the perch); however, it is recommended that all owls should be kept off tether in aviaries, even if they are flown.

Pigeons

Racing pigeon lofts should be well ventilated and easily cleaned. They should be insulated to protect from cold. There is often grilling/grating above the floor to prevent the pigeons from walking in and pecking at their own excrement. Within the loft, age groups are segregated. Compartments are provided, with perches or nest boxes for each bird or pair. Openings from the loft are often adjustable, allowing entry but preventing exit.

For non-racing pigeons, an outdoor flight/aviary with an insulated shelter is recommended. The sheltered section should be easily cleaned. Numerous natural branch and shelf perches should be available in the aviary. A square mesh should be used. If breeding, an appropriately sized cupped plastic or clay nest pan should be provided in a nest box, and nesting material should be placed in the aviary for gathering and building.

Poultry and waterfowl

A coop or hen-house and a predator-proof run are essential. The coop should be easily cleaned, well ventilated and offer nest boxes and perches for roosting. It should be insulated to protect from cold. Substrates that are useful include chopped cardboard, shredded paper, chopped straw (not hay) and hardwood shavings (not sawdust). The run should be as large as possible. The perimeter should be secured against predators by burying wire to prevent 'tunnelling in'.

Fresh water should always be available. Feeders and drinkers should be regularly cleaned and moved around the run to prevent the build-up of pathogens. Swans and geese will benefit from shelter; this can be provided by bushes and shrubs or open-fronted housing. Environmental enrichment should focus on allowing natural behaviour to be exhibited, including foraging and swimming for aquatic species. A pond with a flow of water through it is ideal. Some keepers find a paddling pool is sufficient for small numbers of ducks; this water should be readily changed. A still pond will need to be pumped regularly to prevent overgrowth of pathogens.

Behaviour

A detailed discussion of bird behaviour is far beyond the scope of this text. In most cases problems arise when species are prevented from expressing natural behaviours or when species exhibit modifications of behaviours they would be performing in their natural state. Such examples include foraging for food items in captive parrots, which would occupy a significant proportion of their waking hours, or flying and hunting in captive raptors. In addition, the practice of hand-rearing in certain avian species can result in 'human imprinting', where innate behaviours such as

protection of territory, a mate or food items (often with quite dramatic displays of aggression) can become directed at people. Especially where aggression is involved, such behavioural issues are best addressed by either specialist avian veterinary surgeons or behaviourists.

Acknowledgments

The authors would like to extend their sincerest thanks to Nic and Andy Gilbert and to Brian Stockdale.

References and further reading

Carpenter JW (2005) *Exotic Animal Formulary*. Elsevier Saunders, St. Louis
Chitty J and Lierz M (2008) *BSAVA Manual of Raptors, Pigeons and Passerine Birds*. BSAVA, Gloucester
Clark P, Boardman W and Raidal S (2009) *Atlas of Clinical Avian Hematology*. Wiley-Blackwell, Oxford
Duncan JR (2003) *Owls of the World: Their Lives, Behaviour and Survival*. Firefly Books, Buffalo
Ferguson-Lees J and Christie DA (2001) *Raptors of the World*. Christopher Helm, London
Harcourt-Brown N and Chitty J (2005) *BSAVA Manual of Psittacine Birds, 2nd edn*. BSAVA Publications, Gloucester
Harvey R (1993) *Practical Incubation*. Hancock House, Surrey
King AS and McLelland J (1984) *Birds: Their Structure and Function*. Baillière Tindall, London
Luescher AU (2006) *Manual of Parrot Behaviour*. Blackwell, Oxford
Ritchie BW, Harrison GJ and Harrison LR (1994) *Avian Medicine: Principles and Application*. Wingers, Lake Worth
Whittow GC (2000) *Sturkie's Avian Physiology*. Academic Press, San Diego

Self-assessment questions

1. You are presented with an umbrella cockatoo with a red iris. Can you determine the gender without diagnostic testing and, if so, what sex is it?
2. What colours do carotenoid pigments produce?
3. It produces a holocrine lipid secretion via a nipple-like papilla, which commonly has a tuft of down feathers at the tip. What is being described?
4. How many cervical vertebrae do birds possess?
5. Parrots have two digits directed cranially and two digits directed caudally; what is the term used to describe this foot shape?
6. Which portion of the intestine do the bile and pancreatic ducts empty into?
7. What is the main difference between mammalian and bird tracheas?
8. Where are the sclera ossicles found?
9. Name two foods that should never be offered to parrots.
10. What shape mesh would you recommend for use on an aviary?

4

Reptiles: biology and husbandry

Matthew Rendle and Jon Cracknell

This chapter is designed to give information on:

■ The common species of reptile seen in practice
■ Anatomy and physiology
■ Sexing
■ Nutritional considerations and long-term effects of poor nutrition
■ Housing requirements

The study of reptiles and amphibians is known as herpetology and an individual who studies these animals is called a herpetologist. Owners tend to be either hobbyists or herpetoculturists. The hobbyist has a few reptiles, which tend to be housed in decorative vivaria, have individual names and are much loved pets. Herpetoculturists are interested in all aspects of the reptiles they keep, including behaviour, reproduction and status in the wild. They often have large collections, housed using husbandry techniques that may appear unnatural or inadequate but provide all of the animals' basic needs while enabling the collection to be maintained effectively and efficiently. Examples of both set-ups can be seen in Figure 4.1.

The care of reptiles is a holistic interplay between providing a suitable environment and microhabitat and correct nutrition. Although this is also true for other vertebrates such as mammals and birds, it is even more important for reptiles, due to a general lack of knowledge among owners. In reptiles, incorrect environment, microhabitat or nutrition will result in aberrations in the individual's physiology, leading to pathology and disease. Often the sick reptilian patient has a legacy of months to years of failed husbandry. Thus, in order to provide the best care possible, it is essential that the veterinary nurse has a basic understanding of the correct requirements for each individual species.

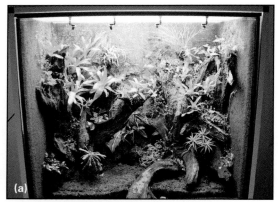
(a)

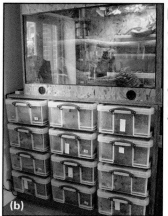
(b)

4.1 The hobbyist herpetologist vivarium **(a)** can be very different to the set-up used by a professional herpetoculturist **(b)**, with different husbandry-related problems seen as a result.

Common species seen in practice

There are over 9000 recognized species of reptile and 6700 species of amphibian, compared with only 5000 species of mammal; however, only a few types of the more common species held in captivity are likely to be seen in practice. These are species that are popular or do well in the reptile pet trade but, as trends change, it is possible that more unusual species will be seen from time to time, some of which may be wrongly identified and may produce venom that is harmful to humans. Common species that may be seen in practice include, but are not limited to, those shown in Figure 4.2a.

There is a current trend for breeding animals that have a genetic predisposition for colours and patterns that can be dramatically different from those of wild-type animals, and these mutations can command high prices. This type of breeding can, however, encourage inbreeding and so lead to congenital abnormalities or other diseases, as well as devaluing the natural wild-type form of the species.

Native reptiles

All native UK reptiles (Figure 4.2b) and amphibians are protected by law from deliberate killing and from sale or trade. In addition, the smooth snake, sand lizard, natterjack toad, great crested newt and pool frog are European Protected Species (EPS); it is illegal

Species	Description	Vivarium	Nutrition
Lizards			
Bearded dragon	An easy-to-keep medium-sized (20–30 cm) species. Become very tame when well handled. Bred in many colour and pattern mutations. Aggression can be a problem if juveniles are kept in groups and can also be a problem with males.	Require a hot spot of 30–35°C. Need a high level of UVB lighting.	Omnivores, they tend to eat mainly insects by choice, but should be encouraged to take greens regularly. Care must be taken not to offer too large a food item to juveniles as there have been anecdotal reports of neurological issues after attempting to swallow oversized items. Will eat small rodents, but these should be given very infrequently if at all. Supplementary dusting of food with vitamin and mineral powder is advised.
Green iguana	Bright green 10–15 cm hatchlings turn into 5 kg, 1 m long, paler green (often brown) adults. Can be very aggressive as adults. Gloves and towels must be used when handling to prevent bites, scratches and whips from their long tails. They make poor pets and are seldom bred in captivity, tending instead to be imported as captive-farmed or wild-caught hatchlings.	Require a hot spot of 30–35°C. Require a high level of UVB lighting.	Herbivores throughout all lifestages, they should be fed a wide range of leafy greens with minimal fruit. They can grow fast and are prone to metabolic bone disease (MBD), Supplementary dusting of food with vitamin and mineral powder is advised.
Panther chameleon	A highly sought-after species of chameleon from Madagascar, with widely variable colours. Females are smaller and tend to be various shades of brown.	Require a hot spot of 27–30°C ideally provided by a spotlight bulb. Require UVB lighting.	Insect feeders, starting with fruit flies as hatchlings and progressing to locusts as adults. They obtain their water by licking leaves after rain or early morning dew. In captivity they require spraying or misting twice daily, as they can become dehydrated very rapidly. They are fast-growing and prone to MBD. Supplementary dusting of food with vitamin and mineral powder is advised.
Leopard gecko	An easy-to-keep small species. Tend to be very tame. Autotomy is used as a defence mechanism but rarely happens in captivity. They come in many colour and pattern mutations. They are sexually mature within 1–2 years and can live for >20 years. They are easy to breed.	They require a hot spot of 28–32°C, with a cooler temperature at night. A warm dry hide and a moist hide or moss box should be provided.	Insect-feeders, which take a wide variety of invertebrate food items in the wild. Avoid feeding waxworms as geckos will often become fixated on them, refusing to eat anything else. Supplementary dusting of food with vitamin and mineral powder is advised.

4.2 **(a)** Common reptile and amphibian species seen in practice. (continues) ▶

Species	Description	Vivarium	Nutrition
Lizards (continued)			
Madagascar day gecko	A wall-climbing species that is bright green with red flashes on the dorsum. Not suitable for handling as they have very delicate skin, which can be torn during restraint.	Require a hot spot of 27–30°C. Will benefit from the provision of UVB light.	Insect-feeders, but will take nectar mixes. Take a wide variety of invertebrate food items in the wild. Supplementary dusting of food with vitamin and mineral powder is advised.
Savanna monitor	Usually imported as tiny wild-caught babies. Can become a very tame pet, despite their stocky adult size of up to 1 m. Tend to be good natured. Seldom breed in captivity.	Require a hot spot of 30–35°C. Will benefit from the provision of UVB light. Require a large enclosure to encourage activity.	Will take insects as hatchlings, and progress on to a rodent diet as adults. They favour eggs and chicks, etc. but are prone to obesity, so must not be overfed or maintained on an excessively high-fat diet.
Snakes			
Californian kingsnake	Come in many colour and pattern mutations. Sexual maturity is within 1–2 years. Lifespan may be >20 years. Adult size is up to 1 m; males are smaller. Can be feisty and fast as hatchlings but calm down quickly with handling.	Require a hot spot of 24–28°C. Hatchlings do best in small enclosures (boxes) with a selection of hides. Will benefit from an annual hibernation (brumation). Very good at escaping. Known to eat other snakes in the wild so best housed alone.	Mice of appropriate size, starting on pinkies as hatchlings and progressing to full-sized mice as mature animals. Males require more infrequent meals.
Cornsnake	An easy-to-keep species that comes in many colour and pattern mutations. Sexual maturity is within 1–2 years. Lifespan may be >20 years. Adult size is approximately 1 m; males are smaller.	Require a hot spot of 24–28°C. Hatchlings do best in small enclosures (boxes) with a selection of hides. Will benefit from an annual hibernation.	Mice of appropriate size, starting on pinkies as hatchlings and progressing to full-sized mice as mature animals. Males require more infrequent meals.
Garter snake	Often purchased as a first snake as relatively small and cheap. Several species and subspecies available. Average lifespan of 10–15 years. Tend to be wild-caught. Females grow to 45 cm on average; males are much smaller.	Require a hot spot of 24–28°C. Active snakes do best with water body within enclosure. Most species will benefit from annual hibernation.	Wild diet is very varied and can include earthworms, tadpoles and small fish. In captivity they are mainly fed rodents, a diet that is thought to shorten their lifespan. Supplementary dusting of food with vitamin and mineral powder is advised.
Mangrove snake	A rear-fanged species that is now not covered by the Dangerous Wild Animals Act (DWAA). Captive-bred juveniles tend not to be aggressive. Adults can reach 2 m and can be feisty. Wild-caught adults tend to be infested with parasites and seldom feed. This species can give a painful bite, which may result in hospital treatment being necessary. A species to be aware of as they are becoming more popular.	Require a hot spot of 28–32°C. Captive-bred juveniles are easily cared for, requiring an arboreal vivarium with high humidity. Wild-caught animals can be very difficult to acclimatize.	Natural diet includes mainly lizards and frogs, but in captivity will accept rodents well; the long-term effects of this diet are as yet unknown.

4.2 (continued) **(a)** Common reptile and amphibian species seen in practice. (continues) ▶

Species	Description	Vivarium	Nutrition
Snakes (continued)			
Common boa	Numerous mutations are available. Males are sexually mature within 2 years; females take on average 3 years. Average lifespan of 20 years. Average length of 2 m but may reach up to 3 m; males usually smaller. Can be feisty when newborn but generally easy to maintain.	Require a hot spot of 28–32°C. Hatchlings do best in small enclosures, with a selection of appropriate hide boxes. Adults require large enclosure with appropriate hides.	Will take small mice as their first meal. Tend to be good feeders; difficult feeders can normally be encouraged to eat by 'scenting' rodents with the yolk of a chick or a few downy feathers. They can progress on to rabbits or chickens, but are often maintained on large rats. Males tend to be more prone to periods of non-feeding, often in correlation with a night-time temperature drop and reproductive activity.
Royal python	Captive-bred hatchlings generally feed and thrive in captivity. They come in a vast array of colour and pattern mutations. Males are sexually mature within 2 years; females take >3 years. Average lifespan is 20 years but have been recorded as living to 40 years. Adults are stocky and may reach >1 m in length.	Require a hot spot of 22–28°C. Hatchlings do best in small enclosures, with a selection of appropriate hide boxes. Wild-caught animals can be problematic to acclimatize and are best avoided.	Start on small mice as hatchlings (anecdotally they seem to favour dark-coloured mice), and will progress on to small rats. A good-sized adult female will happily take an adult rat. Feeding should be fairly infrequent to mimic the wild diet, and periods of non-feeding can be common in some individuals.
Chelonians			
Red-eared terrapin	An invasive feral species, with small populations throughout the UK. Bright green 2–3 cm hatchlings grow into 600–900 g adults within 3 years. They are no longer imported, but this has only resulted in altering the species collected. Other sliders, such as the yellow-bellied slider and hieroglyphic turtle or river cooter, are imported instead and are equally invasive.	Require a dry hot spot of 28–30°C and a water temperature of 24–26°C. Need a large aquatic set-up with powerful external filtration. Will benefit from UV light.	Omnivores, they will eat anything they find. There are some very good pelleted complete diets available. Providing the appropriate variety of food can be very problematic. In addition, any uneaten food will rapidly decompose, promoting bacterial growth and compromising water quality.
Spur-thighed tortoise Hermann's tortoise	These two species are now CITES (Convention on International Trade in Endangered Species of wild fauna and flora) listed, so the number traded has reduced and those traded are generally farmed or captive-bred. Hatchlings can be problematic initially but do well once established. Can be reluctant to breed in captivity and complications in association with reproductive activity are common. Their longevity is well documented (>80 years).	Require a dry hot spot of 28–30°C. Need to be housed in a vivarium or tortoise table for the first few years of life. Can be put outside when temperatures are 20°C or above; when outside they need to be housed in a secure run to prevent escape or predation from foxes and birds. Require a high level of UVB lighting. Should be hibernated from year 3 depending on size and weight.	Herbivores, although in the wild would be opportunistically omnivorous, eating occasional carrion and mammalian faeces. Should be fed a wide range of leafy greens (ideally, home-grown weeds). Prone to MBD and too rapid growth resulting in pyramiding. Supplementary dusting of food with vitamin and mineral powder is advised.

4.2 (continued) **(a)** Common reptile and amphibian species seen in practice. (continues) ▶

Species	Description	Vivarium	Nutrition
Chelonians (continued)			
Horsfield's tortoise	An Asiatic species of wide distribution. It is not CITES listed and is imported in large numbers. They can be problematic in captivity. When males are reproductively active they display very aggressive courtship behaviour towards anything and everything and can inflict serious bite wounds, especially to other tortoises.	Require a dry hot spot of 28–30°C. Need to be housed in a vivarium or tortoise table for the first few years of life. Can be put outside when temperatures are 20°C or above; when outside they need to be housed in a secure run to prevent escape or predation from foxes and birds. Require a high level of UVB lighting. Do better in a more arid environment. Should be hibernated from year 3 depending on size and weight. Tend not to make good pets.	Herbivores, although in the wild would be opportunistically omnivorous, eating occasional carrion and mammalian faeces. Should be fed a wide range of leafy greens (ideally, home-grown weeds). Prone to MBD and too rapid growth resulting in pyramiding. Supplementary dusting of food with vitamin and mineral powder is advised. Prone to prolonged periods of not eating, often misinterpreted as illness rather than normal behaviour. Often these episodes are in correlation with reproductive activity, but not always. Careful monitoring of weight loss and activity levels can determine whether inappetence is due to the presence of a disease process.
Red-footed tortoise	A medium-sized tortoise from the forests and savannah of South America. Can grow to >40 cm. Very colourful as hatchlings and imported to supply the demand for tortoises.	Require a dry hot spot of 28–30°C. Require UVB lighting. Do well in large greenhouse type enclosure, with plenty of cover. Require high humidity, which can be provided by shallow trays of water. Need heat all year round as do not hibernate.	Omnivores, they will eat anything they find, with carrion making up approximately 25% of their diet and the rest being leafy greens with occasional fruit. In captivity, carrion can be replaced with soaked dry dog food or occasional rodents. They are fast growing so can be prone to MBD. Supplementary dusting of food with vitamin and mineral powder is advised.
Amphibians			
White's tree frog	Also known as the 'dumpy tree frog', this is a hardy species that is well established in captivity despite being challenging to breed. Some farmed animals are still imported from Indonesia. Mainly nocturnal. Lifespan around 16 years.	Require a large, well ventilated paludarium (part terrarium, part aquarium) that provides high humidity and climbing opportunities for the frogs but also enables thorough cleaning on a regular basis. Rarely swim but will soak and defecate in shallow water, which must be changed daily. Room temperature is adequate but a warm area of around 28°C will help increase humidity and can be provided by a small heat mat mounted on the outside of the enclosure at one end.	The natural diet includes insects; in captivity they should be fed live food such as crickets and mealworms. Obesity is a common problem, often associated with overfeeding, or a diet of waxworms or pinky mice, which should be avoided. Supplementary dusting of food with vitamin and mineral powder is advised.
Horned frog	Often referred to as the 'pacman frog', these sedentary carnivorous tropical frogs are equipped with powerful jaws and relatively large teeth for holding prey, which is then swallowed whole. They may grow to 15 cm and can live 7–10 years.	Require daily misting and deep damp substrate to bury in, and a large shallow water bowl. They like to change position within an enclosure, especially after defecation, which is infrequent and substantial. Regular removal of faecal matter is essential; poor hygiene can lead to ulceration of the ventrum, especially the hindfeet. This can be problematic to treat. A temperature gradient of 24–28°C should be provided using a small wall-mounted heat mat.	Diet in the wild would be an array of invertebrates and vertebrates, including other frogs. In captivity, juveniles will eat live food such as small earthworms, mealworms and crickets. Adults will also eat larger prey such as locusts, cockroaches, defrosted pinky and fuzzy mice, feeder fish, slugs and snails. Overfeeding on rodents may cause obesity. Supplementary dusting of food with vitamin and mineral powder is advised.

4.2   (continued) **(a)** Common reptile and amphibian species seen in practice.

Species	Description	Housing
Native reptiles		
Common lizard	Small, slender, active lizards, typically 12–15 cm long. Live in a wide range of habitats including moorland, scrub and woodland edge. Very variable colouring from red-brown to olive green, with fine speckled or striped markings. Give birth to live young in July to August. Will shed the tail voluntarily if it is seized.	Temporary housing: Provide a dry quarantined vivarium with plenty of hides and drinking water.
Slowworm	Cylindrical, legless lizards with shiny smooth scales, giving a varnished appearance. Up to about 40 cm total length. Unlike snakes, they have eyelids. Secretive, spend most time beneath stones, log piles and leaf litter, sometimes basking early in the day. Wide range of habitats – quite common in rural gardens, although not often seen. Give birth to live young in late August to September. Will shed the tail voluntarily if it is seized. May live 50 years.	Temporary housing: Provide a dry quarantined vivarium with deep substrate for burrowing and plenty of hides, including a cool moist hide (moss box). Water should be provided in a shallow dish.
Sand lizard	The rarest British lizard species, fully protected by law. Only present in heathlands in Dorset, Hampshire, Surrey and West Sussex, and on some sand dunes in Merseyside and North Wales. Larger than the common lizard (15–20 cm), with a chunkier build and striking chocolate brown and cream 'leopard spot' markings; males develop brilliant green flanks in spring. Eggs laid May to June.	Temporary housing: Provide a dry quarantined vivarium with plenty of hides and drinking water.
Grass snake	A shy, alert, active snake. Females may reach 130 cm. Usually olive green or greyish-green, with dark vertical bars and spots along their sides. Almost all have a yellow 'collar', with two black side patches behind the head. The eyes have round pupils. When captured, they often emit a foul-smelling anal secretion and may feign death. Fine swimmers, usually found in marshy areas or near rivers or ponds. Eggs laid June to July, often in compost heaps.	Temporary housing: Provide a quarantined vivarium with deep substrate for burrowing, plenty of hides and a large water bowl for soaking and drinking.
European adder	Our only venomous snake, shy but can be aggressive when threatened. Instantly recognizable from the dark zigzag along their back. Slit pupils. Heavier build than grass snake and usually shorter, around 40–50 cm. Usual habitats are scrub, dry moorland or heath. Live young are born in August to September.	WARNING: VENOMOUS SNAKE Temporary housing: Provide a quarantined vivarium with plenty of hides and drinking water.
Smooth snake	The rarest British snake, fully protected by law. Only present in heathlands in Dorset, Hampshire, Surrey and West Sussex. Superficially resembles a grass snake but has paired or barred markings along neck and back, and no yellow collar behind head. Up to 65 cm long. Give birth to live young in August to September.	Temporary housing: Provide a quarantined vivarium with plenty of hides and drinking water.

4.2   **(b)** Native reptile species in the UK.

to disturb them in their habitat, capture them or have them in one's possession without a licence from Natural England, Countryside Council for Wales or Scottish Natural Heritage. However, an exemption applies to a person rescuing an EPS wildlife casualty and taking it to a veterinary surgery; and likewise it is legal for the veterinary surgeon to provide treatment to an injured EPS animal, although expert help should be sought afterwards regarding their rehabilitation and release into the wild.

Any native reptile or amphibian may be presented as a wildlife casualty. Immediate veterinary treatment should be provided for obvious wound and trauma, with administration of analgesia as appropriate, but these animals require specialist care.

Initially, the animal should be kept in quarantine in a suitable enclosure. Handling should be kept to an absolute minimum to avoid stress. Enclosures must be secure to prevent escape, particularly of snakes. Suitable warmth is important in these species to speed the healing process; appropriate temperature gradients should be created, along with adequate hiding places, offering a range of micro-environments. Water must be provided, in a suitable container. A high-humidity area is essential for amphibians.

Strict quarantine is vital when dealing with wildlife, to avoid any possibility of their being contaminated with non-native pathogens, which they could take back into the wild when they are released, with possibly devastating results on native populations.

Accurate identification of the species is absolutely essential. If there is the slightest possibility that the casualty is an EPS, the Amphibian and Reptile Conservation Trust (http://www.arc-trust.org) should be contacted and an appropriately licensed expert will be able to identify the species and organize collection and its longer-term quarantine, rehabilitation and (hopefully) release. On admission, a note should be made of the location where the animal was found and contact details for the person who has brought it in; this should enable the animal to be released back into its own environment, if at all possible.

Taxonomy

The three main reptilian orders (and sub-orders) are:

- Squamata
  - Sauria (lizards)
  - Serpentes (snakes)
- Chelonia (tortoises, turtles, terrapins)
- Crocodilia (alligators, crocodiles).

Each species has a scientific name that is specific to that individual species; for example, *Python regius* is the royal python. It is important to be aware that owners will sometimes present their animals with both a common name and the species' scientific name; this is especially important where a species has multiple common names, e.g. the royal python is also known as the ball python but is always *Python regius*.

Anatomy and physiology

Nursing the reptilian patient requires an understanding of the animal's intimate physiological processes. The veterinary nurse should have an understanding of the general anatomical and physiological differences between reptiles and other vertebrates, as well as the differences between reptilian taxonomic groups (Figure 4.3). With over 9000 species of reptile, there are many anatomical and physiological adaptations to specific environments, with different feeding techniques employed; these species-specific differences are beyond the scope of this chapter. Readers are advised to research individual species as they are presented.

Musculoskeletal system and dentistry

Lizards, chelonians and crocodilians are generally more similar to mammals in their skeletal anatomy than snakes are. Snakes have ribs attached to all vertebrae apart from the coccygeal vertebrae. Ventrally, the coccygeal vertebrae contain the coccygeal artery and vein, and this is a common site for venepuncture

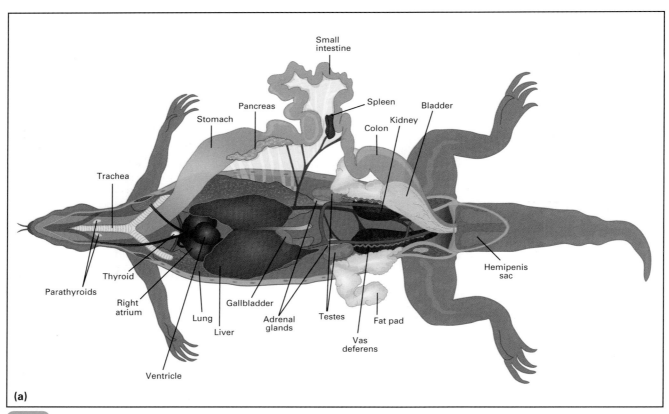

(a)

4.3   (a) Lizard anatomy. (Re-drawn after Mader DR (1996) *Reptile Medicine and Surgery*) (continues) ▶

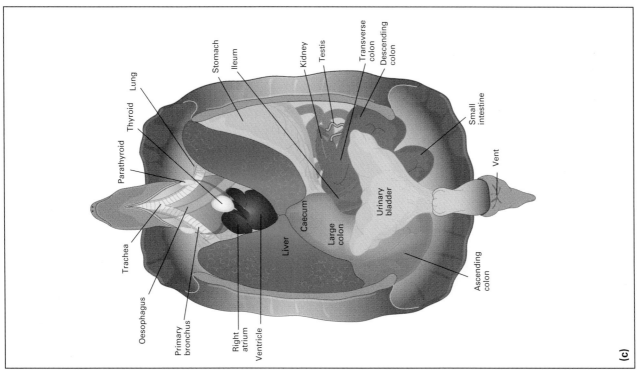

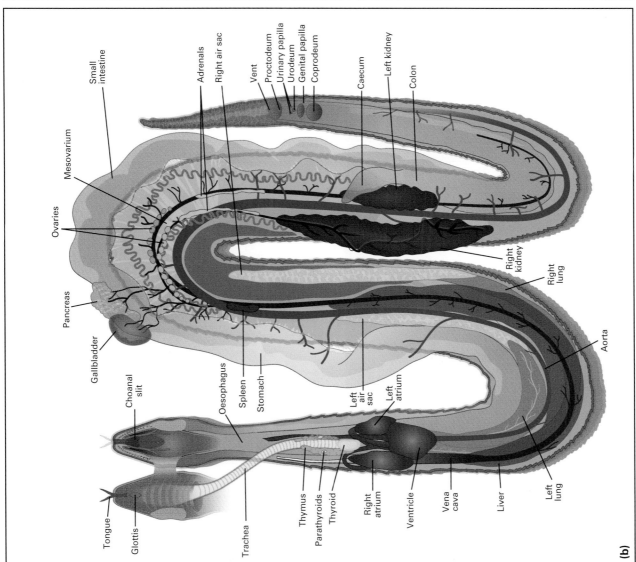

4.3 (continued) **(b)** Snake anatomy. **(c)** Tortoise anatomy Re-drawn after Mader DR (1996) *Reptile Medicine and Surgery*)

(Figure 4.4) and intravenous injections. Care must be taken not to damage the reproductive organs, which are located caudal to the cloaca.

The snake skull has a small cranial cavity. In most snakes the maxilla has four rows of teeth and the mandible has two rows (Figure 4.5). The mandible is loosely attached at the symphysis and the two halves can be moved forward independently, aiding in manipulating prey. Snakes (and some lizards) have adaptations to support their venom apparatus; these range from simple grooves on the teeth through to highly adapted tubular systems within teeth. Typically, snakes

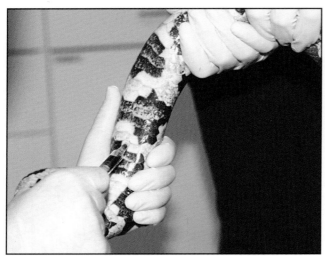

4.4 The coccygeal vein is a useful site for blood sampling.

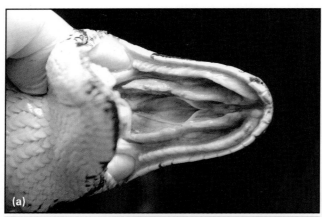

(a)

(b)

4.5 Open-mouth views of a snake showing teeth in the (a) upper and (b) lower jaw. The tubular larynx and the forked tongue within its sheath can also be seen.

are classed as front-fanged or rear-fanged, depending on the location of the venom system. In most species the teeth are shed and replaced continually.

WARNING
NEVER open the mouth of a snake as a means of identification.

Unlike lizards, snakes and crocodilians, tortoises do not have teeth but instead have a tough keratin beak. This can become overgrown and so it is sometimes necessary to burr the beak back to normal apposition using a dremmel drill. Chelonians also have well developed fore- and hindlimb musculature, which provides them with powerful limbs; this must be borne in mind during handling, as they can kick the handler's fingers or crush them against the edge of the carapace.

Respiratory system

Nostrils

Reptiles have paired nostrils that open into the roof of the oral cavity. There is no hard palate (except in crocodilians). Some species have nasal salt glands. Excess salt can appear as nasal exudate but is actually normal, e.g. in the green iguana.

Larynx and trachea

The larynx sits directly below the opening of the nares (Figure 4.6). It is simple and, in some lizard and chelonian species, vocal folds are also present, which allow vocalization. Snakes and lizards have a combination of C-shaped and complete cartilage rings along the trachea.

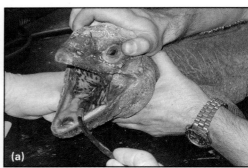

(a)

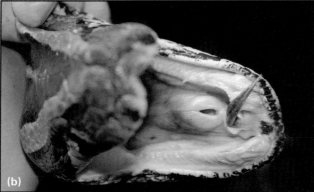

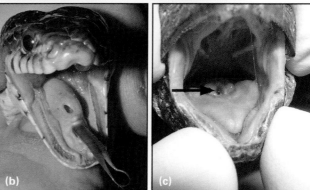

(b)

(c)

4.6 (a) Demonstration of the simple intubation technique in an iguana. (b) The larynx of a cornsnake. (c) The larynx of a tortoise (arrow indicates opening (glottis)).

In snakes the larynx lacks an epiglottis, is extremely mobile and consists of firm rings that prevent compression when the snake is swallowing prey items. Intubation is thus relatively straightforward in snakes and can be performed in conscious animals (see Chapter 7). Uncuffed or Cole's tubes are preferred, due to the presence of some complete rings in the rostral trachea.

In chelonians the trachea has complete cartilage rings; this is an adaptation to allow the animal to breathe when the head is pulled into the shell.

Lungs and respiration

The reptilian lung varies in complexity but is often a vascularized air sac (Figure 4.7), which is very different in morphology from the mammalian lung.

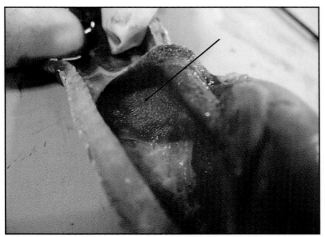

4.7 The lung of a cornsnake (arrowed). The reptilian lung is often a very simple bag-like structure.

Lizards and chelonians have paired lungs, whereas in the majority of snakes the right lung is the major lung, with the left lung remaining as a vestigial structure. The exception is the boids, in which both lungs are of equal size. The lungs are found in the cranial half of the middle third of the body.

There is no diaphragm in any of the reptile species, although crocodiles have a pseudo-diaphragm. The lack of a diaphragm means there is no thorax and abdomen; the whole body cavity is called the coelom or coelomic cavity. Inspiration is due to the expansion of the ribcage or, in chelonians, to the movement of the legs and head. The stimulus for respiration is a lowered partial pressure of oxygen and not an increase in the partial pressure of carbon dioxide; hence intermittent positive pressure ventilation (IPPV) with 100% oxygen will not stimulate a reptile to breathe as it would a mammal. In fact, many chelonians can survive for several hours without breathing at all.

Cardiovascular system

Heart

The heart has three chambers: one ventricle and paired atria (Figure 4.8). However, it functions in a similar fashion to a four-chambered heart, with the

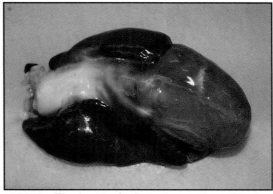

4.8 The heart of a Burmese python. The reptilian heart has a single ventricle and two atria. However, it functions as if it were four-chambered due to the presence of muscular flaps within the ventricle.

ability to separate oxygenated and deoxygenated blood in the single ventricle with little mixing.

The heart lies within a pericardial sac. As a general rule, monitoring heart rates is not as useful in reptiles as it is in mammals. The range of 'normal' heart rates varies considerably for a species, due to a combination of factors including environmental and metabolic processes and health status; hence there are rarely 'normal' values for a given species. However, knowing how to measure heart rate is essential to be able to monitor a patient under anaesthesia or to assess whether or not a patient is dead. Doppler probes, with copious amounts of ultrasound gel, are very useful for locating and monitoring the heart.

- In lizards, a lateral approach either cranial or caudal to the forelimb is useful.
- In snakes, a ventral approach is useful (Figure 4.9). The heart can also often be located by visual assessment of the ventral aspect, where a slow-beating pulsatile movement of the skin can be seen in the proximal third.

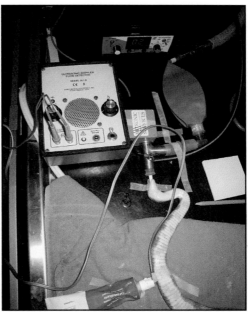

4.9 Doppler ultrasonography can be extremely useful when assessing the heart rate of a reptile patient, such as this cornsnake.

■ In chelonians, placing the Doppler probe between the neck and forelimb, aiming caudally (see Figure 7.19), is optimal. Auscultation is possible with the aid of a stethoscope; however, it can be difficult to listen over the scratching of the scales on the stethoscope diaphragm. A damp cloth can be applied over the scales or scutes to overcome this problem.

> ⚠️ **WARNING**
> **The heart is usually found in the caudal half of the proximal third of the body and is extremely mobile on palpation. This is a relatively common site for venepuncture and has been used for cannulation in sick patients. Care must be taken as it is possible to cause severe pathology if the phlebotomist is unfamiliar with this technique. The tail vein is often a safer route for blood sampling.**

Renal portal system

Reptiles possess a renal portal system, whereby blood drains from the hindquarters directly through the kidney vasculature. It is often advised that injections should not be given in the caudal half of the body as renal clearance of the drug may occur. Current thinking suggests that this is not the case; however, it may be prudent to limit injections of therapeutic agents excreted via the renal system to the cranial half of the body until conclusive evidence emerges.

Digestive system

Oral cavity

The majority of lizards, and all chelonians, have a large fleshy tongue that is used for food manipulation. The tongue is located rostral to the larynx. Chameleons show the most complex form of adaptation with their unique tongue anatomy (Figure 4.10). A hyaline rod supports the relaxed, concertinaed tongue, which has a prehensile tip. This can be fired at prey and then flipped back into the mouth. There are cases where chameleons have ingested their own tongues, leading to death or the need for euthanasia.

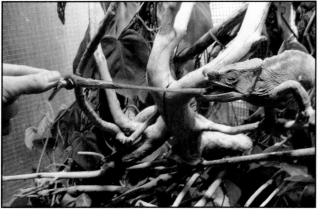

4.10   The chameleon tongue has adapted to be fired over a long distance and is prehensile, aiding in capture of prey.

In snakes, the tongue sits in a sheath at the rostral end of the oral cavity. This can be protruded even when the mouth is shut, through a notch in the lower jaw. In snakes and some lizards (e.g. monitor lizards) the tongue is not used for the prehension of food but is instead used to detect prey and pheromones. The tongue presents odours to the vomeronasal organ, located in the roof of the mouth, which is part of the olfactory system.

Venom

Recent research in reptiles indicates that the majority have venom glands but the venom is often not harmful to humans as it has evolved for the reptile's specific prey choices. Venom is species-specific in its composition and has many different components, with the aim of subduing prey or aiding digestion. In snakes, venom is an essential component of enzymatic digestion, acting within the food item simultaneously with the more routine digestive juices that break down food from the outside; this in part replaces the role of mastication, as snakes swallow prey items whole.

> ⚠️ **WARNING**
> **Do not assume that venomous species will not be presented in the practice. Some relatively common species do not require a Dangerous Wild Animal Licence. If in doubt, always ask the client for more information about a species when it is presented.**

Gastrointestinal tract

Lizard gastrointestinal anatomy, like that of mammals, varies depending on diet. Herbivores tend to have a relatively short small intestine, while carnivores and insectivores have more complex and longer small intestines. The opposite is true of the large intestine, which becomes more complex in herbivores as the reptile relies on hindgut fermentation of herbivorous diets. The liver is often bilobed and the majority of lizards have a gallbladder. Biliverdin is the dominant bile pigment in reptiles, whereas in mammals it is bilirubin.

In snakes the gastrointestinal tract is a relatively simple but distensible and muscular tube. In general terms, the oesophagus is located in the cranial third, the stomach in the middle third, and the small and large intestines in the middle to caudal third of the snake's body. The liver is long and thin, and is found caudal to the heart but cranial to the stomach. A gallbladder is present in most snakes. A pancreas is found in all snakes; in some species it is incorporated with the spleen in an organ called the splenopancreas.

In chelonians the stomach is large and mobile, often occupying the left mid-coelomic cavity. When stomach-feeding medicine or supportive nutritional foods, feeding tubes can be measured to the caudal edge of the pectoral scutes; this equates to approximately one-third of the length of the plastron. The caecum can be large in herbivorous chelonians (some are carnivorous; several are omnivorous). A large bilobed liver is found dorsal to the gastrointestinal tract but ventral to the lungs. A gallbladder is often present.

Faeces

Reptile faeces are often mixed with urates but can be passed separately, as both the gastrointestinal and urogenital tracts empty into the common cloaca. Faeces are dark to black in colour, while urates are the white and sometimes watery component of the droppings (Figure 4.11).

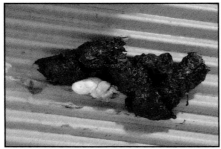

4.11 Reptiles have a common opening of the gastrointestinal and urogenital tracts. Waste is passed separately or sometimes together. Dark matter is faeces from the gastrointestinal tract, while the white matter is urates and of urinary origin.

Urinary system

Lizards and chelonians have paired small kidneys, which are often found within the pelvis, sometimes projecting cranially into the coelom. Snakes have paired elongated kidneys located in the caudal third of the body, the right being more cranial then the left.

Lizards possess a bladder-like part of the cloaca, which is absent in snakes. Chelonians have a large urinary bladder, which is important in fluid management.

Reptiles are uricotelic. This means that unlike mammals, where urea is the primary nitrogenous waste product, most reptile species produce uric acid (some aquatic species excrete ammonia). Uric acid is a relatively insoluble material and it is thought that this is an adaptation for conserving water. The white material, often mistaken for faeces, is the urate (Figure 4.11). In renal disease or dehydrated animals this material can be laid down in tissues and result in the clinical signs of gout (see later).

Reproductive system

Males

Male lizards and snakes have paired testes located just cranial to the kidneys and adjacent to the adrenal glands. These can increase in size considerably during the breeding season. Seminal fluid is produced by a reproductive part of the caudal pole of both kidneys.

Lizards and snakes have paired hemipenes located in the tail (Figure 4.12). These lie in an inverted state, causing outpouchings of the caudo-ventral aspect of the cloaca, just ventral to the anal glands. During mating, the engorged hemipenes evert and pop out of the cloaca; semen drops from the cloaca and runs along the outside of the hemipenes, along grooves, into the female's cloaca. The hemipenes have no role in urination. The inverted hemipenes are used to tell males from females when 'probing' snakes (see later).

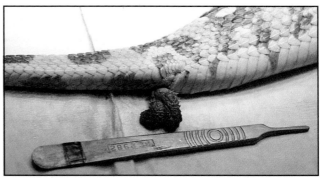

4.12 Hemipenes are the paired, male reproductive organs in snakes and lizards. They play no role in urination, only delivery of sperm, generally along external grooves on this organ.

Chelonians have a single phallus and cannot be 'probed'. The phallus operates functionally in a similar fashion to the hemipenes of the other reptiles.

In certain circumstances the phallus or hemipenes can become damaged; amputation is compatible with life, but if bilateral (or unilateral in chelonians) will prevent breeding.

Females

Female reptiles have paired ovaries. They adopt one of three reproductive strategies:

- Oviparous species lay eggs (e.g. the Burmese python)
- In ovoviviparous species, membranous egg-like structures 'hatch' inside the snake and are passed at birth with the young (e.g. the boa constrictor)
- Viviparous species give birth to live young with no egg-like structures as part of the reproductive strategy (e.g. the common lizard)

Reproductive strategies vary considerably between species. In some, the temperature of incubation will alter the sex ratio of the offspring produced. If unsuitable husbandry, environmental or nutritional conditions are provided, reptiles can exhibit follicular stasis or other reproduction-related disease. Ultimately, this can be life-threatening, and management is aimed at treating the husbandry issues, providing medical and nutritional support of the underlying pathophysiology or, in most cases, undertaking an ovariectomy.

External anatomy

Integument

In snakes, the skin has similar layers to those of mammals and contains folds of epidermis that form the scales (Figure 4.13). Dorsal scales are often smaller than ventral scales and are varied in appearance; some are smooth and others have a keel (a ridge along the axis of the scale). The scales ventrally are the width of the snake and are often referred to as scutes. They are useful in locomotion. Caudal to the cloaca, ventral scales often become paired along the ventral aspect of the tail.

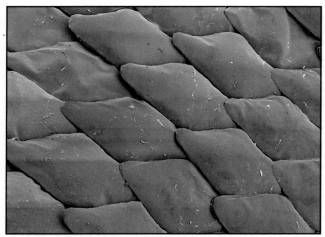

4.13 Scales of a snake as seen using electron microscopy.

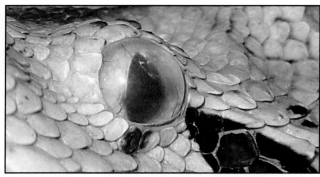

4.14 The spectacle is a single, clear scale that has replaced the eyelid in snakes. This often becomes opaque prior to ecdysis. Sloughed skins should be inspected for the presence of spectacles.

Adaptations

- **Lizards:** Certain lizard species have spikes and raised projections along their backs. These have a dual function as they provide defence from predators and also increase the surface area for basking. With the onset of maturity, crocodilians and many lizards develop osteoderms, which are bony plates within the skin that can be used for protection and heat absorption; these can cause artefacts on radiographs.
- **Snakes:** The eyelids of snakes have become fused to form a single scale over the eye, called the spectacle. Some species of snake also have labial pits running along the dorsal aspect of the upper lip. These are used as heat sensors in prey acquisition.
- **Chelonians:** The most impressive external reptile adaptation is arguably the shell of the chelonians. The shell is dermal bone, which is fused to the spine and covered with keratinized epidermis. It consists of a dorsal carapace and a ventral plastron. The pillars (the thickened part of the bone, where the carapace and plastron join) can be used for placing intraosseous needles for fluid therapy (see Chapter 6).

Ecdysis

Reptiles regularly shed their skin in a process called ecdysis; if abnormal, this is termed dysecdysis. Snakes shed their entire skin, while chelonians shed scutes of the shell, and lizards shed in a piecemeal fashion. Ecdysis is a complex process and is dependent on many factors, such as age, growth, time of year, environment and nutritional status.

In the snake a new layer of skin forms below the old one. Once complete, an enzyme-containing lymphatic fluid is secreted between the two layers; this can be seen as the snake becoming dull in colour and the spectacle covering the eye changing to a white-blue opaque colour (sometimes termed 'in milk') (Figure 4.14). This fluid aids separation and is reabsorbed once separation is completed, with the spectacles often returning to normal. The snake will start to rub at the corners of its mouth, over the head and slowly along the length of the body. In the normal ecdysis process the snake should shed the skin in one single piece, including the spectacles.

If dysecdysis occurs it can be managed with soaking, which has the benefit of aiding rehydration. Soaking in a warm bath for an hour will soften the skin, and the snake can often then remove the skin if given suitable cage furnishings, e.g. cork bark has a rough surface, which enables the sloughing skin to be caught and removed. Alternatively, the skin can be removed manually with a soft towel or a gloved hand. Extreme care must be taken not to scrape or tear off the shedding skin as this can lead to damage or scarring of the new layer of skin, predisposing the animal to chronic dysecdysis.

Special attention should be given to the spectacles of snakes; these are prone to retention and forcibly removing them is bad practice. Soaking or the daily use of a topical paraffin eye ointment (e.g. Lacri-Lube) will rehydrate and soften the scale. The removal of retained spectacles is often not a quick procedure and it may take several sessions of soaking to allow them to come away safely.

Other external features

The cloaca

Reptiles have a single external urogenital/gastro-intestinal opening, termed the cloaca. This is found ventrally at the base of the tail. The cloaca can assist in fluid therapy by allowing the absorption of water from the bladder and across the skin and mucosa. It is also clinically useful for some methods of sexing reptiles (see later).

The tail

The tail is a site of fat storage in some reptiles such as the leopard gecko and can be useful when assessing the body condition of these species. Certain reptile species may use their tails as whips; tails should therefore be secured when handling larger species such as the green iguana. Some lizards exhibit autotomy, which is the process of shedding the tail, through fracture sites in the distal tail, as an adaptation to escape predators. It is important to be aware that poor handling may induce autotomy; however, the tail will grow back in most species. The new tail does not always contain bone and will appear smaller and stunted compared to the original tail. When shed, the tail piece can be propelled a fair distance and will convulse to distract predators from the rest of the animal. This can be distressing for owners if they are not expecting it.

Vestigial limbs

All true snakes lack external limbs, with the exception of some pythons and boas (boids), which retain vestigial limbs in the form of spurs just cranial to the cloaca (Figure 4.15).

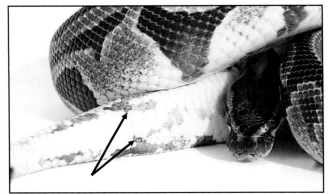

4.15 Snakes lack limbs; however, some pythons and boas have vestigial limbs close to the cloaca, called spurs (arrowed). These can sometimes be helpful for sexing.

Body temperature

Reptiles are ectotherms, meaning they rely on external sources to supply body heat. Reptiles mostly obtain heat from the environment through radiation (sunlight) and conduction (contact with warm surfaces). As with other vertebrates, the correct body temperature is essential for biological processes such as digestion, correct immune function and other metabolic processes. In sickness, reptiles will increase basking times to induce a 'behavioural fever'. Providing a range of temperatures in a vivarium is essential to allow the reptile to manage its own body temperature. Most species have defined preferred optimum temperature ranges (POTRs), which should be provided in their microhabitat. The animal's behaviour and response to temperature will change depending on multiple factors, such as activity levels, digestion, reproductive state and illness. A failure to provide suitable temperature ranges (either too cold or too hot) is one of the leading factors underlying reptilian medical problems.

Thermogenesis

Some female snakes have evolved a thermogenic ability to aid egg incubation. If the environmental temperature drops below that which is optimal for incubation, the female will twitch her whole body, generating heat and increasing the temperature of the egg clutch. This behaviour can be misinterpreted as a sign of an illness such as hypocalcaemia. Such thermogenic behaviour is commonly observed in many nesting pythons such as the green tree python, diamond python and Burmese python.

Sexing

Accurate sexing of captive reptiles is an essential part of examination for both medical and husbandry reasons. The owner may be convinced that an animal is male and yet on initial examination it shows all the classic signs of follicular stasis; in this case, it is important to be able to confirm the sex of the animal in a timely manner. When mixing two animals that are wrongly sexed (especially if both are male) the result can be violent territorial fighting, with extensive injures to one or both animals or, in some cases, death. The male reticulated python is equipped with teeth designed purely for fighting other males. Even in some species of tortoise such as the Horsfield's tortoise, males will attack almost anything they suspect to be a rival male and can inflict some surprisingly extensive bite wounds.

Until recently, 'probing' was the only method used for sexing snakes, and some lizards were said to be impossible to sex until they had reproduced. As knowledge has developed, the profession has developed alternative modalities. It is important to know which method works best for individual species; confidence in the use and interpretation of the different methods is also important when selecting which one to use. Advice and practical teaching can usually be obtained from experienced veterinary surgeons or from local herpetology groups.

Lizards

Probing

Probing is possible in lizards but is not recommended due to subtle differences in the anatomy of the hemipenes; alternative methods are recommended.

Femoral pores

Many lizard species have obvious femoral pores on the ventral surface of the thighs. These are much larger and more obvious in mature males and are absent or very small in females. The function of these pores is thought to be related to pheromone communication. The pores are clearly visible in species such as the bearded dragon and the green iguana. The presence/absence and size of femoral pores is not a definitive method of gender identification, as in some species it can be very subjective. However, it is made easier if there are several animals to compare and it should be used in combination with other factors. The location of the femoral pores can vary. For example, in the leopard gecko they are cranial to the cloaca and in adult males form a very clear 'arrowhead' row of pores (Figure 4.16); the enlargement of these pores in the males of this species starts at around 3 months.

Sexual dimorphism

Gender identification can be straightforward in some species such as the veiled (or Yemen) chameleon, where the male has an extra digit on the hindlimbs that is present from hatching (Figure 4.17). As adults, most male lizards show male characteristics, such as stockier bodies and bigger heads compared to

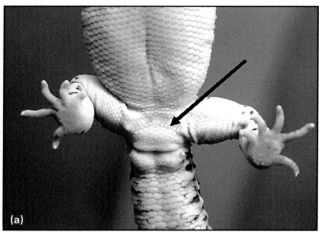

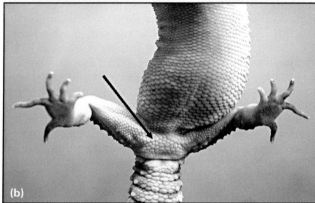

4.16 Femoral pores (arrowed) can be useful in some species for gender identification but can be very subjective in others. **(a)** Male leopard gecko. **(b)** Female leopard gecko.

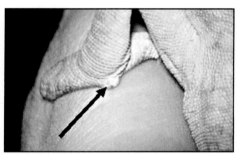

4.17 Sexual dimorphism is exhibited in some species such as the veiled chameleon, where the male has an additional digit on his hindlimbs; this is lacking in the female.

females; this, combined with interactive behaviour between lizards, can allow gender to be assigned quickly in some lizards such as the bearded dragon. In normal pairs of bearded dragons, during a reproductive introduction the male will puff out his 'beard' and turn it black to show his dominance. In return, a receptive female will display a slow wave with one of her forelimbs. Non-reproductive or gravid females will mimic males by puffing out a less impressive black 'beard', which can lead to confusion. In the past it was thought that female green iguanas became green and the males became orange during the breeding season. However, gravid or non-reproductive females will turn orange as well, to avoid harassment from amorous males.

Snakes

Probing

This is a tried and tested method that has been used for decades. Ideally a specifically made snake probe is used; these are stainless steel rods of various sizes with an atraumatic, rounded end. Plastic dog or cat urinary catheters can be a useful substitute if specialist probes are not available. The probe is lubricated with a water-based lubricant (e.g. K-Y Jelly, Johnson & Johnson). The probe is inserted into the cloaca, parallel to the body wall, in a caudal direction. In the male, the probe will pass a distance of approximately 12 to 15 scales into one of the inverted hemipenes; in the female, the probe has no structure to enter and touches the side of the cloaca, a distance of only two to five scales (Figure 4.18). The probe should require only minimal pressure. This technique needs practice to be carried out with minimal stress.

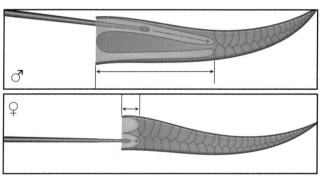

4.18 Probing is a popular method for sexing snakes. The male can be probed deeper then the female, due to the presence of the inverted hemipenes.

Probing is not without its risks, especially in young delicate species such as the green tree python and the emerald tree boa.

- The snake must be restrained firmly; inevitably this requires an assistant to control the rest of the body, leaving the person who is doing the probing free to restrain just the tail.
- It is important to hold the probe such that if the snake starts to move there is no risk of the probe being forced unnaturally deep into the hemipenis; if the delicate thin walls of the hemipenis are punctured, this can result in compromised erectile function and potentially lasting reproductive failure. At the time of probing the snake, all that may be noted is minor bleeding when the probe is removed, but in the long term the snake may be prevented from breeding.
- Probing needs to be undertaken in a delicate manner; female snakes are often thought to be males due to overzealous probing. In these cases, the probe tends to enter the subcutis in the ventral tail, potentially causing severe damage. This can be avoided with good restraint, an understanding of the anatomy of the tail and, most importantly, experience.

Popping

If done correctly and with experience, popping can be carried out quickly and safely, with no risk to the snake. The method here is to apply pressure with a thumb to the ventral aspect of the tail, just caudal to the cloaca, and, with a rolling action, push towards the cloaca (Figure 4.19).

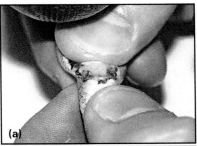
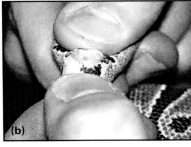

4.19 Popping is a safer method for sexing snakes but requires more experience. The hemipenis, if present, is rolled out of the cloaca. **(a)** Male python. **(b)** Female python.

- In young (less than a month old) members of the family Colubridae (approximately two-thirds of all snake species), this will cause the hemipenes to evert and, once pressure is released, they will return. This should only be done briefly; if the hemipenes do not appear then the animal is likely to be female.
- In older animals, it is not possible or safe to evert the hemipenes. Therefore the nurse should look for the subtle anatomical differences between the male and female, such as the presence of the bright red hemipenal veins.

This method should be safe, although there are reports of cases of spinal trauma resulting from excessive force being used.

Pinging

Pinging is the newest technique for sexing snakes and is widely used by herpetologists. This method is one best taught in a practical demonstration by a competent herpetologist; it is the author's (MR) preferred method. Again, it is best carried out with an assistant restraining the rest of the snake. A thumb is placed on the ventral aspect of the tail just caudal to the cloaca and, with slight pressure applied, the thumb is run along the tail towards the tip. If the snake is

male, the hemipenes are effectively pulled caudally and can be felt 'pinging' past the thumb; with a female nothing is felt. Once practised, this is safe, effective and quick, and no specialist equipment is needed.

Sexual dimorphism

Sexual dimorphism is less common in snakes than in lizards and chelonians but, when present, is mainly size-related, with females tending to be larger, more bulky animals (e.g. the boa constrictor). Pelvic spurs are present in only the males of some species, such as the Kenyan sand boa, but in the royal python spurs are present in both males and females (although they tend to be larger in males).

Chelonians

Sexing chelonians can be very challenging, especially in juveniles. Tail length is the most reliable method: mature males often have very long tails compared to females, but if examining a single tortoise this is not always easy to judge.

Concavity of the plastron is often thought to indicate that an individual is male, with the alleged advantage of providing more stability when mounting the female. However, this method of sexing is not reliable: plastron shape is highly variable, even in the same species, and there is no correlation between concavity and a male's ability to mate.

Aggression between male terrestrial tortoises is very common and is often misinterpreted as overzealous mating behaviour rather than a fight between two males. These encounters can result in serious injuries.

Sexual dimorphism

- Males and females of certain species differ in size; knowledge of the species is important.
- Red-eared terrapin males have very long front claws (Figure 4.20), which are used during courtship with the female.
- In box turtles the male has bright red eyes and females have orange eyes.

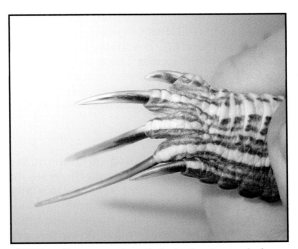

4.20 Some species of chelonian have obvious sexual dimorphism. This is especially true in the red-eared terrapin, which has extremely long nails for use in courtship. Knowing the individual species differences is important.

Other technologies

Ultrasonography

Ultrasound examination can be very useful for sexing lizards such as the green iguana, the bearded dragon and the Gila monster and for most chelonians. Scanning aims to detect the presence of follicles on the ovaries; if these cannot be visualized in a mature animal it is likely to be male. Testes in reptiles outside the breeding season tend to be small and not visible, hence this method is not always conclusive; however, it is non-invasive and often does not require sedation. Reptile scales trap air, which can make ultrasound imaging difficult. One solution is to place the reptile in a water bath and scan its abdomen under the water, ensuring that the animal's head is above the water.

Laparoscopy

When carried out under sedation/anaesthesia by an experienced veterinary surgeon, endoscopy is 100% conclusive and has been carried out on even the smallest of hatchling chelonians.

Diet

General considerations

The long-term effects of poor nutrition include: abnormalities in homeostasis; compromised immune function; aberrations in organ function; a failure to develop; dysecdysis; and many other clinical manifestations. The requirements for good reptile nutrition are generally easily achieved and it is often a case of giving less rather than more.

In times of low food availability (often a normal part of the year), healthy snakes will use up energy stored as fat and then progress to absorb the myocardium and the villi in their gastrointestinal (GI) tract. When the snake next ingests a meal these structures rapidly return to their optimal state to enable the processing and absorption of the meal.

There is a massive biodiversity within the reptiles, with a variety of different dietary preferences represented between the different species; providing a balanced diet is therefore not always as straightforward as it would first appear. The terms herbivore, omnivore and carnivore are not clear cut, as a reptile's dietary requirements may alter depending on physiological states such as reproduction and growth.

Omnivores

Omnivores are widely distributed throughout the taxonomic groups of reptiles (although there are no omnivorous snakes). Diet can alter seasonally throughout the year as a reflection of what is available to eat, or may vary as a life-stage adaptation. For example, the young giant Amazon river turtle is a true omnivore but as it reaches adulthood its large size and sedentary lifestyle mean that it requires fewer calories and it is too large to hunt. It is then mainly herbivorous but would eat, for example, a carcass should one come its way.

Herbivores

When feeding herbivorous reptiles, especially the terrestrial chelonians, there are many more challenges than with insectivores and carnivores. In the wild, herbivores would see a seasonal variation in the volume and type of food available. At certain times during the year it is likely that there would only be a single, nutritionally poor food source available, whereas at other times there would be a wide variety of highly calorific fungi and plants, including shoots; these nutritionally rich foodstuffs are likely to result in significant increases in body fat that may well be the precursor to reproductive activity. In captivity, however, reptiles are often given the same foods every day, with little variation, and owners then become distressed when food is not consumed with vigour every day of the year. How fortunate would a wild Hermann's tortoise be to feed well once a week, let alone once a day? In addition, males and females of the same species may vary dramatically in their dietary requirements and appetite throughout the year; owners often find this hard to grasp.

The food provided for herbivorous reptiles should be fresh enough for human consumption. There is a fine line between ripe and rotten, but the nutritional content of the latter is going to be poor. No one item provides all of the nutritional requirements for a given species and a range should therefore be offered (Figure 4.21). Seasonal produce that is locally grown is likely to be of better quality. There are also brands of 'tortoise grass' available that contain varieties of leafy greens and can be grown and harvested by owners, guaranteeing freshness.

Plant	Comments
Dandelion	A common weed that is a rich source of vitamins A, B complex, C and D, as well as minerals such as iron, potassium and zinc. The yellow flowers are highly palatable for even the most debilitated herbivorous reptile. A reptile super food!
Clover	A very common member of the pea family. Fast-growing and rich in protein, as well as vitamins and minerals. Ideally needs to be fed in a mix rather than exclusively
Greater plantain	Very common weed, which has tough leaves and a bitter taste but is eaten readily by most herbivorous reptiles. Rich in vitamins and minerals
Smooth sow thistle	Common, fast-growing weed. Rich in calcium, vitamins and minerals. Highly palatable to most herbivorous reptiles

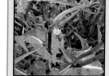 **4.21**   Common food items for herbivorous reptiles.

There is some debate as to whether to grate or chop up the leafy greens or just to give larger items that the animal has to work at to eat. Providing whole foods can be enriching, but it can be very difficult to convince owners that if a new food is not devoured instantly then this does not mean the animal will not eat it eventually; if nothing else is offered then it will usually, in time, be eaten. Tortoises can become fixated on fruit, and owners like to feed it as the animals will always eat it; however, due to its sugar content, high fruit consumption can lead to obesity and nutrition-related disease in the long term.

Carnivores

Rodent-feeders

Rodent-feeding carnivorous reptiles also tend to be poorly fed in captivity; a wild field vole has a percentage body fat of 15%, whereas the percentage body fat of a farmed mouse produced to feed a reptile is a worrying 47%. Obesity is now a real problem in all types of reptile, and this is especially true of carnivores.

The source of rodents also requires careful consideration (Figure 4.22). There are different methods

Item		Comments
Mice		
	Pinkies	Newborn mice weighing approximately 1–1.5 g. Nutritional content is very variable, depending on when the pinkie last suckled. If they have not fed they can be very low in calcium and should be supplemented
	Mouse fluffs	Approximately 3–5 g mice. Higher in calcium and lower in fat
	Small mice	Approximately 5–10 g
	Adult mice	Approximately 25–35 g
	Giant or jumbo mice	Approximately 40–60 g. Large adults tend to be ex-breeding stock and can offer low nutritional value
Rats		
	Rat pups	Newborn rats weighing approximately 8–10 g. Nutritional content is very variable, depending on when they last suckled. If they have not fed they can be very low in calcium and should be supplemented
	Rat fluffs	Approximately 30–50 g. Higher in calcium and lower in fat
	Weaner rats	Approximately 50–70 g
	Small rats	Approximately 70–100 g
	Medium rats	Approximately 100–200 g
	Large rats	Approximately 250–350 g
	Giant or jumbo rats	Approximately 400–700 g. These very large adults tend to be ex-breeding stock and can offer low nutritional value
Birds		
	Chicks	Hatchling chickens. Low in calcium and high in fat, but useful for tempting reluctant feeders
	Quail	Approximately 200–250 g adult birds. Farmed for human consumption and are fairly balanced nutritionally. Males can have large spurs, which may need removing before feeding
Fish		
	Many species available	Freshwater farmed fish are now readily available in a variety of sizes from fishing tackle shops; they should be used in preference to marine fish wherever possible for freshwater reptile species

4.22 Common food items for carnivorous reptiles.

of euthanasia and storage, all of which have an impact on the nutritional value of the final meal. The preferred method is to use either carbon dioxide or carbon monoxide as the method of euthanasia, followed without delay by blast-freezing in small batches. This stops any autolysis in these food items and should maintain their nutritional value.

The welfare of the rodents and other vertebrates must always be considered; for instance, if they consistently have obvious broken necks one has to question this and review the source.

How to defrost rodents and other vertebrate food items causes much debate in the herpetological world. The author's (MR) preferred choice is to submerge the frozen food item in warm water; once it is completely defrosted and at a roughly mammalian body temperature (this will require the water to be changed and replaced with warm water several times), the item is roughly dried and given to the reptile without delay. The key point is that the water should be warm, not boiling, and it can take a little while. Ideally, the defrosting process should not take place in the room where the reptile is housed, as the smell will be obvious and may cause the reptile to become hyper-alert; in large snakes and monitor lizards it can cause a premature 'food reaction', which can lead to serious bites, even when just trying to open the vivarium.

An alternative is to remove the rodents from the freezer and allow them to defrost at room temperature; however, this takes a long time and they can be exposed to flies and autolysis. Once defrosted, they are often fed without any extra warming. This method also has the potential for increased risk of bites, even with the use of long feeding tongs; if the feeder's hand is warmer than the food being offered the reptile may well strike and bite it, even if it is 50 cm further away.

> ⚠️ **WARNING**
> **Never underestimate how fast reptiles can react and move when trying to catch their prey – or what they think is prey!** Reptiles rely on rudimentary signals to tell them how to react. If you give one or more signals that you might be food (e.g. smell, temperature, movement), a reptile will react and may well inflict a serious injury.

Piscivores

Maintaining a consistent food supply for fish-eating reptiles is very difficult. Feeder fish often contain high quantities of thiaminase, an enzyme that destroys vitamin B1 (thiamine). The clinical signs of hypovitaminosis B1 can be as subtle as swollen eyelids, ranging through to neurological tremors, convulsions and death. Treatment is not without its problems, as indicated by the number of cases of iatrogenic hypervitaminosis B1. As always, prevention is better than cure and defrosting the feeding fish in hot water destroys the thiaminase.

Piscivorous reptiles should be fed similar fish to those they would eat in the wild (e.g. terrapins would not eat marine fish). Fish stocks would also vary considerably over the course of a year, and this should be reflected in the diet given to piscivorous reptiles.

Insectivores

Insectivorous reptiles in the wild would feed on many different types of insect (Figure 4.23) and other invertebrates and there would be clear seasonal variation in availability. As one would expect, these prey items would be full of their own ingested food and water (invertebrates on average contain 65–75% water). The invertebrate's own gut contents supply additional nutritional value that is often overlooked.

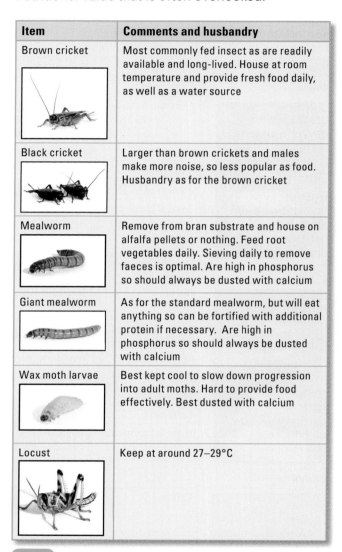

Item	Comments and husbandry
Brown cricket	Most commonly fed insect as are readily available and long-lived. House at room temperature and provide fresh food daily, as well as a water source
Black cricket	Larger than brown crickets and males make more noise, so less popular as food. Husbandry as for the brown cricket
Mealworm	Remove from bran substrate and house on alfalfa pellets or nothing. Feed root vegetables daily. Sieving daily to remove faeces is optimal. Are high in phosphorus so should always be dusted with calcium
Giant mealworm	As for the standard mealworm, but will eat anything so can be fortified with additional protein if necessary. Are high in phosphorus so should always be dusted with calcium
Wax moth larvae	Best kept cool to slow down progression into adult moths. Hard to provide food effectively. Best dusted with calcium
Locust	Keep at around 27–29°C

4.23   Common food items for insectivorous reptiles.

Gut loading

Gut loading simply requires the invertebrate prey to be fed on a good diet before it is offered to the reptile. In the pet trade there are very few types of insect reliably available. The common species include black crickets, brown crickets, mealworms and giant mealworms. Traditionally, these are fed on bran, which serves to increase their phosphorus level and therefore reduce their already poor calcium to phosphorus ratio further. These food items should always be assumed to be dehydrated and in a poor nutritional state, and will offer very little to the reptile in the way of energy, vitamins and minerals. Gut loading was the first stage towards improving the nutritional value of the invertebrate food items; good nutritional care of invertebrates results in optimal nutrition for the reptile that subsequently eats them.

Gut loading traditionally involved feeding the invertebrates a few hours before offering them to the reptiles, but is now achieved by feeding them for 2–3 days before offering them. After purchasing invertebrate food items they should be placed in a well ventilated, escape-proof container of a suitable environmental temperature and fed a suitable calcium-rich diet. Ideally this diet should be naturalistic, so dark leafy greens such as watercress, kale and rocket are useful. Crickets are omnivorous scavengers and will eat most organic matter. Powdered commercial invertebrate diets are popular, as they are simply mixed with water into a paste and then fed. Water should also be provided to the invertebrates in an appropriate fashion, which tends to be via either moist cotton wool or an invertebrate water gel.

Dusting

Dusting is used to improve the calcium content of invertebrate prey. The animals are covered in a calcium-based powder by adding some to the feeding container (i.e. the container holding the invertebrates) and shaking it. The invertebrates must be given to the reptiles immediately, before they clean themselves and remove the powder. Dusting can be a useful adjunct to gut loading but should not be seen as an alternative.

Calcium metabolism and disease

Calcium is an essential macromineral that plays a role in many metabolic processes, especially in bone formation and muscle function. Calcium deficiency is a common problem in most reptile diets, except that of carnivores fed whole carcasses. Typically, poor bone calcification (with or without hypocalcaemia) can result due to:

- Deficiency of vitamin D (or its metabolites)
- Deficiency of calcium or excess phosphate in the diet
- Deficiency of vitamin A, C, or K
- Alterations in the hormones of calcium homeostasis
- Excessive production of oestrogen (e.g. for egg-laying)
- A combination of several of these factors.

Metabolic bone disease

Metabolic bone disease (MBD) is a term often used to describe the loss of calcium from bone; however, it is not a disease in itself but rather a clinical sign (Figure 4.24).

The most common underlying pathophysiology of MBD is nutritional secondary hyperparathyroidism (NSHP), although there are other possible causes, including:

- Renal secondary hyperparathyroidism
- Hypertrophic osteopathy
- Chronic osteomyelitis.

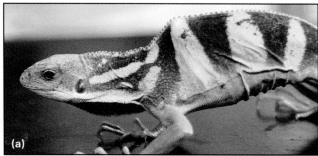
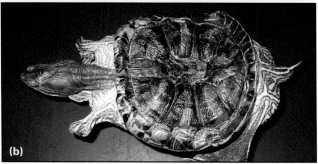

4.24 Metabolic bone disease (MBD) is a common presentation in poorly managed reptiles. This is a clinical sign and not a disease in itself. It can present in many different ways. **(a)** Lordosis and scoliosis of the spine can be seen in this Fijian iguana. **(b)** Deformed carapace in a terrapin.

A combination of the provision of suitable UVB light, adequate calcium in the diet (with a calcium to phosphorus (Ca:P) ratio of 1.5–2:1) and a good plane of nutrition, hydration and growth will prevent MBD in the majority of reptiles. The Ca:P ratio is especially important in herbivorous and insectivorous diets, as phosphorus is extremely common in plants and invertebrates.

Phosphorus and calcium utilize the same hormonal mechanisms for absorption, except the elements that increase uptake for one tend to promote excretion of the other. Therefore, in the case of diets with excessive phosphorus and low calcium, the body responds to the low serum calcium by stimulating the parathyroid gland. Parathyroid hormone restores serum calcium levels by mobilizing calcium from the bones, if insufficient calcium is available from the diet. Vitamin D3, either synthesized in the skin under UVB light or obtained from the diet, is also essential for calcium absorption from the gut. So in vitamin D deficiency, serum calcium levels are also lowered, stimulating the parathyroid gland with similar results.

If left long enough even the calcium reserves in the body are exhausted and the animal will start to develop clinical signs associated with hypocalcaemia, while the parathyroid gland hypertrophies, resulting in NSHP. Symptoms include anorexia, weight loss, tremors, seizures, weakness, fractures, ovostasis and possible death. MBD is uncommon in snakes and carnivores fed whole carcasses as they contain sufficient calcium and vitamin D3; however, some animals are fed on meat diets such as heart and this can lead to MBD. There are many other nutrition-related diseases of reptiles, but NSHP is the most common and illustrates the close relationship between husbandry, nutrition and reptilian diseases.

Housing

General considerations

A reptile tank is called a vivarium. When planning a vivarium for the first time it is important that due attention is paid to the requirements of the individual species (see Figure 4.2), e.g. somewhere to climb, or a desert or aquatic environment (Figure 4.25). There is no such thing as a generic reptile vivarium design. It is impossible to replicate all the variation found in the wild but all efforts should be made to provide a varied, enriching environment that meets the following essential requirements.

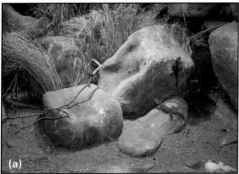

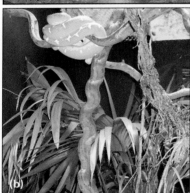

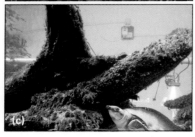

4.25 Reptile preventive medicine consists of providing adequate husbandry and nutritional needs for each species, meeting their individual requirements through the development of varied microhabitats. These are examples of vivaria for desert **(a)**, arboreal **(b)** and aquatic **(c)** species, each supplying different needs but using similar underlying principles of habitat design.

Containment

A vivarium should provide a suitable microhabitat that meets the needs of the reptile. It is essential that the vivarium is secure to prevent the animal from escaping into the local environment, which is unlikely to provide for the needs of the species and may be detrimental to the animal's health, as well as being distressing for the owner or neighbours.

The use of plastic boxes for keeping reptiles provokes controversy but, with some thought, they can provide everything a reptile needs and are easily cleaned and maintained, making them ideal for use for hospitalization or for managing large, professional collections (Figure 4.26). Within these fairly bland environments, enrichment can be provided by alternation of several types of hide boxes, the use of different type of substrate, etc.

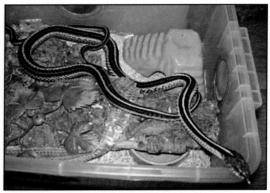

4.26 A box set-up (lid removed), which meets the basic requirements of the snake.

Temperature

It is important to consider how ectothermic animals behave in the wild. Each reptile species has a preferred optimum temperature range (POTR) at which it functions best physiologically (see earlier).

Constant heat is generally not good for reptiles, and does not mimic the natural situation. In the wild, most reptiles avoid the hottest part of the day, often hiding in burrows or under rocks to escape the excessive heat. They are usually most active in the morning as the sun rises, when they can be seen basking. A reptile will alter its behaviour to accumulate heat in order to meet its needs as they occur.

A range of temperatures must be provided in the vivarium (a thermogradient) to allow the animal choice and the ability to manage its own requirements.

Reptiles tend to obtain their heat in two ways, commonly using a combination of both.

- **Heliotherms** are the basking reptiles that obtain warmth directly from the sun's radiant heat. The bearded dragon and snakes such as the Boelen's python exhibit typical heliotherm behaviour. Heliotherms tend to seek out a basking spot, periodically moving away to hunt for food and returning when their core temperature decreases. They do not normally spend hours basking. If a captive heliotherm is seen sitting (basking) under its heat source for the entire day, this is a sign that an inadequate temperature is being provided by the vivarium's 'hot spot'. If the radiant heat is being provided by a basking lamp that is also the source of ultraviolet (UV) light, this might also raise concern that the animal is being exposed to an abnormally excessive amount of UV light. The bearded dragon and snakes such as the Boelen's python (*Morelia boeleni*) exhibit typical heliotherm behaviour.
- **Thigmotherms** obtain their heat via conduction, often by lying under rocks or in shallow sand, seldom venturing into full sunlight. It is likely that these animals would be exposed to limited UV light in the wild and may even be nocturnal, but warm up during the day due to the increase in ambient temperature. The leopard gecko and the royal python exhibit this type of behaviour.

Most reptiles use a combination of these methods to obtain heat and it is important that their captive husbandry reflects this. A thermal gradient must be provided in the vivarium, with a hotter and a colder end. The thermal range within the vivarium should enable the reptiles to use the whole of the environment. There are many equipment options that will provide a thermal range, often using a source of background heat (for providing the minimum environmental temperature) in combination with specific heat sources that provide the higher temperatures of the POTR. All heat sources should only be used in combination with a good quality thermostat.

Thermostats

Thermostats control the environmental temperature automatically within specified ranges. There are three types:

- **On/off** thermostats simply switch the heat source on or off, with maximal output during the 'on' phase until the set temperature is reached, followed by zero output until the temperature falls sufficiently to trigger a restart. This can result in swings of temperature within the vivarium as it cools before the thermostat turns back on (±2–5°C) and cannot be used with a light-emitting heat source, as the constant switching is disturbing and also shortens bulb life.
- **Pulse proportional** thermostats (Figure 4.27) are often the preferred option for non-light-emitting heat sources such as ceramic heaters, but are more expensive. They alter the flow of electricity to the heat source and modulate the vivarium temperature, by pulsing it at a rate which depends upon the vivarium temperature, providing much tighter control (±0.5°C) within the specified range. However they also switch the heat source on and off, albeit in very rapid pulses, which would cause light bulbs to flicker.
- **Dimming thermostats** are the only type suitable for light bulbs, but can also be used for most other heaters. Like pulse proportional thermostats, they alter the flow of electricity but they do this by reducing the current, so there is no flicker. Control is very accurate (±0.5°C) within the specified range.

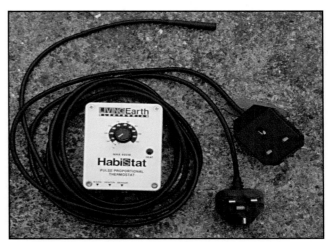

4.27 Thermostats, such as this pulse proportional thermostat, are essential for maintaining preferred optimum temperature ranges (POTRs).

Sources of heat

Heat mats

Heat mats are typically low wattage heaters that come in a range of sizes and wattages; this makes them very versatile. However, they often can't produce the basking tempreatures required for heliotherms. They are not recommended for in-vivarium use for any large reptiles, either, as a large body lying on the mat may not absorb the heat as fast as it is produced (i.e. thermal blocking) and the heat build-up under the body may reach hazardous temperatures. Debilitated reptiles that do not have enough strength to move off the heat mat can also overheat easily and, in these cases, other heat sources are more suitable. Thermal blocking can also occur if thick substrate is used over the mat; which can cause excessive heat under the substrate.

Positioning of heat mats varies; they may be placed external to the container (e.g. under boxes with a shallow substrate) but can also be applied internally (e.g. to the back wall of a vivarium). The positioning is very much dependent on the individual set-up of the container. The mats radiate heat to objects or animals that are close to them and conduct heat to objects in contact with them. They are often used under plastic boxes to provide a 'hot end' that is fairly natural for a thigmotherm; they should be controlled by a thermostat with its sensor probe resting on the surface directly over the mat. True heliotherms may experience problems, however, as they have evolved anatomically to obtain heat from above. For example, the heliothermic bearded dragon senses heat and light on its back and uses this to position itself for basking, and has evolved spines on its dorsum that increase surface area, combined with the ability to spread its ribs out to widen the area that can be warmed, and it uses chromatophores to darken its skin and absorb more heat.

'Hot rocks'
'Hot rocks' are plastic rock-shaped heaters that contain a heating element or coil. They often produce an unpredictable and excessive amount of heat and have the potential to cause horrendous burns to reptiles. They are therefore not recommended.

Lamps and bulbs
Lamps and bulbs are useful for providing heat and light; however, it is often not possible to rely on one bulb to provide both. At night the animal requires the light to be turned off and this results in loss of the heat source as well. The selection of bulb types, the role they provide and the suitability for the individual species can be a complicated business and is constantly changing as new bulb technology becomes available. It is often simpler to have a range of different bulbs in a single vivarium in order to provide 'sunlight' (heat, light and UV) in a suitably large 'basking spot'. It is important to provide species-appropriate levels of heat, light and UV. The choice and maintenance of bulbs, lamps, light and heat is an ongoing process that is a critical aspect of husbandry yet is a factor that is often misunderstood by herpetologists, especially new hobbyists.

It has recently become apparent that certain UV lights, depending on the wavelengths of light they emit, may even be harmful to reptiles. This is a complicated issue and further advice may be obtained from www.uvguide.co.uk.

Ceramic lamps
Ceramic lamps come in a wide range of wattages (40–300 W) and shapes, and will provide high levels of heat (which is actually long-wavelength infrared radiation). When using ceramic lamps consideration must be given to the safety of the personnel that handle them. Ceramic heaters must always be used with a thermostat. They must be wired by a qualified electrician to a high-quality ceramic bulb-holder with a heat-proof cable, and they must have a suitably low-amp fuse in the plug. Protection for the animal is also of paramount importance; these heaters must either be housed outside the vivarium or, if in the vivarium, placed in a non-conductive protective guard. The reptile must never be able to come into contact with ceramic lamps as they can cause severe burning on contact. They also tend to produce a very dry heat and so do not work well in environments that require high humidity. Ceramic lamps do not produce any visible or UV light.

Incandescent light bulbs
There are two types of incandescent light bulb: tungsten filament lamps (standard 'light bulbs') and halogen lamps. The spectrum of both types is similar: no UVB and only small amounts of UVA. Some species of reptile favour visual 'hot spots' that can be produced using a standard spotlight bulb. If used correctly, these produce a small area of light and heat that the animal can venture into; again, they should be used with a dimming thermostat, as discussed earlier. They should only be turned on during the day, so must be used in combination with another heat source for nocturnal temperature management if this is required.

Photoperiod and quality of light
Quantity and quality of light is very important for reptiles; they need a photoperiod that is controlled and mimics daily variation in their natural environment. The use of a plug-in timer is essential so that the standardization of the photoperiod is not reliant on someone remembering to switch the light on and off on a daily basis. Information on daylength around the world is widely available and must be considered. When attempting to breed reptiles, alterations may be made to the photoperiod (as well as to temperatures) to try and reflect natural seasonality and hopefully stimulate reproductive activity.

Light intensity is a separate issue. Desert diurnal species, such as the Saharan spiny-tailed lizard, although not always spending vast amounts of time out in the heat of the day, still benefit from bright lighting that is not associated with heat. Nocturnal species would obviously not be used to such bright light and would actively avoid it. Species such as the leopard gecko would rarely venture into full sunlight in the wild and so this needs to be taken into account in captivity. The basic anatomy should be considered: reptiles with large eyes or pale, delicate skin tend to have evolved to be nocturnal. The presence of heat-sensing labial pits in snakes can also be a good indicator that the snake has evolved to survive in low levels of light.

Ultraviolet light
UV radiation is essential for many reptiles, not only for the production of vitamin D3 and subsequent metabolism of calcium and immune function (UV light in the B spectrum, UVB) but also for normal colour vision, important for mating displays as well as food

recognition (UV light in the A spectrum, UVA). UV light in the C spectrum (UVC) must never be present as it is harmful to reptiles as well as people.

Reptiles have evolved with sunlight providing optimal UVB levels but as soon as an animal is placed in a vivarium the levels of natural UV radiation that reach it are reduced to virtually nil; it is well documented that most types of glass and plastic filter out UV light, and even mesh screening will significantly reduce the amount that reaches the reptile. For most captive reptiles it is therefore essential to provide these wavelengths of light, to ensure that basic husbandry and welfare needs are met.

UV-emitting bulbs

There are many brands of UV-emitting light bulbs, which vary widely in the quality and quantity of UV emitted. Manufacturers' claims regarding the

spectrum, output and longevity are not always supported by independent trials. It is advised that any serious herpetologists purchase a good quality UVB meter (e.g. the Solarmeter 6.5 UV Index Meter, Solartech Inc). This enables accurate measurement of the UV index (UVI) output of a bulb at any given time and location within the vivarium. In some practices clients can leave a deposit and, for a small fee, take the meter home for a day to take readings from their lamps. UV index charts can be drawn up for various bulbs, showing the output at a range of distances within the vivarium (Figure 4.28). The UV requirements of different species vary depending upon their habitat and behaviour in the wild. For example, many heliotherms bask in morning sunlight with a UV index of around 3–5; but shade-dwelling thigmotherms may never expose themselves to a UV index higher than 0.5–1.

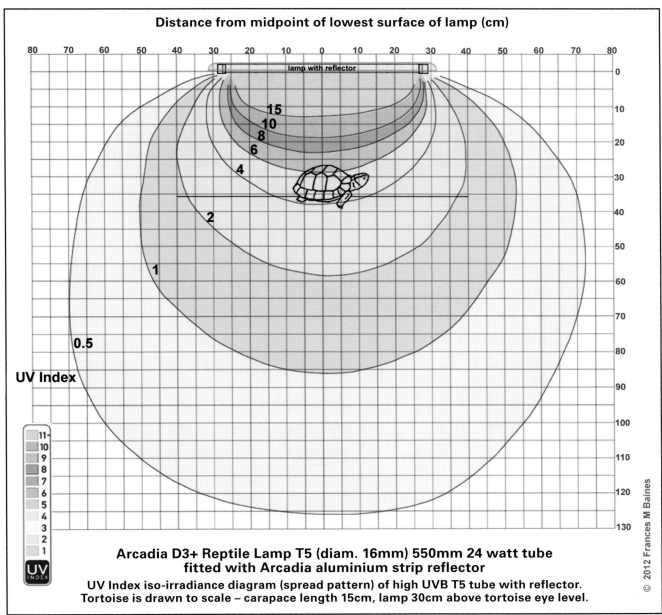

Distance from midpoint of lowest surface of lamp (cm)

Arcadia D3+ Reptile Lamp T5 (diam. 16mm) 550mm 24 watt tube fitted with Arcadia aluminium strip reflector
UV Index iso-irradiance diagram (spread pattern) of high UVB T5 tube with reflector.
Tortoise is drawn to scale – carapace length 15cm, lamp 30cm above tortoise eye level.

© 2012 Frances M Baines

4.28 UVB is extremely important for any vivarium. There are many different lights available and knowledge of the types of UVB, the amount emitted and the distances that the UVB reaches are all important. Here, three different lamps are assessed using a UVB meter to produce UVB charts. (© 2011, 2012 Frances M Baines) (continues) ▶

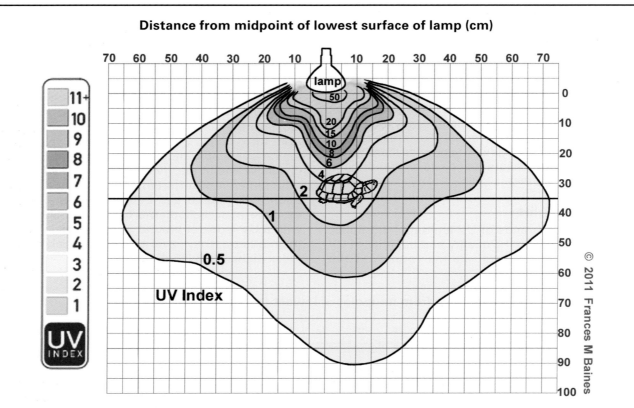

Distance from midpoint of lowest surface of lamp (cm)

Arcadia D3 Basking Lamp 160 watt Flood Mercury Vapour Lamp
UV Index iso-irradiance diagram (spread pattern) of high UVB wide floor lamp.
Tortoise is drawn to scale – carapace length 15cm, lamp 30cm above tortoise eye level.

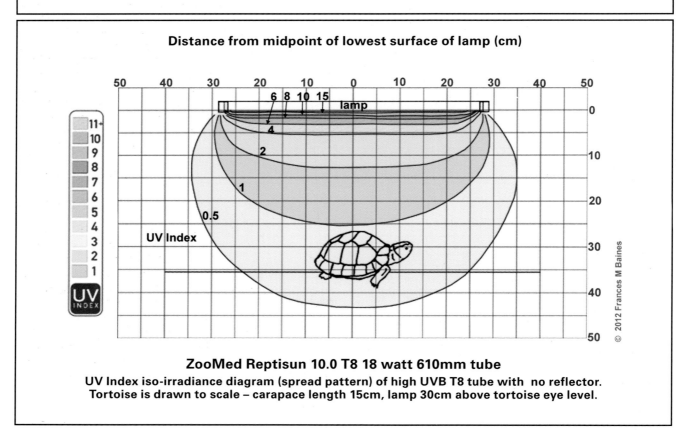

Distance from midpoint of lowest surface of lamp (cm)

ZooMed Reptisun 10.0 T8 18 watt 610mm tube
UV Index iso-irradiance diagram (spread pattern) of high UVB T8 tube with no reflector.
Tortoise is drawn to scale – carapace length 15cm, lamp 30cm above tortoise eye level.

4.28 (continued) UVB is extremely important for any vivarium. There are many different lights available and knowledge of the types of UVB, the amount emitted and the distances that the UVB reaches are all important. Here, three different lamps are assessed using a UVB meter to produce UVB charts. (© 2011, 2012 Frances M Baines)

In most husbandry-related disorders it is a lack of UVB that is the problem. However, overzealous provision of UVB can lead to multiple health issues. Unnaturally intense or prolonged exposure can cause eye damage (photokerato-conjunctivitis) and even serious skin burns, especially if the lamp spectrum contains unnaturally short-wavelength UVB or UVC.

Care must be taken if the UV-emitting lamp is providing the reptile's only source of heat because, as previously stated, if that lamp is not providing sufficient warmth across a large enough 'hot spot' then the animal will spend too much time basking and may be at risk from localized thermal or even UV burns.

It is sometimes believed that excessive UVB may lead to overproduction of vitamin D3, leading to 'vitamin D poisoning'. This is not possible in natural sunlight, since vitamin D3 synthesis is self-limiting with the solar spectrum. However, there is some evidence that certain lamps (e.g. some mercury vapour lamps) have spectra that distort this process, enabling much higher levels of vitamin D3 to build up. Surprisingly, in normal reptiles this seems to cause few problems, but some, possibly those with pre-existing NSHP, may develop calcium deposition in the tissues, termed metastatic calcification, which can in turn lead to disease and even death as a result of haemorrhage from friable vessels.

UV-emitting lamps come in two main types: high-intensity discharge (HID) lamps and fluorescent UVB-emitting tubes.

High-intensity discharge lamps

HID lamps include mercury vapour lamps and metal halide lamps. These emit heat, light and UV from an inner arc tube, which is contained within a reflector bulb which spreads the beam. The front glass allows heat, light, UVA and UVB to pass out but blocks hazardous UVC. Arc tubes require a ballast, a device intended to limit or control the amount of current passing through the lamp and prevent it failing or exploding. Internally ballasted lamps (e.g. self-ballasted mercury vapour lamps) use an ordinary incandescent filament as a ballast; this also adds to the heat and light. Due to the construction of HID lamps, they cannot be dimmed in any way. This can be restricting, as they tend to be of high wattage and produce high levels of heat; they are unsuitable for small vivaria.

Due to the construction of these lamps, they cannot be dimmed in any way. In a domestic environment this is very restricting, as they tend to be of high wattage and produce high levels of heat. Externally ballasted bulbs (e.g. metal halide lamps) are fairly new to the market. They are controlled by a small electronic ballast normally placed outside the vivarium. Metal halide bulbs emit extremely bright visible light and minimal heat, and are also available in low wattages, which makes them very useful for smaller environments, although they still cannot be dimmed.

As with all UV-emitting devices, they need to be used with care. Consistent monitoring of the reptile's behaviour within its environment is often very informative.

Fluorescent UVB-emitting tubes

Fluorescent UVB-emitting tubes are often the ideal compromise for the hobbyist or veterinary practice. These are available either as linear tubes, which require a fixture and ballast controller (just like household fluorescent tubes) or as compact fluorescent lamps, which are small coils or bars, with a miniature ballast built into the base. They produce low- to mid-range levels of UV with practically no heat. There are many sizes and brands on the market, of varying quality and output. The use of a reliable UV index meter is essential.

The amount of UV produced by some brands of linear tube decreases fairly quickly, requiring replacement within 6 months, but this is variable and can only be assessed with a UVB meter; some may retain their output for a year or more. Compact lamps on the whole decay more rapidly, and produce a much smaller UV zone than linear tubes. Some new 'T5' slim linear tubes have a much higher UV output, even rivalling mercury vapour lamps if fitted with an aluminium reflector.

Water and hydration

All reptiles should have access to clean water. Chronic dehydration, often in association with kidney disease, is the most common cause of dysecdysis and is common in sick reptiles, in which it can further exacerbate pathological processes. This dehydrated state normally starts with poor provision of water in combination with other inadequate husbandry.

Provision of drinking water is not straightforward for all reptiles. Many lizards, such as chameleons, iguanas and geckos, have evolved to obtain their daily fluid intake by licking foliage after rain or when it is covered in early morning dew. These species often do not recognize a bowl of still water as being a source of water; thus, it cannot be assumed that because a water bowl is present a reptile is not dehydrated. In captivity, misting, spraying or the provision of water drippers (which can be made from used fluid therapy giving sets) is essential to allow some species to maintain their hydration.

Snakes like to drink freshly poured water and will often show no interest in a half-full water bowl that has been standing for a period of time. It is important to change the water daily, as snakes will often drink as soon as the fresh water is put in the vivarium. Some of the desert species are adapted to obtain all of their water needs through the diet. It is important to look at a species and consider its environmental niche and subsequent adaptations when considering fluid requirements and how to provide water.

Aquatic reptiles such as terrapins tend not to become dehydrated if housed in water of an acceptable quality, but the onset of dehydration can be rapid if they are forced to be housed in an arid environment. See Chapter 5 for more information.

Chronic dehydration

Anecdotally, herpetologists often talk of a syndrome in which a debilitated snake that has not fed for a worrying amount of time finally feeds and then dies shortly afterwards. It is hypothesized by Mader (2005) that the underlying reason for this is a lack of protein, which restricts the ability of the snake's organs to absorb the meal. However, it is more likely that the snake's death is due to chronic dehydration and that it is lacking the essential electrolytes needed for digestion and haemopoiesis.

From a nursing perspective, one must always rehydrate chronically debilitated reptiles before even considering assisted- or tube-feeding. The choice of fluids for rehydrating reptiles is fairly wide; Lectade (Pfizer) or lactated Ringer's solution work well, either given orally or used as a warm bath, where it can be absorbed via the cloaca as well as stimulating drinking. Care should be taken with debilitated patients when bathing them. Baths should be shallow, to prevent possible drowning, and should be warmed to the POTR of the animal. Baths have other benefits compared to parenteral fluids: they promote the expulsion of often desiccated faeces and urates; and absorption of water via the gastrointestinal tract is rapid.

> **WARNING**
> **Cloacal enemas should not be used, as they can cause retrograde flushing of faecal matter into the urogenital and/or reproductive tract.**

Visceral gout

Dehydration can also result in uric acid becoming concentrated in the blood to such a high concentration that it forms crystals within the highly vascular organs. This is termed visceral gout and can be quickly terminal if this crystallization process prevents a major organ (such as the brain, kidneys or liver) from working, through obstruction of its blood circulation. In such cases the animals usually have highly elevated blood uric acid in preprandial blood samples.

Patients with less severe disease are very difficult to diagnose and often present with chronic ill-health, seem unable to maintain their hydration, often regurgitate, and fail to grow or breed. These clinical signs are not pathognomonic for visceral gout but rather tend to be part of all reptile disease processes.

Treatment for gout is palliative at best. Methods of monitoring and assessing renal function are still evolving but are not as simple as in mammals. Iohexol clearance testing looks likely to be a useful diagnostic tool, but finding a veterinary laboratory to screen for iohexol levels in the UK can be problematic and costly.

Humidity

Some species of reptile will require a high level of humidity and it may be fundamental in maintaining their hydration; however, it is not straightforward to provide the correct level. Provision of heat, the presence of water and a reduction in ventilation will increase humidity, but will also cause a 'stale air' microhabitat that promotes the growth of moulds and fungi, some of which can be pathogenic. Generally, the consideration given to humidity should be similar to that given to heat, in that a gradient should be provided. In practical terms, this is almost impossible in a small vivarium, so best practice is often to provide opportunities for the reptile to seek out a higher

humidity area within the vivarium. This can be achieved simply, using a plastic tub or nest box that contains some moist moss or peat and has small entrance holes. This gives the reptile the chance to be in a high-humidity zone without compromising the general environment. At certain times, such as during sloughing, this high level of humidity is essential for good health.

Substrate

The substrate in a vivarium must be non-toxic, non-irritant and easy to clean. Substrate choice is dependent on the species being housed and its normal behaviour:

- Does the animal burrow?
- Is it arboreal, terrestrial, aquatic or semi-aquatic (Figure 4.29)?
- What behavioural needs does it have and what implications will the substrate have?
- How will it interact with the substrate?

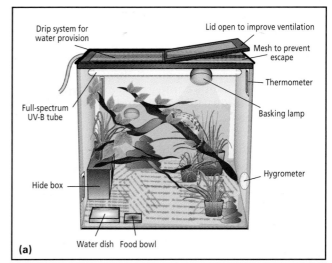

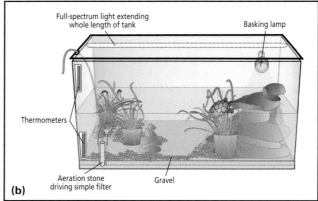

4.29 Naturalistic reptile environments. **(a)** Arboreal. **(b)** Semi-aquatic. (Reproduced from the *BSAVA Textbook of Veterinary Nursing, 5th edn*)

Several types of sand and gravel are commonly used for terrestrial and aquatic species but care must be taken as this can be inadvertently ingested when eating prey. Hypocalcaemic reptiles may deliberately ingest substrate to try and obtain vital minerals, leading to intestinal obstruction. Wood chips or shavings and small pebbles can result in similar problems. Alfalfa pellets are a good absorbent substrate and will not lead to impactions. Topsoil or coir-type substrates can be useful, as they can be moistened and used to maintain high humidity. Excessively rough surfaces should be avoided as they can cause abrasions, especially when rubbed against while trying to slough skin. Newspaper, although not aesthetically pleasing, is extremely useful, especially in hospital cages.

Behavioural enrichment

When considering enclosure size for adult reptiles, as long as an appropriate thermal gradient can be provided, the bigger the environment the more enriching it can be. Thought must be given periodically to enriching it further by adding novel substances or smells, such as leaves or diluted essential oils. Hiding places should be provided for all except arboreal species, both for privacy and as a retreat from the heat (Figure 4.30). The use of live plants can be enriching but care must be taken with herbivorous species to ensure that the plants are not toxic.

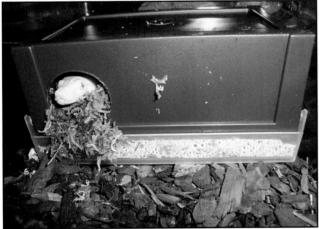

4.30 A hiding place is provided both for privacy and as a retreat from the heat.

Further husbandry advice

Owners often seek guidance from shops and suppliers but the best sources of information are breeders, local clubs, national societies (such as the British Herpetological Society (BHS) and the International Herpetological Society (IHS)) and reliable reptile forums, such as www.kingsnake.com.

Amphibians

The popularity of amphibians as pets is on the increase. Unfortunately, some people are drawn to a species by its appearance without giving enough thought to the complexity of its husbandry. Water quality is often paramount in keeping these animals in good health. This, combined with the difficulties in providing them with an appropriately varied diet, means they should never be taken on lightly. They tend to make poor pets as they often do not cope with being handled on a regular basis. When a physical examination is unavoidable, it must be kept as brief as possible. Powder-free gloves should always be worn and moistened with appropriate water (e.g. that in which the individual lives). For small frogs and newts, examination can often be carried out by briefly placing them in a clear sandwich-type bag (Figure 4.31).

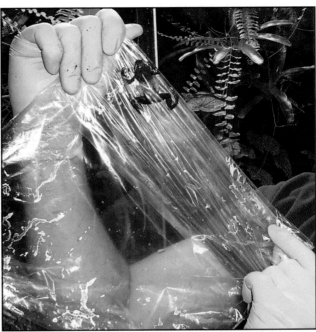

4.31 A clear bag can be very useful for a brief examination of small amphibians.

Chytridiomycosis

It would be inappropriate not to mention chytridiomycosis, which is an emerging infectious disease of amphibians caused by the fungus *Batrachochytrium dendrobatidis*. The disease is associated with widespread global amphibian decline and species extinction; however, the principal factors that underlie the emergence of this disease remain unclear. Current evidence implicates the worldwide trade in amphibians for its rapid spread. It is important to be aware of its occurrence in common amphibian pet species and to prevent any possible spread. Treatment is uncomplicated in pet amphibians and involves the administration of readily available anti-fungal medication. Every effort should be made to treat these pets, not only for their own welfare but also to prevent any possible spread of the disease into native populations.

References and further reading

Girling S (2003) *Veterinary Nursing of Exotic Pets*. Wiley-Blackwell, Oxford

Mader D (1996) *Reptile Medicine and Surgery*. Saunders Elsevier, St. Louis

Mader D (2005) *Reptile Medicine and Surgery, 2nd edn*. Saunders Elsevier, St. Louis

McArthur S (2004) *Medicine and Surgery of Tortoises and Turtles*. Wiley-Blackwell, Oxford

Meredith A and Johnson-Delaney C (2010) *BSAVA Manual of Exotic Pets, 5th edn*. BSAVA Publications, Gloucester

Ross R and Marzec G (1990) *The Reproductive Husbandry of Pythons and Boas*. Institute for Herpetological Research, California

Self-assessment questions

1. What are the limitations associated with breeding animals that have a genetic predisposition for colours and patterns?
2. What is the preferred optimum temperature range (POTR) and why is this important?
3. What is thermogenesis?
4. How can the reptilian cloaca assist in fluid therapy?
5. How does a reptilian heart differ from that of a mammal?
6. Name the three different types of reproduction adopted by female reptiles.
7. What is the significance of ultraviolet light in the A spectrum (UVA) and ultraviolet light in the B spectrum (UVB) in terms of reptile husbandry?
8. Define the term dysecdysis. Identify the most common cause of this process and how to prevent it.
9. What does 'gut loading' mean and why would this be advocated?
10. What is metabolic bone disease (MBD)? Identify the possible underlying pathophysiology and explain how this condition can be prevented.
11. Reptiles rely on external sources to supply body heat. Which one of the following terms describes this process?
    a. Heliotherms
    b. Thigmotherms
    c. Ectotherms
    d. Endotherms
    e. Thermogradient
12. When stomach-feeding a chelonian, feeding tubes can be measured to the:
    a. Caudal edge of the pectoral scutes
    b. Cranial edge of the pectoral scutes
    c. Pillars of the shell
    d. Axillary notch
    e. Axillary buttress
13. Which one of the following is the dominant bile pigment in reptiles?
    a. Ammonia
    b. Biliverdin
    c. Bilirubin
    d. Nitrate
    e. Urea
14. Which one of the following is not a function of a snake's tongue?
    a. Prehension of food
    b. Detection of prey
    c. Presentation of odours to the vomeronasal organ
    d. Detection of pheromones
    e. Sampling the chemical environment
15. Which one of the following food items provides a rich source of protein, vitamins and minerals for herbivorous reptiles?
    a. Smooth sow thistle
    b. Greater plantain
    c. Clover
    d. Dandelion
    e. Orchard grass

5

The hospital ward

William Lewis, Lyndsey Stanton and Sarah Flack

This chapter is designed to give information on:

- The facilities and equipment required in the exotic pet ward
- Housing and nutritional requirements of the hospitalized exotic and wildlife patient
- Care of orphaned mammals, birds and reptiles
- Cleaning and disinfection of hospital accommodation and equipment
- Zoonotic and anthropozoonotic diseases
- The health and safety aspects associated with nursing exotic pets

---

Ward design

An exotic pet ward will always require compromise: a wide range of species with differing needs must be accommodated and the natural predator–prey relationships between them taken into consideration (see also Chapter 1). University teaching hospitals, large referral centres and wildlife rescue centres have the space and resources to allow for the building of separate wards for different species (Figure 5.1). Most small animal practices, however, will have to adapt to different requirements as and

5.1 A ward for avian and reptilian patients.

when they arise. Practices should have some basic facilities and equipment available that will cater for the majority of situations.

Common sense must be used when deciding where to house a patient. This will depend on whether there are other patients of a similar species being housed, the danger of transmission of disease, and the presence of other patients in the hospital that may be viewed as potential predators. For example, if the cat ward is empty then this may be an ideal place to house rabbits or other small mammals. If a species is presented for the first time then staff will need to be creative when deciding how to house the patient until it can be either referred on or returned to the owner.

Mammals

Rabbits, guinea pigs and chinchillas should ideally be housed in an area that is the least stressful at the time of admission, as far away from dogs, cats and ferrets as is practical. Guinea pigs need to be kept warmer than rabbits and chinchillas. It may be possible or practical to have a small area set aside with two or three cages for rabbits that would cater for the average caseload seen in a small animal practice.

Smaller mammals such as mice, rats, hamsters, gerbils and degus may be housed in their own cages, in an area away from predator species such as dogs, cats and ferrets. Ferrets should ideally be housed away from dogs and cats, but this is rarely possible.

Birds

Birds may be housed in incubators, which can be moved around to different areas of the practice, depending on where is most appropriate at the time of admission. Psittacine and passerine birds that are in reasonable health may be housed in their own cages. They should be housed in a quiet area of the practice or in an isolation area if a zoonosis such as psittacosis is suspected (see later).

Poultry and peafowl may be housed in dog and cat kennels. Walk-in kennels are useful for larger patients such as emus and turkeys.

Raptors have very specific housing and dietary requirements and may be best kept in their travelling boxes, and hospitalized for as short a period as possible, before returning them to their owners or referring them to a specialist centre. If they are hospitalized then it might be useful to have a bow perch and a block to cater for the different species (see later). Smaller species such as barn owls may be easier to accommodate.

Reptiles

It would be useful to have one or two vivaria of different sizes if reptiles are seen on a regular basis. It may then be possible to meet the specific temperature and humidity requirements of different species. A small plastic tub resting on a heat mat (see Figure 5.9) is an acceptable compromise for short-term hospitalization or if all available vivaria are full, especially for smaller snakes and lizards.

Tortoises may be housed in open table-top style enclosures with appropriate heating, lighting and ultraviolet (UV) lamps.

Reptiles carrying infections that may be contagious should be housed in isolation, which creates another level of logistical problems. Special thought must be given to disinfection of vivaria and facilities after hospitalization of such cases. Use of F10 foggers (Figure 5.2) may be suitable (see Figure 5.18 for more information).

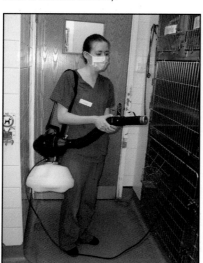

5.2 A commercially available fogging machine can be used with F10 Biocare to disinfect the environment.

Large and potentially dangerous reptiles such as pythons, boas and crocodiles will require very secure housing to protect staff. Venomous reptiles create a whole new dilemma and serious consideration would have to be given as to whether or not to hospitalize these patients (see Chapter 1).

Wildlife

Wildlife patients are best referred to a specialist wildlife centre as soon as possible. Smaller mammals (including bats) and birds can be housed in cages in a quiet area and covered with towels to reduce stress.

Larger and potentially more aggressive species such as foxes and badgers pose more of a problem and will need to be dealt with on an individual basis, attempting to keep stress to a minimum and prevent injury to staff involved in their care. Badgers are very powerful and have a very dangerous bite. They should always be treated with great care. Nets such as those used by anglers may be used to capture badgers. Alternatively, a board may be used to encourage them into a transport box or dustbin. Severely injured or moribund badgers may be gripped by the scruff of the neck, taking care to support the body. Gloves offer no protection from bites and are not recommended under any circumstance. Baskerville muzzles may be useful when examining badgers. If wire baskets are used to transport badgers they should be covered with a blanket or towel to provide a feeling of security. Members of the public who find an injured fox or badger should be directed to local wildlife organizations or the RSPCA if possible (see Chapter 1).

Equipment

For a very small financial investment, an array of equipment specific for exotic pets may be purchased (Figures 5.3–5.5), which will go a long way towards helping to manage an exotic pet ward more efficiently.

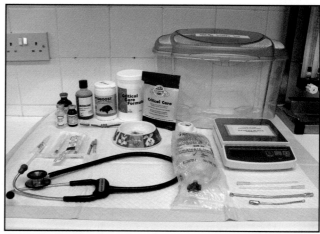

5.3 A selection of equipment necessary to perform daily inpatient checks, feeding and medication. Equipment shown includes: commonly used drugs; Tamodine scrub and toothbrush; Reptoboost; Critical Care Formulas for both reptiles and herbivores; weighing tank and digital scales; variety of crop/feeding tubes; fluids; Durapore tape; stethoscope; bowl; heparin flush; and a variety of needles and syringes.

Equipment	Uses/description
Gram scales	Should measure to 1 gram
Vacutainers	Useful for diluting injectable drugs to lower concentrations (Figure 5.5)
Dropper bottles	Each drop delivers 0.05 ml so oral drugs can be diluted to provide accurate dosing
Crop needles/feeding tubes	These tubes are used for crop/gavage-feeding. They can be re-used and sterilized if appropriate
Recovery aids	Foil blankets, bubble wrap and hot water bottles
Nebulizer	Useful for delivering drugs directly to the respiratory system, particularly to avian patients with aspergillosis
Gags/specula	Protect tubes when feeding psittacine birds
Feeding formulas	Useful for force-feeding. Various different types of food are available depending on species and stage of recovery
Foods/supplements	Suitable foods required for common species

5.4 List of equipment useful for an exotic pet ward.

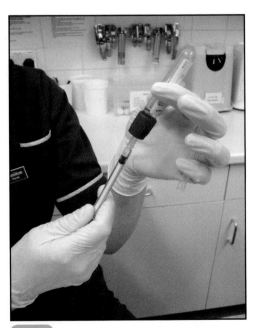

5.5 Vacutainer for diluting medication.

Small syringes, feeding tubes, weighing scales, blood collection tubes, dropper bottles and a calculator are essential items.

In many situations, equipment that is used for dogs and cats can be utilized or adapted for use with exotic pets. A little lateral thinking is sometimes required to cope with an unusual situation. Crush cages, incubators and critical care units, intravenous catheters, feeding tubes, mouth gags and various other pieces of standard equipment can be adapted to house various species and aid with feeding, endotracheal intubation and dental work.

Requirements of the hospitalized patient

The requirements of different species need to be considered, as well as the medical reason for hospitalization. A seriously ill parrot will have different temperature requirements from those of a completely healthy parrot that is being hospitalized for an elective procedure. Thought will need to be given to each individual case and a plan created to cope with the specific circumstances that may arise.

Housing requirements within the hospital

Cages and cage furniture should be cleaned and fresh bedding provided daily. To prevent cross-contamination, cage furniture should be disposed of appropriately when the patient is discharged.

Wild animals that no longer require ongoing intensive veterinary treatment should be moved to a wildlife rehabilitation centre, where larger, more appropriate accommodation can be provided prior to release.

Mammals

For all species, water should be available at all times and food left in the cage for the animal to consume unobserved.

Rabbits, guinea pigs and chinchillas

Rabbits (wild and domestic), guinea pigs and chinchillas can be housed in proprietary veterinary cages. They should have good quality mould-free and dust-free hay for bedding. Some hay may be offered from a height to encourage the animal to stretch up to reach it. Guinea pigs and chinchillas require a 'house' (a cardboard box will suffice) to hide in when they feel threatened; this should also contain some hay. Guinea pigs are particularly sensitive to changes in housing and the resultant stress will at best impair recovery and at worst lead to deterioration in health.

For long-stay rabbit and guinea pig patients, providing an outdoor exercise area should also be considered. However, one should be mindful of the following.

Considerations for rabbit and guinea pig outdoor exercise areas

- The run must be weather-proof and predator-proof (to airborne predators such as sparrowhawks and buzzards as well as to terrestrial predators).
- There must be adequate shelter within the run and additional boxes or piping to hide in.
- The run should not be situated in direct sunlight, as rabbits and guinea pigs are sensitive to heat stress.
- The run should be escape-proof.
- Water must be provided.
- Rabbits or guinea pigs with open wounds or diarrhoea/urine scalding should not be allowed outside due to the risk of myiasis.
- The risk of theft should be considered.

Providing different heights in the cage of a chinchilla will encourage exercise, and non-toxic branches/wooden toys can be provided for gnawing. Plastic items, including bowls, must be avoided as these can be chewed and ingested. A dust bath can also be offered for a few minutes each day.

Rabbits and chinchillas should not be kept too warm as they are unable to sweat and can therefore overheat easily; the ambient room temperature should be no higher than 21–23°C. Provision should, however, be made for critically ill patients or those that have undergone surgical procedures and may be hypothermic. Heat mats, lamps, hot water bottles and incubators may all prove useful in these circumstances.

Mice, rats, hamsters and gerbils

These species are best housed in their own cages, with familiar smells and bedding. A few spare cages may be useful in situations where patients are brought into the practice in a box or carry case. Small rodents require housing in purpose-built non-toxic wire cages, to prevent escape. Only gerbils should be housed in plastic or glass tanks as they require deep substrate for burrowing. The poor ventilation and accumulation of ammonia in tanks results in respiratory problems in the other species.

Hamsters are prone to climbing wire cages and falling; a cage with a deep plastic tray is therefore recommended. Most rodents like to burrow, so an area of deep substrate should be provided. Sawdust makes an ideal substrate due to its high absorbency, but where open wounds are present or the patient has respiratory problems, shredded paper can be considered. Cardboard boxes and rolls can be used as hiding places and chewing material. Solid exercise wheels are also useful.

A temperature of approximately 21–23°C should be aimed for. A small incubator may be useful for critically ill patients or those that may be hypothermic following long surgical procedures.

Ferrets

Ferrets can be hospitalized in metal dog and cat cages or in rabbit or guinea pig cages but, instead of hay, a towel or blanket should be provided, which the ferret will use to sleep on or under. If they are staying in hospital for some time, an outdoor run would be beneficial.

Temperatures of approximately 21–23°C should be adequate unless the patient is critically ill.

Wild mammals

Foxes and badgers are best housed in walk-in kennels (preferably in an isolation ward) with a bed of hay or straw for warmth and comfort (unless contraindicated by injury, in which case polyester bedding (e.g. Vet bed or Pro Fleece) may be used). The kennel door should be covered with a towel to reduce stress.

Hedgehogs and squirrels can be kept in proprietary veterinary cages lined with newspaper and containing a towel under which they can sleep. Bats require a container that is a minimum size of twice the wingspan in all directions.

Care must be taken when housing the small mustelids (including stoats and weasels). These species must be housed in escape-proof hamster or small bird cages, with bars that are close together. Extra vigilance should be exercised when closing the doors and checking the cage for signs of damage. If these species escape in an exotic pet ward, they are capable of entering other cages and killing the other patients (a tiny weasel can bring down an adult wild rabbit).

The housing requirements of wild rabbits and rodents are the same as those of the domestic species.

The particular temperature, humidity and lighting requirements for the different wildlife species will vary tremendously. See the BSAVA *Manual of Wildlife Casualties* for further information.

Orphans

Orphans should be contained in the same way as puppies and kittens. An incubator should be provided or, where this is not possible, a heat pad, hot water bottle or microwavable heat pad (such as a Snuggle Safe) covered with fleece blankets would also be appropriate. As the orphans become more mobile and independent, their housing can be modified accordingly.

Birds

Unless it is necessary to keep a bird confined in a smaller space (e.g. to restrict movement of injured limbs), the cage should be large enough to allow the bird to extend its wings in all directions. Stainless steel cages are ideal for most bird species, but smaller species such as budgerigars, canaries, sparrows and finches will need to be housed in purpose-built bird cages.

For most species (excluding ducks, geese and swans), at least one perch should be available, of a diameter suited to the size of the bird's feet. The perch should be positioned such that the bird will not foul its food and drinking water. The material of the perch should be wood or natural branch for most species, attached to two blocks of wood, which will raise the bird high enough to keep its tail off the floor. Perches should be thoroughly cleaned and disinfected prior to use. Sandpaper covers should not be used as they traumatize the base of the feet. Bowed perches should be provided for hawks (to mimic branches) and flat blocks should be provided for falcons (to mimic cliff edges). These should be covered with artificial turf to prevent pressure sores on the feet, which could lead to bumblefoot.

Most bird species can be offered food and water in plastic or stainless steel bowls; the exception are species (including parrots) that may gnaw at plastic. If fouling of the water occurs, the bowl should be washed and fresh water offered.

To provide enrichment for psittacine birds, a variety of fruits can be offered on a skewer. Smaller pet birds are usually admitted in their own cages, so may have appropriate toys such as bird mirrors, bells and ladders. Passerine birds can be provided with pieces of hollowed-out wood containing various food items such as seeds and mealworms.

Poultry and anseriforms (ducks, geese and swans) will appreciate a bed of good-quality mould-free hay. Ideally, cages of adult anseriforms should be fully waterproof and should contain as large an area of water as possible, for feeding and bathing. This can be a large cat litter tray filled with water, preferably sourced from a pond, which should be changed regularly throughout the day to prevent bacterial growth.

All adult birds can be given a bath of warm water (35–40°C) (Figure 5.6); this helps them to maintain good feather condition. Some birds may enjoy being 'misted' with water from a spray gun; the client should first be asked whether the bird is misted at home as, if not, this may be stressful.

A decision will need to be made as to whether the patient can be housed in a conventional cage or a hospital cage, or whether it requires additional heat or oxygen, in which case it would be best housed in an incubator or avian-specific hospital cage. Many of these cages are thermostatically controlled so that temperatures can be more easily managed. Humidity is much harder to regulate and may not be critical for short-stay patients. For the majority of psittacine and passerine birds, a temperature of approximately 27–30°C should be adequate.

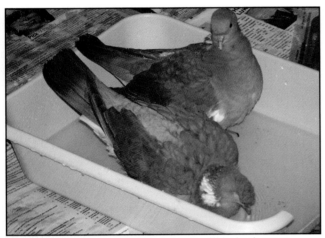

5.6 Birds appreciate a bath; it will help them to keep their feathers in good condition, as well as providing enrichment activity.

Wild birds

The housing principles given above can also be applied to wild birds. However, it is worth bearing in mind that adult wild birds will likely be too stressed in the veterinary practice to appreciate much in the way of enrichment. It is most important that they are housed somewhere quiet (preferably in a ward of their own) and away from their natural predators and referred on to a specialist centre as soon as possible. Where space is at a premium, however, the cage can be covered with a towel.

Orphans

Altricial orphaned birds (those born naked, with closed eyes and unable to ambulate) have no feathers and will therefore lose heat very quickly. They should ideally be kept in an incubator at around 25°C until fully feathered, but where this is not possible a heat pad will suffice. A 'nest' can be constructed using a woolly hat or fleece material wrapped into a ring

shape and lined with kitchen roll. If an incubator is used, a faecal sample pot containing water, with holes in the lid should be placed inside to increase the humidity. Perches are not required until about 10–14 days of age. If perches are introduced when the bird is too young, injury may result.

Precocial orphan birds (those born fully feathered with their eyes open and able to ambulate, such as ducklings, goslings and cygnets) should have a mop head suspended from the wall or ceiling of their incubator (Figure 5.7), simulating the presence of the mother, which they can huddle under.

Items of the bird's natural diet should be made available once its eyes are open. Live food should not be given and the items of food should not be so large that the bird has trouble swallowing them. This will encourage it to start picking up food for itself. Where possible, orphans of similar age and species should be housed together as this will enable them to develop much more quickly and successfully than if reared in isolation.

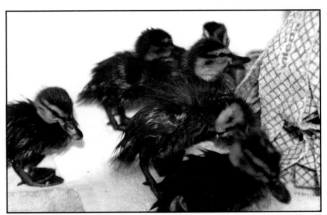

5.7 A mop head suspended from the wall or ceiling of the incubator simulates the presence of the ducklings' mother. (Courtesy of the Wildlife Aid Foundation)

Reptiles and amphibians

All reptile species should be housed in a vivarium, with a heat lamp and UV lamp overhead (see Figure 5.1). If a purpose-built vivarium is not available, a makeshift one can be constructed using a plastic tank covered with wire mesh, with a heat lamp and UV lamp suspended above and, where appropriate, a heat mat placed underneath. Furniture in the vivarium should reflect the habitat of the particular species and should be disposed of when the patient is discharged.

- Desert, terrestrial species such as the bearded dragon should have cardboard boxes arranged to resemble large flat rocks, so that they can climb and bask on the surfaces or shelter beneath them.
- Tropical, arboreal species such as the green iguana and pythons should have plastic tubes or cardboard rolls arranged to mimic branches for climbing. These must be strong enough to support the weight of the reptile. It may be necessary to cover the plastic tubes/cardboard rolls with tea-towels, to provide a surface that can be gripped.

- Semi-aquatic species (such as the red-eared terrapin) and amphibians should have a litter tray or plastic tank incorporated into the vivarium, containing aged water (tap water that has been allowed to stand for 24 hours to allow chlorine to escape and the temperature to equilibrate to that of the environment) and stones or rocks arranged to allow the animal to climb in and out of the water with ease. Amphibians should also be provided with a damp environment, which can be achieved by using peat or sphagnum moss as the substrate for the tank or vivarium.

Newspaper is the most hygienic lining for a vivarium. Sand should be avoided, as this may be consumed and could potentially lead to intestinal impaction.

Tortoises and iguanas like to bathe and this encourages defecation, urination and drinking, as well as absorption of water via the cloaca. Where possible, iguanas should be offered a bath deep enough to swim in. Fresh aged water should be offered daily for bathing, and should also be changed throughout the day if it is fouled.

A separate feeding tank for semi-aquatic reptiles and amphibians should be used, as the food will contaminate the water, encouraging bacterial growth. This water should be aged or, if ageing is not a viable option in practice due to pressure on space, the temperature can be equilibrated by adding warm water and the water can then be dechlorinated using a proprietary aquarium water conditioner.

Chameleons and many other reptiles tend to consume water by licking water droplets; for these species, the vivarium should either be misted or a 'dripper' set up (using a used fluid therapy giving set), to provide a constant dripping supply of water.

It is important to have some knowledge of the individual temperature and humidity requirements of the reptile species that may be hospitalized (Figure 5.8). If more unusual species are presented then the owners may be able to provide husbandry details. If not, useful websites include the Tortoise Trust (www. tortoisetrust.org), Melissa Kaplan's website for iguana care (www.anapsid.org) and the Exotic DVM website (www.exoticdvm.com). More information is also provided in Chapter 4.

Correct temperatures should be fairly easy to achieve using heat mats (Figure 5.9), heat lamps and thermostats (see Chapter 4).

Most snake species do not require UV light; it is of most importance to lizards and tortoises. However, provision of UV light is not essential for healthy reptiles that are undergoing elective procedures. UV lights should be replaced on a regular basis or the lights should be tested to assess their UV output. Most lights degrade with time and need to be replaced every 6–9 months. Further advice may be obtained from www.uvguide.co.uk.

Daylength should mimic that of the wild situation and can be controlled using light bulbs, UV lamps or room lights. If uncertain, a daylength of approximately 12 hours should be provided. It is important to provide hides, especially for nocturnal species such as the leopard gecko.

Species	POTR (°C)	Relative humidity (%)	Requires UV light?
Green iguana	25–35	75–100	Yes
Bearded dragon	25–35 (basking area 38–42)	30–40	Yes
Leopard gecko	25–30	30–40	No
Asian water dragon	24–30	80–90	Yes
Savannah monitor	26–38	20–50	Yes
Veiled chameleon	21–38	75–80	Yes
Cornsnake	25–30	30–70	No
Common boa	28–30	50–80	No
Royal python	25–30	50–80	No
Burmese python	25–30	50–80	No
Mediterranean spur-thighed and Hermann's tortoises	20–28	30–50	Yes
African spurred and leopard tortoises	25–35	40–75	Yes
Red-footed tortoise	21–27	50–60	Yes
Yellow-footed tortoise	25–27	75–80	Yes
Red-eared terrapin	20–24	60–90	Yes

5.8 Temperature, humidity and UV light requirements of the reptile species seen on a regular basis by the average small animal practice. POTR = preferred optimum temperature range.

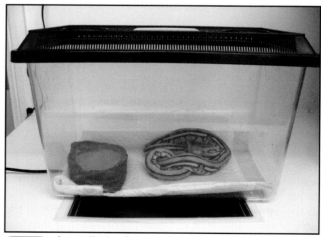

5.9 A small plastic container placed on a heat mat can be used for temporary housing of small reptiles.

Humidity may be more difficult to fine tune at short notice, but the use of large water bowls and misting with a spray bottle may help to raise the humidity and create a suitable environment for those species that require a higher level.

Nutritional requirements

This section is concerned with meeting the nutritional requirements of *hospitalized* exotic and wildlife patients that are able and willing to feed themselves, as well as the requirements of orphaned animals. Supportive feeding for sick and convalescing species is covered in Chapter 6. See also Chapters 2, 3 and 4.

It is advisable for the practice to possess a small selection of the foodstuffs of the more commonly seen exotic pet and wildlife species. Day-old chicks and mice are purchased frozen and are very cheap, so can be stored for some time in the freezer. Live foods such as maggots and mealworms are more expensive and have a shorter shelf-life; however, in practices where a lot of exotic species are being seen regularly, a small supply should be considered, which can be stored in the refrigerator. Alternatively, many owners will be prepared to bring food in for their pets.

All dried food should be kept in airtight containers in a cool dry place, and fresh fruit and vegetables should be kept in a refrigerator. Day-old chicks and mice should be kept in a freezer and defrosted on demand (see Chapter 4).

Mammals

Small mammals have a rapid metabolic rate and so tend to eat continuously while awake. It is therefore essential that fresh food and water are always available. Both water bowls and bottles should be offered, to cater for differing preferences. Bowls should be heavy enough to resist tipping and the sippers of water bottles should be cleaned and checked for patency daily. Very small mammals, such as mice, shrews and bats, should have a piece of tissue saturated with water to serve as a source of water, as this will guard against accidental drowning.

Figure 5.10 summarizes the natural diet of small mammals and suitable hospital alternatives that may be offered. It is not an exhaustive list but is designed for use in an emergency.

Rabbits and guinea pigs

Rabbits and guinea pigs should be offered only a small amount of species-specific complete pellet (approximately 1 tablespoon), with the majority of their diet being a mixture of good quality hay (e.g. Timothy), fresh grass and dandelions, plus a mixture of fresh green leafy vegetables, such as cabbage, broccoli, carrot, kale and spring greens.

Guinea pigs digest fibre more efficiently than rabbits and so require less hay; it is therefore more important that this species consumes pellets. Guinea pig pelleted foods are supplemented with vitamin C and so should be stored in cool, dry, airtight containers and used quickly, as the vitamin levels will rapidly decrease. As vitamin C is a water-soluble vitamin and excess is excreted in the urine, it is advisable to give all guinea pigs a vitamin C supplement, even if they receive a complete pelleted diet. Guinea pigs should receive the vitamin C (ascorbic acid) supplement at a rate of 10 mg/kg/day (20–30 mg/kg/day for pregnant females). This can be added to the water, but it breaks down very quickly (a new solution must be mixed daily) and will also react with stainless steel water bowls and bottles; it is therefore preferable to administer the tablet directly.

Grass clippings should not be offered to rabbits or guinea pigs as they start fermenting, causing gastrointestinal upset. Food should be offered at room temperature and checked for signs of mould before feeding.

Mice, rats, hamsters and gerbils

Mice, rats, hamsters and gerbils have similar nutritional requirements. They should be offered species-specific pelleted food in hospital, as offering commercial seed mixes leads to selective feeding.

Species	Natural diet	Hospital alternatives	Orphan feeding
Rabbits and guinea pigs	Mainly grasses but also crops, some flowers, bark, some seeds and grains	Primarily hay, grass, leafy green vegetables plus a small amount of complete pelleted food. Guinea pigs should also be given a daily dose of vitamin C (10 mg/kg)	Rabbits: As for wild rabbits and hares (see below). Hay from 3 weeks, then solid food introduced. Fully weaned at 6–7 weeks Guinea pigs: Eating solids from day 3. Between 12 hours and 3 days, milk replacer (e.g. Esbilac) at 2-hourly intervals initially, gradually reducing frequency as solids introduced. Fully weaned at 3 weeks
Rats, mice, hamsters and gerbils	Grains, plant seeds, plant parts, worms, snails and insects	Commercial pelleted complete food (preferable) or commercial seed mix, vegetables, fruit, insectivorous bird food	As for wild mice and voles (see below). Fully weaned at 3–4 weeks
Chinchillas and degus	Grasses and bushes (bark, leaves and fruit)	Grass-based chinchilla pellets and hay	Milk replacer (e.g. Esbilac) at 2-hourly intervals initially, introducing solids from 10 days. At this time, a probiotic and vitamin supplement can be added to the milk. Fully weaned at 7–8 weeks
Ferrets	Fresh whole rodent and rabbit	Day-old chicks, dry kitten food (can be moistened) but preferably dry complete pelleted diet	Milk replacer (e.g. Esbilac) at 2-hourly intervals initially, reducing to 3–4 times daily by 3 weeks. Weaned from 5 weeks, once eating solids in sufficient amounts
Wild mammals			
Foxes	Small mammals, earthworms, birds	Dog/cat food, day-old chicks, mice	Goat's milk or milk replacer (e.g. Esbilac) 4–5 feeds daily. Wean on to dog food, mice and day-old chicks

5.10   Diets of various commonly seen mammals and suitable hospital alternatives. (continues)   ▶

Species	Natural diet	Hospital alternatives	Orphan feeding
Wild mammals (continued)			
Badgers	Earthworms, slugs, snails, carrion, vegetation	Earthworms, day-old chicks, mice	Goat's milk or milk replacer (e.g. Esbilac) 4–5 times daily. Wean on to dog food, mice, day-old chicks and earthworms
Hedgehogs	Earthworms, slugs and snails	Non-fish dog/cat food, chopped day-old chick, mealworms	Milk replacer (e.g. Esbilac) 4–5 times daily. Wean on to puppy/kitten food (covered with a cat milk substitute, e.g. Cimicat)
Squirrels	Nuts, acorns	Muesli, rabbit mix, chopped fresh and dried fruit	Goat's milk or milk replacer (e.g. Esbilac) 4–5 times daily. Wean on to a variety of muesli, rabbit mix, chopped fresh and dried fruit
Rabbits and hares	Grass, hay, dandelions	Grass, hay, dandelions	Milk replacer (e.g. Esbilac), twice daily (morning and evening). Wean on to dandelions and clover
Stoats and weasels	Mice, voles, rabbits	Dead mice	Goat's milk or milk replacer (e.g. Esbilac), 4–5 times daily. Wean on to chopped mice
Mice and voles	Mice: Berries, shoots, (various depending on species) Voles: Vegetation	Mice: Digestive biscuit crumbs, fruit, table scraps Voles: Dandelions	Milk replacer (e.g. Esbilac), hourly during daylight hours, at 2-hourly intervals during the night. Wean on to crumbled digestive biscuits for mice or dandelions for voles
Water vole	Vegetation	Leafy twigs, buds, hay, grass, leafy green vegetables	Milk replacer (e.g. Esbilac), hourly during daylight hours, at 2-hourly intervals during the night. Wean on to dandelions
Shrews	Insects and larvae	Insectivorous bird mix with maggots and mini-mealworms or waxworms	Milk replacer (e.g. Esbilac) offered on a paintbrush, hourly during the day, at 2-hourly intervals overnight. Wean on to mini-mealworms and maggots
Bats	Insects on the wing	Decapitated mealworms, innards squeezed into bat's mouth. If old enough, well enough and no open wounds, leave bowl of whole live mealworms in cage	Milk replacer (e.g. Esbilac), at 2-hourly intervals over a 16-hour period, using a bat pipette or paintbrush. Wean on to mini-mealworms

5.10   (continued) Diets of various commonly seen mammals and suitable hospital alternatives.

Feeding can be supplemented with vegetables such as broccoli, cabbage, kale, carrots, etc., and fruit such as apples and pears, as well as insectivorous bird mixes.

Chinchillas and degus

Chinchillas are best fed on chinchilla pellets, along with a plentiful supply of good quality hay. Raisins are a favourite of chinchillas and are ideal for use when giving medication orally, but should be limited to a maximum of two per day. Additional supplementation with fresh vegetables and fruit, such as celery, carrots, apple and cranberries, should be no more than twice weekly, with only very small amounts offered.

Degus can be fed chinchilla pellets or a 50:50 mixture of chinchilla and guinea pig pellets (which should be molasses-free). They should have good quality hay available at all times, which must be mould-free and must have been stored in a cool, dry place.

Ferrets

Ferrets are obligate carnivores and it is essential that their diet contains animal protein. A number of proprietary complete foods are available and this is the diet of choice. Where this is not possible, dry kitten food may be offered, moistened if necessary. Day-old chicks may also be fed whole, but this diet is messy and will not contain the full range of vitamins and minerals provided by a complete food.

Water bowls will require frequent cleaning and replenishing, as ferrets tend to play in their water.

Wild mammals

- Foxes and badgers can be fed whole day-old chicks, mice and worms twice daily. Foxes may also be offered tinned dog food.
- Hedgehogs can be offered tinned dog food, although this should be of a non-fish variety.
- Other carnivorous mammals such as stoats and weasels do well with mice and day-old chicks.
- Very small mammals such as mice, shrews and bats have high metabolic rates and should have food and water available at all times, to facilitate *ad libitum* feeding; fresh food should be provided at least once daily and refreshed if fouled, or if all has been consumed.
- Wild mice will generally make use of any food offered to them, from biscuit crumbs to fruit.
- Voles and other herbivorous wild mammals should be offered hay, grass, dandelions and leafy green vegetables.
- Shrews are insectivorous, so can be offered insectivorous bird mix, along with small mealworms, waxworms and maggots.

- Squirrels can be offered a proprietary rabbit mix or muesli (preferably with no added sugar), along with chopped fresh fruit, such as apples and, if available, acorns.
- Debilitated bats can be offered the innards of a decapitated mealworm, squeezed directly into their mouths, or can be offered whole mealworms using tweezers. Eventually, it may be possible to leave a bowl of whole live mealworms, but this must not be done in situations where the bat has an open wound, is very sick or very young, as the mealworms may attempt to feed on the bat. Keeping a bat warm during feeding facilitates digestion.

Orphans

Guidelines for suitable milk substitutes and the frequency and delivery of feeds for the various different species are given in Figure 5.10.

The first feed for any orphaned mammal should be a suitable electrolyte solution. As the patient is likely to be somewhat dehydrated on admission, an electrolyte solution will help to replenish fluid and electrolyte losses. It will also give the patient a chance to get used to feeding from a teat; aspirating some electrolyte solution is much less likely to do any harm than aspirating milk.

The type of vessel used for feeding the patient should be determined by their size; puppy and kitten bottles are suitable for large mammals such as foxes, badgers and deer; 1 ml syringes with a soft teat on the end are more suitable for rabbits, guinea pigs, rats, ferrets, chinchillas, degus, squirrels, hedgehogs and stoats. Very tiny mammals such as mice, voles, weasels, shrews and bats should be offered milk on a paintbrush or with a bat pipette or a small intravenous catheter attached to a syringe.

Hygiene is of utmost importance when feeding young mammals. The same bottle/syringe/brush and teat should be used for the same patient and between feeds, after rinsing, should be stored in a baby feed bottle disinfectant.

Milk should be freshly made up and should be warm to the touch when it is fed; not only does this aid digestion, but some patients will refuse milk that is offered at the incorrect temperature. This means that reheating may be necessary during the feed; it is preferable to do this by placing the milk in warm water but a microwave may be used, taking care to ensure there are no hotspots.

Toileting should be undertaken both before and after feeding: the anogenital region should be gently dabbed with dampened cotton wool until urine/faeces have finished passing.

Birds

The potential variety of birds presenting at a veterinary practice is vast and so are their nutritional requirements. Figure 5.11 summarizes the dietary requirements of the species most likely to be presented at the practice. It is impractical to provide a diet identical to the natural diet of each species; suitable alternatives have therefore been listed and, if these are not already kept in the practice, a local supplier should be identified so that food can be purchased as needed.

Psittacine and passerine birds

Large parrots should preferably be fed a complete pelleted diet, supplemented with fruit and vegetables. The complete pellet should comprise at least 50% of the daily diet. If birds are not fed a complete pellet at home, there may be some difficulty weaning them off a commercial seed mix (see Chapter 3). If birds refuse to eat a complete pellet, they should be offered the diet they are familiar with, along with fruit and vegetables.

Small psittacine birds and granivorous passerine birds should preferably be fed as for parrots, although feeding a good quality seed mix in these species does not appear to have such a detrimental effect on their health. They should also be offered fresh leafy green vegetables.

Budgerigars frequently suffer from iodine deficiency. If the diet provided does not contain an iodine supplement, commercial iodine blocks should be provided.

Species	Examples	Natural diet	Hospital alternatives	Orphan feeding
Parrots	African grey, Amazon, cockatoo, parakeet	Fruit, pollen, nectar, some seeds, some insects	Commercial seed mixes or complete pellets, leafy green vegetables	Granivorous bird rearing mix, e.g. Tropican or Kaytee Exact (species specific formulas are available), Harrison's Juvenile and Neonate formulas
Escaped parakeets	Ring-necked parakeet	Seed, fruit	Parrot mix	Granivorous bird rearing mix, e.g. Tropican, Kaytee Exact or Harrison's Neonate or Juvenile Formulas
Small psittacine and passerine birds	Budgerigar, cockatiel, canary	Fruit, vegetables, seeds, insects	Commercial seed mixes or complete pellets, leafy green vegetables	Granivorous or insectivorous bird rearing mix, depending on species, e.g. Tropican, Kaytee Exact or Harrison's Juvenile Formula
Finches and sparrows	Greenfinch, goldfinch, bullfinch, tree sparrow, house sparrow, starling	Insects, larvae, grains and seeds	Wild bird seed, chopped/live maggots	As for insectivorous garden birds above, but add in some good quality seed mix or preferably insectivorous bird rearing mix, e.g. Harrison's Recovery or Neonate Formulas, at 1–2-hourly intervals (half-hourly for birds less than 5 days old)

5.11 Diets of various commonly seen birds and suitable hospital alternatives. (continues) ▶

Species	Examples	Natural diet	Hospital alternatives	Orphan feeding
Insectivorous garden birds	Blackbird, thrush, robin, dunnock, tits, wren, goldcrest	Earthworms, insects, larvae	Chopped/live maggots, mealworms, earthworms	As for corvids below, but for the smaller species, leave out the cat food and ensure maggots and mealworms are finely chopped, or preferably insectivorous bird rearing mix, e.g. Harrison's Recovery or Neonate Formulas, at 1–2-hourly intervals (half-hourly for birds less than 5 days old)). Syringe a small amount into the bird's mouth and allow it to swallow
Corvids	Magpie, jay, crow, jackdaw, rook	'Roadkill', baby birds, small mammals, eggs	Chopped day-old chicks, cat/dog food, insectivore mix	Mashed cat food mixed with chopped maggots/mealworms and insectivore mix via tweezers/spoon/paintbrush, on gaping, at 2–3-hourly intervals
Woodpeckers	Green woodpecker, greater spotted woodpecker, lesser spotted woodpecker	Insects, insect larvae, other arthropods, fruit, tree sap	Mealworms	Mealworms with heads removed. If refuse to gape, crop-feed mashed cat food or preferably insectivorous bird rearing mix, e.g. Harrison's Recovery or Neonate Formulas, at 4-hourly intervals. Amounts determined by size of crop and crop-emptying time
Hirundines	Swift, swallow	Insects	Waxworms	Chopped waxworms, mealworms or maggots if gaping, offered on paintbrush, otherwise, crop-feed insectivorous bird rearing mix, e.g. Harrison's Recovery or Neonate Formulas, at 4-hourly intervals
Hawks	Sparrowhawk, goshawk	Small garden birds	Day-old chicks	Chopped day-old chicks, at 3–4-hourly intervals initially
Falcons	Kestrel, peregrine falcon	Small mammals. Large falcons will hunt pigeons	Dead mice, dead pigeons, day-old chicks	Chopped dead mice, pigeons and day-old chicks, at 3–4-hourly intervals initially
Owls	Barn, tawny, short-eared, long-eared and little owls	Mice, voles, shrews	Dead mice	Chopped dead mice, at 3–4-hourly intervals initially
Gulls	Herring gull, blackcap gull, kittiwake	Various sea fish	Whitebait with thiamine supplement	Hand-feed whitebait, fed head first
Swans, geese and ducks	Mute swan, Canada goose, mallard duck	Insects, snails and water plants, seeds, roots	Mixed corn, chick crumbs and a litter tray of water for dabbling, wholemeal bread (last resort)	As for adults; feed independently
Herons and egrets	Grey heron, egret	Freshwater fish, water voles	Whitebait with thiamine supplement	Hand-feed whitebait, fed head first
Moorhens and coots	Moorhen, coot	Small freshwater fish, leaves, berries, snails	Maggots, whitebait with thiamine supplement	Chopped maggots and small pieces of whitebait offered on tweezers
Kingfishers	Kingfisher	Small freshwater fish and aquatic insects	Whitebait with thiamine supplement	Hand-feed whitebait, fed head first
Columbiformes (pigeons and doves)	Woodpigeon, stock dove, rock dove, feral pigeon, collared dove, turtle dove	Grains, seeds, leafy green vegetables, elderberries	Wild bird seed, mixed corn, chick crumbs, broccoli	Granivorous bird rearing mix, e.g. Tropican or Kaytee Exact, at 2-hourly intervals when very young (less than 5 days old), 4–6-hourly when older (five days to three or four weeks). Amounts will vary between less than 1 ml to up to 20 ml per feed depending on age and size; size of crop and crop-emptying time should guide amounts offered
Poultry, peafowl and other gamebirds	Chicken, bantam, pheasant	Corn, seeds, vegetation, insects (small reptiles and amphibians, in the case of peafowl)	Chick crumbs, mixed corn	Chick crumbs

5.11 (continued) Diets of various commonly seen birds and suitable hospital alternatives.

For the majority of granivorous garden birds, a good quality wild bird seed mix (BTO or BSA accredited) should suffice for a few days. It is important that the seed is stored in a cool, dry, airtight container and discarded after a period of 3 months, to prevent fungal growth. Fresh seed should be offered daily and any uneaten food discarded.

Insectivorous species should be offered a soft-bill mix containing dried insects, mealworms, dried fruit and seed. These are often advertised as 'robin mix' and suchlike, and are commercially available from wild bird food retailers and garden centres. Live foods such as earthworms, mealworms and maggots can be offered where possible. Species such as woodpeckers and swifts are notoriously difficult to feed in captivity and appear to prefer live mealworms and waxworm larvae, respectively. These can be purchased either through wild bird food retailers or from shops selling supplies for reptile keepers.

Both granivorous and insectivorous birds may appreciate the addition of suitable fruit and vegetables to their diet, such as leafy green vegetables (e.g. kale, cabbage and broccoli), peas, elderberries, pyracantha berries, etc.

Corvid species such as jays, jackdaws and crows can be offered wet cat or dog food, but if their stay in hospital is to amount to a few days, they should be offered chopped day-old chicks and/or mice. Contrary to what was believed in the past, the yolk-sacs of day-old chicks need not be removed, as the Ca:P ratio is good.

Day-old chicks should also be the food of choice for hospitalized birds of prey (although they should be de-yolked if fed to merlins). Prime cuts of meat are unsuitable, as they do not provide the wide range of nutrients that can be found in an entire carcass. Whole carcasses promote good gastrointestinal health due to the mechanical effects of fur and feathers on the proventriculus and crop. Uneaten food should be removed after a few hours.

Fresh drinking water should be available at all times, although insectivorous and carnivorous birds are likely to consume far less water than granivores, due to the higher water content of their diet.

It is also necessary to provide a vitamin and mineral supplement to birds that are hospitalized indoors. Calcium metabolism is regulated by vitamin D3 and many birds produce a precursor to this vitamin (provitamin D3) in their preen gland. They spread this precursor across their feathers during preening and it is activated to previtamin D3 by the action of UV light. It is then ingested, where it is metabolized by the liver and kidneys, producing vitamin D3, which regulates the absorption of calcium. If birds do not have access to unfiltered UV light, the result can be hypocalcaemia. Suitable daily supplements are available that include vitamin D3 as well as other essential vitamins and minerals (e.g. Avimix and Nutrobal, Vetark), and these should be thoroughly mixed into the food offered.

Providing fine oyster shell grit for each patient not only offers another source of dietary calcium but also aids the grinding of food in the gizzard.

Waterfowl

Ducks, geese and swans are occasionally brought into the practice. They will usually take chick grower pellets soaked in water, ideally sourced from a pond. A litter tray of water should be made available for 'dabbling'. Wild waterfowl may be less likely to consume commercial pelleted food and in some cases, particularly where they are brought in from an area frequented by people feeding them, it may be necessary to offer wholemeal bread, although fresh vegetable scraps and seeds are preferable.

Adult gulls, herons, egrets, moorhens, coots and kingfishers can all be offered whitebait in a bowl of water. It is imperative that a vitamin B7 (thiamine) supplement is added, such as Fish Eaters Tablets (Mazuri Zoo Foods).

Orphans

During the spring and summer months, a wide variety of wild orphaned birds may be presented to veterinary practices. Their nutritional requirements are wide-ranging and it is important that the correct diet is offered. Suggested diets are given in Figure 5.11 for a range of different species. If complete commercial formulas are not being used, vitamin and mineral supplementation should be included in the first meal of the day.

Where crop feeding is being used, care should be taken to ensure that the crop is empty before feeding. The crop should not be filled to capacity and the amount of food given will depend on the species and age of the patient. The process should be carried out slowly, to ensure that food does not come back up the oesophagus, which could result in aspiration, leading to pneumonia.

Frequency of feeding is also age- and species-dependent; however, as a general rule, nestling and fledgling birds will gape until they have consumed enough food and they will begin to chirp when they are hungry. Fresh food should be offered at room temperature and, if using formula food, this should be lukewarm.

Reptiles

Reptiles inhabit a variety of extreme climates and have evolved to feed on the organisms most accessible to them in their environment. They can be divided into herbivores, insectivores, carnivores and omnivores. Their nutritional requirements are summarized in Figure 5.12.

All reptiles require fresh water daily, preferably in a container that is large enough for them to bathe in. Species from sub-tropical regions are more accustomed to licking droplets of water rather than drinking; the vivarium should therefore be misted until droplets form on cage furniture. Water should be aged by leaving it to stand for 24 hours before introducing it to the reptiles; this allows potentially harmful chlorine to escape and the temperature of the water to increase to that of the environment. It is imperative that this is done in the case of aquatic reptiles, such as turtles.

Of the carnivorous reptiles, the majority are snakes. They will eat whole mammalian, amphibian

Dietary group	Examples	Natural diet	Hospital alternatives
Herbivores	Tortoises, iguanas	Vegetation	Dandelions, green leafy vegetables (kale, cabbage, watercress etc), herbs, sweet pepper. Offer fresh food at least daily
Insectivores	Leopard gecko, slowworm, common lizard, chameleon, Chinese water dragon	Various insects, arachnids and molluscs	Locusts, crickets, mealworms, grasshoppers, maggots, waxworm larvae. For slowworms: small grey slugs. Offer food at least daily
Small and medium carnivores	Cornsnake, grass snake, adder, king snake, monitor lizard	Small mammals	Mice (move around on end of stick to simulate live prey; can warm slightly and cut open to release blood scent)
Large carnivores	Pythons, boas	Larger mammals	Rats, rabbits (but only if long-stay, as feed once every 3–4 weeks)
Omnivores	Bearded dragon, box turtle	Vegetation and various insects, molluscs and arachnids. The bearded dragon is predominantly insectivorous initially, but becomes progressively herbivorous with age	Mealworms, maggots, crickets, earthworms, along with fruit and vegetables. Bearded dragons: vegetables daily and insects 2–3 times weekly. Aquatic species: pondfish pellets, bloodworms, *Tubifex* worms, vegetables. Offer fresh food at least daily

5.12   Diets of various commonly seen reptiles and suitable hospital alternatives.

and avian prey. Day-old chicks, rats and mice should suffice during a hospital stay. It is not necessary to provide additional supplements if whole prey is being fed. The width of the prey should be no greater than the width of the central section of the snake or, in the case of carnivorous lizards, half the width of the head. Frequency of feeding is dependent on age and size, varying from every 3 days for young carnivorous lizards, to every 3 or 4 weeks for large snakes. If the food is not consumed within a few hours, it should be removed, discarded and a new food item offered later. Commercial dog, cat and primate diets are unsuitable for reptiles due to their high protein and vitamin D levels.

Insectivorous, omnivorous and herbivorous species require calcium/vitamin D3 supplementation. The food should be dusted with an appropriate powder supplement, such as Nutrobal (Vetark), prior to feeding. In the case of feeding live food, dusting should take place immediately before the food is offered; otherwise much of it will fall off the prey as they move about. Alternatively, live food can be 'gut loaded' with calcium and vitamin D3 by feeding the prey supplemented food, using a feed additive such as Bug Grub (Vetark), for a number of days prior to feeding.

Suitable food for insectivorous and omnivorous species includes crickets, locusts, mealworms, silkworms and waxworm larvae.

Appropriate fruit and vegetables for lizards such as bearded dragons include peppers, salad leaves, broccoli, kale, bok choy (Chinese cabbage) and spring greens. Food for juveniles should be finely chopped. The mix of fruit and vegetables should be such that they provide the correct calcium to phosphorus ratio for each species but this is beyond the scope of this chapter and, for the majority of short-stay hospitalized reptiles, is probably not of great concern.

Amphibians

Suggestions for feeding amphibians in hospital are given in Figure 5.13. Small amphibians are

insectivorous and will target prey moving across their field of vision, so it is important that live food is offered, as most amphibians will ignore dead prey. Amphibians must have their food supplemented by dusting it with a calcium/vitamin D3 supplement.

In their natural environment, most species would be consuming small numbers of insects frequently while awake. It is unlikely that this is possible in a hospital environment, so it is necessary to offer larger prey than would perhaps normally be consumed in the wild.

Examples	Natural diet	Hospital alternatives
Common frog and toad, poison arrow frog, palmate newt, great crested newt, smooth newt	Insects, slugs, snails, woodlice	Live insects or insect larvae

5.13   Diets of amphibians and hospital alternatives.

Daily hospital routines

When looking after any animal in a hospital environment, it is important to develop a routine of inpatient care so that all the necessary checks are carried out. The inpatient checks suggested are a general overview, suitable for most inpatients. Depending on the species in question and the medical condition concerned, some of these may not be as necessary as others, and other checks may be more important to their nursing care.

As exotic species can be very different from cats and dogs in many ways, it is important to have some understanding of what is 'normal' for them. Any changes in behaviour, feeding habits, urine/faecal output, etc., should be recorded (Figure 5.14).

Record-keeping	It is important to keep detailed records for all patients in the hospital, so it is clear to see what treatments and medications have been given and what still needs to be done each day. Careful monitoring and record-keeping is vital, as much can be told from slight changes in behaviour, urine and faecal output and feeding habits
Handling	Try to keep handling to a minimum as most exotic species are prone to stress, especially when in an unfamiliar environment. Many will not be accustomed to handling on a daily basis, and doing so can cause further stress. To reduce handling time, ensure you prepare all equipment needed and any medications that are due before you take the animal from its enclosure. Ensure you have enough people to handle the animal and carry out the necessary checks and procedures. Some animals may be difficult to handle or, in the case of the larger snakes and lizards, may require two or more handlers for health and safety reasons
Treatments and medications	Try to time treatments and medications with any procedures due. If the animal requires a sedation or general anaesthetic during the day, it may be sensible to use this time to examine them thoroughly, clean their enclosure, perform follow-up radiographs and scans, obtain blood samples and administer any injections that may be needed. It is also useful to work as a team so that one person can check the animal over and give medications, whilst another is checking the enclosure, cleaning it and replacing food and water
Infectious patients	Always be sure to treat and clean any infectious patients last or, when possible, have one nurse designated exclusively to working with them to prevent cross-contamination. Any infectious patients should be kept separate from others when possible and any food bowls, bedding, cage furniture and feeding tubes used for them should be carefully labelled and kept exclusively for use by that patient

5.14 Some basic rules that should be considered when nursing exotic species.

General routines

- General ward inspection – All animals should be inspected in a brief tour of the ward. This is to check for any urgent cases that may need immediate attention, and to allow for prioritization of those that need more care.
- Weighing and recording weight – Any increase or decrease should be noted. Weighing should be done on scales appropriate to the size of the animal. Small species such as birds, mice, rats and geckos should be weighed using scales that read to the nearest one-tenth of a gram, as drug doses and feeding rates can change in animals of this size if a very slight weight change occurs. It is usually easiest to weigh small animals by placing them in a small container or box (Figure 5.15). Larger birds and reptiles can be placed in a box or cat carrier to be weighed. Traditional practice scales used to weigh dogs and cats that measure to the nearest 100 g can be used for rabbits, as well as for larger tortoises and lizards. Animals should be weighed at the same time each day before feeding, as bodyweight will fluctuate during the day.

- Respiratory rate should be checked and recorded twice daily. If the patient has respiratory problems, it may be necessary to check more often. It is best to try and measure the respiratory rate by observing the animal carefully while it is still in its enclosure, as any handling will increase the rate. Biological data for selected species can be found in Chapters 2, 3 and 4.
- Heart rate should be checked and recorded twice daily. If the animal is hospitalized for a cardiac problem then this should be checked more frequently. For mammals and birds this can usually be carried out using just a stethoscope, but a Doppler probe (Figure 5.16) is often needed for reptiles. It may be possible to auscultate the heart by placing a damp towel over the area of the heart and using a stethoscope. Biological data for selected species can be found in Chapters 2, 3 and 4.

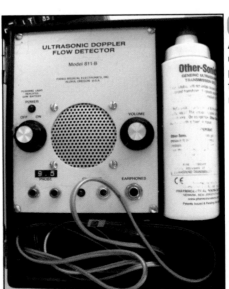

5.16 A Doppler ultrasound probe is used for monitoring reptile hearts.

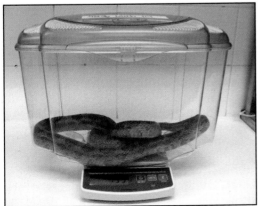

5.15 Smaller species can be weighed in a box or container, to the nearest gram.

- General demeanour – Prey species do not show many outward signs of pain or ill health; it is therefore very important to monitor them closely for any slight changes. (See Chapters 2, 3 and 4 for information on what is 'normal' for each species.)
- Wounds or dressings should be checked daily and cleaned or re-dressed as required.
- Frequency and consistency of urination and defecation should be noted. Samples can be collected if required for microscopy. This is especially important with reptiles as they may not defecate daily and it may be several days before a sample can be obtained.
- Enclosures should be checked and cleaned daily – All waste, bedding and substrate should be removed, the enclosure cleaned with a detergent and left to dry before disinfecting with a suitable disinfectant (see later).
- Any uneaten food should be removed.
- Suitable fresh food and a water source must be provided. The hospital chart should be used to record any food that is given, at what time and how much of it remains, so that even if the patient eats only a small amount, this can be monitored.
- Check patency and flush any intravenous catheters in place – Catheters should be flushed using heparinized saline (unless contraindicated), and re-dressed daily. Sutures holding catheters in place should be checked to ensure they are still in place, and are not too tight.
- Any signs of pain or discomfort must be noted.
- Fluid therapy should be given as directed – This may be intravenous, oral, subcutaneous or intraperitoneal.
- Medications should be administered as directed, with an aim always to give them at the exact time they are due. All medications given and the time of administration should be recorded. If medications are given in food, checks should always be made that the food has been consumed.
- Assisted feeding should take place if necessary.
  - Rabbits, chinchillas and guinea pigs can be syringe-fed fairly easily with a proprietary product.
  - Birds can be crop-tubed using a crop tube of appropriate size.
  - Reptiles can be stomach-tubed using a dosing catheter of appropriate size.
  - See Chapter 6 for feeding methods and more detail on foods available for assisted feeding.

Species-specific routines

Small mammals

Rabbits and guinea pigs

- Daily exercise should be allowed if possible, preferably in a suitable run or in a confined area of the practice. This gives the animals an opportunity to bask in sunlight and synthesize vitamin D, as well as allowing access to grass and other plants. It also helps promote normal gut activity. As rabbits and guinea pigs are prey species, suitable hides must be made available so that animals do not feel too exposed and become too stressed.
- Rear-end checks for any soiling should take place at least twice daily. Any faecal impaction or urine scalding should be treated as necessary.

Chinchillas

- Dust baths should be provided at least twice a week, as this forms a part of a chinchilla's usual grooming routine. Commercially available chinchilla bathing dust should be used, and placed in the enclosure for 20–30 minutes at a time.

Birds

- Misting birds with a spray bottle encourages them to preen their feathers and also helps to keep their skin hydrated. Commercially available misting sprays can be used (Figure 5.17) or, alternatively, tepid, clean filtered water. Misting should be carried out using a spray bottle directed above the bird so that the spray falls like rain and is not sprayed directly at the bird. Misting should take place in the daytime and the bird should then be allowed to dry naturally.

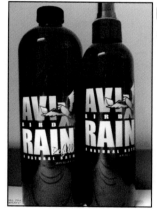

5.17   An example of a commercial misting spray for birds.

Reptiles

- The temperature and humidity of the vivarium should be checked, ensuring it is set to the correct temperature range for the particular species and that a suitable humidity is achieved. If the vivarium does not have a humidity setting, it can be altered by adding a water source to increase humidity or by misting the vivarium with water from a spray bottle.
- UV lighting should be checked, ensuring that the correct type is being used (see www.uvguide. co.uk for further advice), that it is functioning properly, and that it is being turned on for the correct number of hours each day, as this varies with species. UV lights should be replaced every 6–9 months.
- Bathing of tortoises and lizards should be carried out as required in warm water.

Cleaning and disinfection

Exotic species have the potential to spread or carry many types of bacteria and disease; good husbandry in the practice is therefore essential. It is important that a strict cleaning and disinfection protocol is put in place, and that the disinfectants used are appropriate for the type of organism involved.

When it comes to cleaning and disinfection in the wards, it is not only the kennels, cages and vivaria that must be considered; the following are equally important:

- Floors
- Scales
- Substrate
- Work surfaces
- Food and water bowls
- Perches and cage toys/furniture
- Equipment such as feeding tubes, gags and towels
- Hospital equipment such as mops, dustpans and kitchen utensils
- Surgery staff and visitors.

The spread of airborne diseases must also be considered.

General rules

Cleanliness in the hospital environment is important to prevent spread of disease from patient to patient, as well as to prevent nosocomial infections (i.e. those brought into the hospital by patients) and zoonoses.

Three basic steps are required in order for the hospital to be deemed clean:

1. Cleaning should be performed with a cleaning product, not a disinfectant. All cage furniture, bedding and food bowls should be removed from the cage, along with any organic material such as dirt, grease, urine, faeces and blood. Following this, detergent should be used to scrub the cage completely, including the ceiling and doors. Any other items such as food bowls and feeding tubes should be cleaned separately using detergent.
2. The cage and other items should then be dried, either naturally or by using clean paper towel or another appropriate drying method.
3. Once adequately dry, disinfection can begin using a suitable disinfectant.

Disinfectants are denatured by organic material and will not work without prior application of detergent and a period of drying.

Selecting an appropriate disinfectant

The products that are used in practice can be dependent on many factors. These include:

- Target organisms – The types of bacteria that are sensitive to the product
- Ease of use – Many products need to be diluted to a particular concentration
- Intended use – Some disinfectants are suitable for use in kennels, but not for items such as food bowls and bedding
- Contact time – The manufacturer's recommended contact time must always be noted. This may vary depending on the concentration of the disinfectant and the organisms involved. This is vital to the efficacy of the product
- Odour – Birds and small mammals are particularly sensitive to odorous disinfectants and these may cause respiratory problems
- Safety of staff and animals – Ideally, a product that is non-irritant, non-corrosive and non-toxic should be used. An awareness of individual sensitivities to particular products in both patients and staff is necessary.
- Availability of the product
- Economy of use – Many products can be bought in a ready-to-use solution, but this is often not the most cost-effective way to purchase or store them.

> ### Control of Substances Hazardous to Health Regulations 2002
>
> COSHH Regulations require that an assessment is carried out regarding exposure to hazardous substances, such as those in Figure 5.18. The purpose is to identify the hazards and risks and determine whether control measures are adequate.

Figure 5.18 gives some examples of the disinfectants available and their recommended uses.

Disinfectant class	Example of product	Presentation	Recommended concentration	Recommended use and information
Biguanides: Chlorhexidine	Hibiscrub (Mölnlycke)	Concentrate	Use neat or can be diluted	Good for skin and wound disinfection
Cationic surfactants: Quaternary ammonium compounds	Ark-Klens (Vetark)	Ready-to-use, concentrate	10 ml/5 litres (0.025%)	Suitable for disinfection of cages, vivaria, kennels, food and water bowls. Safe for use in incubators. Broad antibacterial activity; recommended against *Escherichia coli*, *Salmonella*, *Chlamydophila*. Virucidal against lipophilic viruses

5.18   Disinfectants and their recommended uses. (continues) ▶

Disinfectant class	Example of product	Presentation	Recommended concentration	Recommended use and information
Cationic surfactants: Quaternary ammonium compounds (continued)	F10 Biocare (Meadows Animal Healthcare)	Ready-to-use, concentrate, aerosol fogger, wipes, hand gel	Gram-positive bacteria: 1:1000 water. Gram-negative bacteria: 1:500 water. Fungi, yeast, moulds: 1:500 water. Fungal and bacterial spores: 1:250 water. Viruses: 1:500 water	Suitable for disinfection of cages, vivaria, kennels, food and water bowls. Safe for use in incubators. Proven effective at safe concentrations against all types of bacteria, viruses, fungi and spores including MRSA, avian influenza and parvovirus. Wide range of products to suit most practice needs, including single-use foggers and aerosol disinfectant
Oxidizing agents	Virkon (Alstoe)	Tablets, powder, concentrate, ready-to-use	1:100 (1% solution) with water	Broad-spectrum disinfectant. Tested and proven effective against all known viral families, most bacteria, fungi and mycoplasma
Alcohol-based	Amprotect Hand Rinse (Vetark)	Gel pump	Ready-to-use	Suitable for use before, after and between patients to prevent disease transmission. Not suitable when handling amphibians, as they can absorb chemicals through skin
Halogens and halogen-containing compounds: Iodophors	Tamodine-E (Vetark)	Concentrate	Walls, floors and surfaces: 45 ml/10 litres warm water (90 ml/10 litres for heavily soiled surfaces). Dishes, utensils and instruments: 30–45 ml/10 litres warm water. Hand dips for personnel: 15–30 ml/10 litres warm water	General purpose disinfection. For animal accommodation or dishes, rinse off before use. Has a built-in colour marker so the user can see where they have treated and also when it is washed off
Halogenated tertiary amine	Trigene (Medichem)	Ready-to-use, concentrate, wipes, hand gel	1:200 for general purpose use in intermediate-risk areas. 1:100 for high-risk areas	Suitable for disinfection of cages, vivaria, kennels, food and water bowls. Safe for use in incubators. Bactericidal, fungicidal, virucidal, mycobactericidal and sporicidal. Suitable for use on most surfaces, chairs, floors, walls and appliances
Chlorine-based	Bleach	Concentrate	Dilute to 10% solution with water	Effective against all pathogens, including bacterial spores. Highly irritant to tissues and is toxic. For use only in the environment for general disinfection. Inexpensive, but limited use

5.18 (continued) Disinfectants and their recommended uses.

Species-specific information

Small mammals

Cages for small mammals should be emptied, wiped down and cleaned at least daily. Between patients (or at least once a week) they should be fully disinfected with a suitable product. Before animals are returned to their cages, they must have completely dried and there must be no odour remaining from the disinfectant used. Small mammals are prone to respiratory problems, which can be aggravated by strong-smelling disinfectants. Any cage furniture and food bowls should be cleaned appropriately.

Birds

Many avian diseases can be spread by airborne pathogens, as well as through direct contact and contamination of the environment. As well as disinfecting the bird's cage and cage furniture, it is therefore also advised to 'fog' the environment between patients, or at least weekly, where possible. Some disinfectant products may be used in a commercially available fogging machine, or alternatively some companies produce single-use fogging canisters (see Figure 5.2). Birds should be removed from the area before fogging is carried out, and any disinfectant particles allowed to settle and dry fully, before returning them to the ward. Ideally, hospitalized birds should be kept isolated, with a separate room and airflow system per bird. However, in most practices this is simply not possible, so infection control is even more important. Owners may be asked to bring in perches, toys and food bowls from home to minimize cross-contamination. Cages should be cleaned out daily, wiped down and disinfected. Between patients (or at least once weekly) the ceilings, floors, walls and windows of the ward should be cleaned and disinfected to minimize environmental contamination.

Reptiles

Particular care should be paid to heated vivaria, as their warm and humid environment is the perfect breeding ground for bacteria such as *Aeromonas*, *Klebsiella* and *Pseudomonas*. Considering the fact that many of the patients in hospital are likely to be stressed and unwell, it only takes a small number of bacteria to lead to an overwhelming infection.

Vivaria should be wiped down and cleaned with a disinfectant such as Ark-Klens (Vetark) at least once daily. The vivarium should be stripped down completely and fully disinfected (e.g.Tamodine-E (Vetark)) between patients (or once weekly for long-term inpatients). Any substrate can harbour disease so this must be disposed of between patients to prevent spread of infection. Cage furniture and water bowls should be cleaned and disinfected in a solution such as Ark-Klens or Tamodine-E (Figure 5.18). Items should be rinsed thoroughly and allowed to dry fully before being used again.

Practice personnel and visitors

Everybody in the practice should play their part in infection control. Before and after handling patients, everyone should be washing their hands with a suitable hand-wash solution to prevent the spread of disease. Disposable gloves may also be worn as an extra measure. Disinfectant foot-baths should be placed outside the wards where any patients with infectious diseases are housed. Consideration should also be given to the use of facemasks and disposable plastic aprons.

Cleaning and disinfection of hospital equipment

Equipment such as mops, buckets and kitchen utensils are often forgotten when it comes to infection control. Although these items are usually washed out after each use, they should also be properly cleaned and disinfected weekly. Any organic material should be removed and the items then cleaned thoroughly using a suitable detergent and left to dry. They should be soaked in disinfectant, and left for the appropriate contact time according to the manufacturer's guidelines. Once soaked thoroughly, they should be rinsed in tap water and allowed to dry before storage. Manufacturer's guidelines should be noted, as some disinfectants are not suitable for use with plastic items such as mop buckets as they can cause corrosion. Extra care should be taken with items such as crop feeding tubes that have a small diameter. It is easy for these to become blocked and also to harbour bacteria. They should be cleaned carefully using a pipe-cleaner and rinsed thoroughly to ensure there is no debris left that may cause a blockage.

Precautions when using chemical disinfectants

- As with any chemicals, handle disinfectants correctly and take care to avoid any spillages.
- Always store products in their original containers.
- Wear gloves to prevent contact with skin.
- Take care to avoid any splashing of chemicals; masks and/or goggles may be worn. ▶

- Only use disinfectants for their intended purpose as recommended by the manufacturer.
- Never mix disinfectants.
- Always take care to follow guidelines and use the correct concentration of disinfectant for the organisms concerned.

Zoonoses and anthropozoonoses

Zoonoses are diseases that are transmissible from animals to humans. It is imperative that staff are constantly aware of the threat posed by zoonoses. Despite the fact that the risk appears to be relatively low, close attention should be paid to ensuring that the risk of staff or clients contracting a zoonosis is kept to a minimum. Special care should be taken with **pregnant women, young children and immune-compromised people.** The two conditions that pose the most likely risk are psittacosis in parrots and salmonellosis in reptiles.

Anthropozoonoses are diseases that may be passed from humans to animals. An example of an anthropozoonosis is human influenza, which may be passed to ferrets, causing upper respiratory disease. Clinical signs may include lethargy, inappetence, sneezing, fever, nasal discharge, epiphora and conjunctivitis. Secondary bacterial infection may lead to pneumonia in kits, which may prove fatal. Staff with influenza should be kept away from ferrets.

Zoonoses fall into one of four categories:

- Viral
- Bacterial
- Protozoal
- Parasitic.

Parasitic zoonoses include both helminth infections and fungal infections such as dermatophytosis (ringworm).

Primates are not frequently seen in private practice but do harbour a huge range of potential pathogens. Great care should be taken when dealing with these patients and it would always be appropriate to wear gloves and masks. Post-mortem examinations also pose a potential risk. The reader is urged to research this topic in more detail if primates are seen on a regular basis.

Figure 5.19 lists many of the known zoonoses of the different species that may be seen in general practice. Huge numbers of species of exotic pet are encountered in private practice and the list of possible zoonoses is extensive. The reader is encouraged to research specific conditions if the need arises.

Psittacosis

All hospitalized parrots, especially those showing respiratory, ocular or gastrointestinal symptoms, should be considered as possible carriers of psittacosis (caused by *Chlamydophila psittaci*). Wherever

Species	Viral	Bacterial	Parasitic/protozoal/fungal
Pet rabbits and rodents	Hantavirus, lymphocytic choriomeningitis (LCM) virus, monkeypox virus, reoviruses	*Bordetella bronchiseptica, Campylobacter jejuni, C. pylori, Corynebacterium kutscheri, Francisella tularensis, Leptospira* spp., *Listeria monocytogenes, Pasteurella multocida, Salmonella* spp., *Streptobacillus moniliformis* and *Spirillum minus* (rat bite fever), *Streptococcus pneumoniae, Yersinia pseudotuberculosis, Y. enterocolitica*	*Cheyletiella parasitivorax, Cryptosporidium, Encephalitozoon cuniculi, Giardia, Rodentolepis* (formerly *Hymenolepis*) spp., *Sarcoptes scabiei, Trichophyton* spp., *Trixacarus caviae*
Foxes	Lyssavirus (rabies) – not yet reported but should be considered as a possible risk for the future	*Borrelia burgdorferi* (Lyme disease transmitted by *Ixodes* ticks), *Campylobacter jejuni, Coxiella burnetti* (Q fever), *Escherichia coli, Leptospira, Mycobacterium bovis, Salmonella* spp., *Staphylococcus* spp., *Streptococcus* (from bites)	*Capillaria, Cryptosporidium, Echinococcus* (potentially), *Giardia, Leishmania* (reported in Jersey), rickettsial infections, sarcoptic mange, *Toxoplasma gondii, Trichinella spiralis, Trichophyton* spp.
Rabbits and hares		*Brucella, Escherichia coli, Francisella tularensis, Leptospira, Listeria*, pseudotuberculosis, *Salmonella*	*Giardia, Toxoplasma gondii*
Hedgehogs			Dermatophytosis (ringworm)
Bats	European bat lyssavirus (EBL 1 and 2), Western equine encepahilitis virus	*Escherichia coli, Salmonella*	*Trichophyton* spp.
Birds	Avian influenza	*Chlamydophila psittaci, Mycobacterium* spp., *Salmonella* spp., *Yersinia pseudotuberculosis, Y. enterocolitica*	*Dermanyssus gallinae*
Reptiles		*Actinobacillus* spp., *Bacteroides* spp., *Citrobacter* spp., *Clostridium* spp., *Corynebacterium* spp., *Coxiella burnetti, Edwardsiella tarda, Escherichia coli, Leptospira* spp., *Mycobacterium, Neisseria* spp., *Pasteurella* spp., *Staphylococcus* spp., *Streptococcus* spp.	Zygomycosis (*Absidia, Cunninghamella, Mucor, Rhizomucor, Rhizopus*)

5.19   Zoonotic infections in commonly encountered species.

possible, they should be housed in isolation and barrier nursed. It is wise to test all sick psittacine birds for psittacosis. All parrots should be considered as potentially contagious.

Salmonellosis

All reptiles should be considered potential carriers of *Salmonella*. Great attention should therefore be paid to careful and thorough cleaning of vivaria with suitable disinfectants (see later). Faecal material and bedding should be carefully disposed of and staff should be encouraged to wash their hands thoroughly after working with reptiles. Work surfaces should also be thoroughly cleaned. Food and water bowls and other furniture should not be kept in sinks that are used to wash crockery and cutlery used by staff. One should also be aware of the possibility of passing on infections to dogs and cats if communal washing facilities are used. Care should be taken when using computers, as pathogens may be harboured on keyboards if hands are not carefully washed after handling patients. Consideration should also be given to ensuring that infections are not transferred to other work surfaces, pens, nail clippers, towels and other items used in a consulting room or hospital setting.

Encephalitozoon cuniculi

This is a potential zoonosis that is commonly encountered in pet rabbits in general practice. It may cause renal failure in immune-compromised humans, although this is rarely reported. It may still be worth mentioning *Encephalitozoon cuniculi* to clients, as people undergoing chemotherapy or who have had organ transplants may be especially at risk. People that are HIV-positive would also be considered an 'at risk' group, as well as those receiving immunosuppressive treatment for autoimmune conditions such as pemphigus.

Rabies

Bats pose a risk of transmitting rabies and great care should be taken when handling these patients. Fatalities have been reported following bat bites. Further information may be sought in the *BSAVA Manual of Wildlife Casualties*.

Other aspects of health and safety

Because of the nature of work in a veterinary practice, staff, visitors and patients are exposed to many potential hazards on a daily basis. When it comes to exotic species, there are the obvious dangers of aggressive animals that may try to bite, scratch, strangle or sting, but the less obvious dangers must also not be forgotten, such as the larger lizards that may whip with their tails, spiders that may shed hair that can cause irritation to the eyes, and amphibians that may produce toxic secretions.

The best way to stay safe in these situations is to know the species that is being dealt with, understand the potential dangers and recognize the signs of threat and insecurity. Particular attention should be paid to safety if venomous species of snake are being hospitalized or larger dangerous species such as crocodilians or the larger primates.

Other issues regarding health and safety in the practice include:

- General maintenance of buildings and equipment – Any cage facilities, wards or areas the animals will be in should be well maintained, secure, and suitable for the species involved. When dealing with birds and reptiles there is always a risk they may escape; they are capable of getting into many small spaces or out of cracks in windows. This could pose a danger to the animal, staff and people in the surrounding area
- Exotic species are prone to a number of diseases, of which the most important are probably salmonellosis and psittacosis (see earlier). These can easily be passed to humans, so good hygiene is very important to prevent disease transmission
- Fire precautions – Precautions should be taken when using heat lamps in vivaria. If not properly maintained, these could catch fire, causing harm to the patient and possibly even staff and premises
- Disinfectants and cleaning products – These should be handled appropriately, taking care to wear protective clothing when necessary (see earlier)
- Waste disposal – Care should be taken when disposing of clinical waste, hazardous waste and any sharps.

Important health and safety legislation:

- Health and Safety at Work etc. Act 1974
- Management of Health and Safety at Work Regulations 1999
- Control of Substances Hazardous to Health Regulations 1999 (COSHH)
- Reporting of Diseases and Dangerous Occurrences Regulations 1995 (RIDDOR).

Any accidents that occur at work should be reported, no matter how small. They should be recorded in the Accident Book for future reference.

References and further reading

Agar S (2001) *Small Animal Nutrition*. Butterworth-Heinemann, Oxford

Bat Conservation Trust, London (2012) *Bat Care Guidelines*. www.bats.org.uk/publications.php

Brash M (2009) The role of fibre in rabbit nutrition. *Veterinary Nursing Journal* 24 (12), 25–27

Brown D (2010) Kitting out an exotics ward. *In Practice* 32, 263–266

Carter W (2008) Toad fact file. *Veterinary Nursing Journal* 23 (5), 40

Chaffin C (2009) Frog fact file. *Veterinary Nursing Journal* 24 (8), 40

Cheeke PR (1987) Nutrition of guinea pigs. In: *Rabbit Feeding and Nutrition*, pp. 344–353. Academic Press, Orlando

Chitty J and Lierz M (2008) *BSAVA Manual of Raptors, Pigeons and Passerine Birds*. BSAVA Publications, Gloucester

Cousquer G (2006) Veterinary care of rabbits with myiasis. *In Practice* 28, 342–349

Cousquer G and Parsons D (2007) Veterinary care of the racing pigeon. *In Practice* 29, 344–355

Divers S (1996) Exotic animal practice: Basic reptile husbandry, history taking and clinical examination. *In Practice* 18, 51–65

Girling S (2003) *Exotic Pet and Wildlife Nursing*. Blackwell Publishing Ltd, Oxford

Girling S and Raiti P (2004) *BSAVA Manual of Reptiles, 2nd edn*. BSAVA Publications, Gloucester

Harcourt-Brown F (2009) Dental disease in pet rabbits: 2. diagnosis and treatment. *In Practice* 31, 432–445

Harcourt-Brown N and Chitty J (2005) *BSAVA Manual of Psittacine Birds, 2nd edn*. BSAVA Publications, Gloucester

King C (2008) Preoperative nursing care of the rabbit patient. *Veterinary Nursing Journal* 23 (12), 27–29

Meredith A and Johnson-Delaney C (2010) *BSAVA Manual of Exotic Pets, 5th edn*. BSAVA Publications, Gloucester

Meredith A and Keeble E (2009) *BSAVA Manual of Rodents and Ferrets*. BSAVA Publications, Gloucester

Roberts R (2004) *Diseases of Free Range Poultry*. Whittet Books Ltd, Stansted

Roberts V (2009) The basics of keeping backyard chickens. *Veterinary Nursing Journal* 24 (9), 18–21

Rowland M (2009) Exotics: veterinary care of bearded dragons. *In Practice* 31, 506–571

Slade R and Forbes M (2008) The importance of the source of fibre in the diet of the rabbit. *Veterinary Nursing Journal* 23 (3), 27–28

Stanford M (2009) Introduction to raptor management and husbandry. *In Practice* 31, 267–275

Stocker L (2000) *Practical Wildlife Care*. Blackwell Publishing Ltd, Oxford

Stocker L (2009) Tip of the iceberg. *Veterinary Nursing Journal* 24 (12), 29–31

Williams A (2008) Wildlife care: the red fox. *Veterinary Nursing Journal* 23 (1), 24–25

Williams A (2009) Care of the juvenile bird. *Veterinary Nursing Journal* 24 (6), 37–41

Useful websites

www.uvguide.co.uk
www.exoticdvm.com
www.tortoisetrust.org

Self-assessment questions

1. Define the term zoonosis and identify two common conditions that pose the most risk from (a) birds and (b) reptiles.
2. Ferrets are obligate carnivores. Explain what this term means and describe a suitable diet for this species.
3. Why must care be taken when hospitalizing small mustelids (including stoats and weasels)?
4. What does the term 'altricial' mean and how does this differ from the term 'precocial'?
5. Identify a suitable enclosure for an orphaned mammal.
6. Identify the most suitable lining for a vivarium and list a substance that would not be suitable, explaining the reasons why.
7. Guinea pigs should receive a vitamin C (ascorbic acid) supplement daily. What are the reasons for this? At what rate should this be given and how?
8. Explain why chinchillas require a dust bath and state how often this should be carried out.
9. Describe crop-feeding and list the key considerations associated with this technique.
10. List the factors that influence selection of an appropriate disinfectant.
11. UV light is essential for production of which one of the following vitamins?
    a. Vitamin A
    b. Vitamin B1
    c. Vitamin C
    d. Vitamin D3
    e. Vitamin E
12. The ambient temperature for hospitalized small mammals should be:
    a. 15–18°C
    b. 18–21°C
    c. 21–23°C
    d. 24–27°C
    e. 27–30°C
13. Budgerigars can suffer from deficiencies of which one of the following dietary components?
    a. Calcium
    b. Iodine
    c. Lysine
    d. Vitamin C
    e. Zinc
14. Which one of the following reptiles does not require UV light?
    a. Leopard gecko
    b. Green iguana
    c. Bearded dragon
    d. Red-eared terrapin
    e. Mediterranean tortoise
15. Which one of the following statements is not correct?
    a. Bearded dragons are omnivorous
    b. Ferrets are obligate carnivores
    c. Tortoises are herbivorous
    d. Iguanas are insectivorous
    e. Rats are omnivorous

6

Nursing hospitalized patients

Richard Saunders and Emma Whitlock

This chapter is designed to give information on:

- Administration of fluids to exotic patients, including different methods of application and rate calculations
- Administration of suitable nutrition to exotic patients, including calculations of energy requirements in different species under different circumstances
- Administration of medications to a variety of different species
- Nursing care plans, their uses and application to exotic patients

---

Fluid therapy

Fluid therapy is one of the most important aspects of treatment in any patient, but is particularly important in exotic species. A combination of frequent poor husbandry and the tendency of these species to mask clinical signs of disease as an evolutionary self-defence strategy often results in chronic and significant dehydration. Many exotic species also have a high metabolic rate, increasing their fluid maintenance requirements (Lichtenberger, 2007).

Fluid therapy is employed if an animal cannot maintain normal hydration by eating and drinking, or where fluid is required because:

- There have been extracellular losses
- Blood pressure/volume is low
- Extra fluids are needed to stimulate diuresis
- Nephrotoxicity is anticipated, e.g. with the use of aminoglycoside antibiotics.

Body fluids: a quick reminder

- The adult animal's body contains approximately 60% water, although it may be as much as 75% in reptiles.
- Fluid is distributed among intracellular and extracellular compartments: approximately 40% is intracellular and 60% extracellular. ▶
- Extracellular fluid is divided into three sub-compartments:
  - Interstitial
  - Transcellular
  - Intravascular.
- The intracellular and extracellular compartments are separated by semi-permeable membranes, which allow fluid to move across the membrane according to the osmotic pressure gradient.
- Dehydrated patients have lost water from the extravascular space.
- When fluids are given intravenously they are re-distributed to the other compartments until solutes are in equilibrium again, thus correcting extravascular losses.
- Fluids are administered not only to correct fluid losses but also to:
  - Correct electrolyte abnormalities
  - Induce kidney diuresis
  - Maintain tissue and organ perfusion before, during and after anaesthesia and/or surgery.

The fluid plan

When administering fluids, a plan should be drawn up to incorporate the type, quantity, route and rate of fluid to be given. The plan should include criteria for assessing the effectiveness of fluid therapy, so that members of the nursing team know when to alert a veterinary surgeon that therapy is not effective, and to ascertain when therapy has been effective and should cease.

A fluid plan, as part of the patient's nursing care plan, will help to encourage and support frequent evaluation of the patient in line with the fluid type, volume and rate administered. The fluid plan will also allow for the effective administration of therapeutics.

The aim of any fluid plan is to use the most appropriate fluid type and volume to match the particular requirements of the animal. While a continuous infusion at the correct rate is optimal, if a larger amount of fluid (as a bolus) will result in decreased handling of the patient, this should be considered to reduce stress. All fluids, regardless of route of administration, should be warmed to approximately body temperature prior to administration. For reptiles (and for birds and mammals with or at risk of hypothermia) it is vital that fluid therapy is carried out in association with steps to maintain normothermia, to avoid poor uptake and to increase efficacy.

Phases of fluid therapy

1. **Resuscitation:** Perfusion deficits are corrected. There is an urgent need to restore tissue perfusion and oxygenation. Initially, the intravascular volume should be replaced. The underlying disease process and the type of shock are used to determine the type, quantity and rate of fluid administered.
2. **Rehydration:** Interstitial deficits are corrected. Re-evaluation of hydration status is necessary before commencing this phase.
3. **Maintenance:** Correct fluid balance is maintained. The maintenance phase replaces ongoing losses with fluids and electrolytes, meets metabolic requirements and restores intracellular fluid balance.

Planning each of the three phases and monitoring clinical parameters will allow the clinical team to deliver and adjust the fluid type, rate and volume throughout the patient's hospitalization.

Fluid types

Parenteral fluids are divided into two types: crystalloids and colloids. Crystalloids pass readily through the semi-permeable membranes between the fluid compartments of the body, whereas colloids (from the Greek 'kolla', meaning glue-like) do not.

Crystalloids

Crystalloids are the fluid type most commonly used in clinical situations. They contain both electrolyte and non-electrolyte solutes, which can move freely between the body's fluid compartments. Crystalloids are categorized depending on their ability to move water across the semi-permeable membrane in between the intracellular and extracellular compartments. Each type of crystalloid has a specific clinical use.

Isotonic crystalloids

Isotonic crystalloids have equivalent osmolality to the patient's intracellular fluid and plasma. They remain in the interstitial space unless intracellular electrolyte abnormalities exist. They are generally used for:

- Routine surgical supportive perfusion
- Volume replacement in dehydration
- Initial fluid support in blood loss (with colloids as soon as possible)
- Chronic hypovolaemia (together with colloids).

The most useful isotonic crystalloids to stock are 0.9% saline and lactated Ringer's (Hartmann's) solution; the latter is preferred where metabolic acidosis is suspected. It is helpful to have a basic fluid mix readily available at all times, at a temperature suitable for administration (37–42°C), especially where many exotic pet consultations will require a short period of anaesthesia (e.g. trimming beaks and nails or taking blood samples).

Anecdotally, a 20% solution of crystalloid and a proprietary electrolyte solution (e.g. an injectable solution of electrolytes, vitamins, amino acids and dextrose, such as Duphalyte, Fort Dodge, UK) has been used with good success and no reported problems. The authors' workplace makes up a basic fluid mix of lactated Ringer's solution and Duphalyte at a 20% dilution in 10 ml and 20 ml syringes, which are stored within a fluid warmer (see below) for any patient requiring immediate and/or basic maintenance fluid therapy.

When making up a basic fluid mix for everyday use, it is best to make up a 500 ml bag (by removing 100 ml of lactated Ringer's solution and replacing this with 100 ml of Duphalyte, to make a 20% solution). The 500 ml bag can then be refrigerated for up to 7 days.

A warm water bath (e.g. a baby's bottle warmer) can be used to store prepared fluids and keep them at a temperature suitable for administration, which may be adjusted prior to administration as necessary. The water bath *must* be kept topped up with enough water and should be kept appropriately clean and disinfected to prevent overgrowth of bacteria within the warm, damp environment. It is also important *not* to place food syringes within the bath, as any food leaking into the water would encourage bacterial growth.

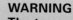 **WARNING**
The temperature of fluids *must* be checked prior to administration as overheating could result in serious thermal damage to the patient.

Hypertonic crystalloids

The osmolality of hypertonic crystalloids is greater than that of the patient's cells and plasma. Consequently, hypertonic crystalloids cause a fluid shift from the interstitial and intracellular spaces to the intravascular space, which means that fluid is replaced more rapidly than if using isotonic crystalloids alone. Hypertonic crystalloid solutions are extremely useful for rapid but transient correction of hypovolaemia in shocked patients, but must be followed up with colloids for maintaining their effects. Hypertonic crystalloids are, however, contraindicated in patients with high sodium levels.

Examples include 7% and 23% hypertonic sodium chloride solutions. The 23% hypertonic saline should be diluted to a 7.5% solution prior to administration.

Hypotonic crystalloids

The osmolality of hypotonic crystalloids is lower than that of the patient's cells and plasma; this results in the movement of fluid from the intravascular space into the cells. Hypotonic crystalloids are therefore useful in patients with electrolyte disturbances such as hypernatraemia, which is generally caused not by an absolute excess of sodium but by a relative deficit of free water within the body.

Examples of hypotonic crystalloids include 5% dextrose in water and 0.45% sodium chloride.

Colloids

Colloids are fluids made up of large molecules that cannot readily pass through the semi-permeable membranes of blood vessels and hence remain within the intravascular space and support the circulation. In other species (e.g. cats and dogs), if blood loss is <5% of the blood volume, no fluid volume resuscitation is necessary because the body is capable of compensation. However, if blood loss is >15% of the blood volume, the intravascular volume must be maintained in order to support cardiac output. An intravenous colloidal solution should be used in this case.

Although crystalloid resuscitation would eventually produce the same volume expansion as colloidal resuscitation, much larger volumes of a crystalloid solution are required to produce the same effect, and electrolyte imbalances, acidosis and interstitial oedema could result.

Colloids may be natural or synthetic. Natural colloids include whole blood and blood products (e.g. red blood cells, plasma and albumin). Blood products (or synthetic haemoglobin-based oxygen carriers (HBOCs), see later) should be used where volume resuscitation alone is not adequate to restore tissue oxygenation.

> ⚠️ **WARNING**
> Colloidal solutions *must not* be warmed up using a microwave prior to administration. There is evidence that the large protein molecules may be damaged and so may not be as effective as they should be at increasing circulating intravascular fluid volume and remaining within the intravascular space.

Blood transfusions

Blood transfusions may be used for exotic patients, with similar indications to those for dogs and cats. Due to the lack of commercial sources, blood transfusion is generally restricted to fresh blood from a healthy donor with a haematocrit of at least 40% that has been appropriately vaccinated and screened for infectious diseases and haematological parameter normality. It is important to note that many exotic pets (especially rabbits) commonly have apparently subclinical anaemia.

Using a related or other in-contact donor minimizes the risk of disease transmission and may have social benefits to the donor in aiding the survival of a bonded companion. Although heterologous transfusions from the most closely related species within a family have been performed and may be the only option in rarer species (e.g. blood from a relatively common blue and gold macaw could be given to the critically endangered hyacinth macaw), homologous transfusions (i.e. from the same species) are preferred.

Indications for blood transfusion

- A haematocrit (packed cell volume, PCV) value of <15%.
- Blood loss:
  - For mammals, a loss of >30% blood volume
  - For birds, a loss of >40% blood volume
  - For reptiles, exact volumes that would necessitate transfusion are not established as these animals are highly resistant to blood loss.
- Ongoing haemorrhage.
- Blood loss associated with collapse.
- A poor response to conventional shock therapies with crystalloids or colloids.

Where blood group characteristics for a species are unknown, or where there have been previous transfusions, cross-matching for agglutination reactions should be performed using scaled-down volumes and a similar technique to that used for dogs and cats. In ferrets, blood groups have not been identified and even repeated transfusions do not require prior cross-matching.

Simplified cross-matching procedure

- Mix two drops of plasma from the donor/recipient with one drop of blood from the recipient/donor on a slide at room temperature. (It does not matter which blood product comes from which animal, as long as one product comes from each.)
- Monitor the slide for 1 whole minute.
- The development of macroscopic agglutination within the mixed samples within 1 minute suggests incompatibility.

Unfortunately, although this procedure predicts potential agglutination, it cannot predict acute haemolytic transfusion reaction (haemolysis), which is the most common fatal transfusion reaction.

Up to 9–10 ml/kg of blood may be safely taken from the donor, under appropriate sedation, using the largest cannula or needle appropriate to the size of the vessel (ideally a minimum of 22 g). Citrate-based (1–7 ml blood) or heparin-based (5–10 units/ml of blood) anticoagulants are used for fresh (within 48 hours) transfusions. Citrate–phosphate–dextrose–

adenine (CPDA) is the preferred anticoagulant for longer-term storage (up to 35 days).

Administration is intravenous or intraosseous, with the blood warmed to body temperature and filtered to remove micro-clots. Sedation is not usually required in the shocked patient. Baseline general health and cardiopulmonary parameters should be assessed before transfusion and then every 30 minutes throughout. Haematocrit and total protein should be measured 1–2 hours after transfusion to assess response.

Synthetic colloids

Synthetic colloids are also known as plasma expanders and include:

- Gelatine solutions, e.g. Haemaccel (MSD) and Gelofusine (B. Braun)
- Etherified starch solutions, e.g. hetastarch and pentastarch
- HBOCs, e.g. Oxyglobin.

Synthetic colloids are used prior to, or in place of, blood transfusions in patients with intravascular losses. They can also be used in patients with an increased risk of third-space fluid accumulation or those that have been given crystalloids but have not been fully resuscitated, e.g. those with severe hypo-albuminaemia. Synthetic colloids draw interstitial fluid into the circulation, requiring additional crystalloids to replace this interstitial fluid.

HBOCs are indicated during the resuscitation phase. They may be used in place of blood transfusions due to their greater availability, long shelf-life, cross-species use, ability to be administered into small blood vessels, and lack of potential transfusion reaction or disease transmission. In addition, their lower oxygen affinity and smaller molecular weight gives them up to ten times the effectiveness of blood in delivering oxygen to the tissues. HBOCs have a moderately short half-life (primary effect lasts for approximately 24 hours, with 90% eliminated from the body within 5–7 days).

Calculating fluid requirements

It is difficult to quantify the fluid deficits of many exotic patients accurately due to unfamiliarity with the species' norms and the confounding effects of the inelastic skin of many species (especially reptiles), emaciation, and generalized illness mimicking the clinical signs of dehydration.

It is most practical to assess percentage dehydration and calculate maintenance fluid requirements with this factor included. When calculating fluid requirements, it is important to ensure replacement of ongoing fluid losses as well as replacement of existing deficits. It is also important to bear in mind that some exotic patients are considerably smaller than dogs and cats, and therefore only small amounts of fluids may be given at any one time. It is very easy to over-perfuse the smaller species, especially if the intravenous or intraosseous route is used. Deficits should be replaced at 50% in the first 24 hours, with the remainder administered over the following 48 hours.

Calculating percentage dehydration

- **5% dehydrated:** No detectable clinical signs. Assume that all patients that are unwell are at least 5% dehydrated.
- **5–6% dehydrated:** Subtle loss of skin elasticity (the skin overlying the pectoral muscles is a good site to assess this in birds), increased thirst, slight lethargy, tacky mucous membranes, increased heart rate.
- **7–9% dehydrated:** As above but with definite skin turgor, anorexia, increased capillary refill time and sunken eyes within orbits (not always obvious).
- **10–12% dehydrated:** Complete loss of skin turgor, dull sunken eyes within orbits, possibly signs of shock and/or alteration in consciousness.
- **13–15% dehydrated:** Dull to comatose, definite signs of shock (imminent death if not corrected).

In birds, it is useful to assess the filling time of the brachial vein on the medial aspect of the wing. If less than 1–2 seconds, this indicates a dehydration level of approximately 7%.

Calculating the fluid deficit

Dehydration % x bodyweight (kg) x 10 = fluid deficit (ml)

Maintenance requirements must be given in addition to the fluid deficit.

For exotic pets, fluid is usually administered as regular intermittent boluses because many animals will not tolerate a giving set; however, if infusing, the calculation for fluid therapy drip rates is as for dogs and cats.

Calculating drip rates where giving sets are used

- Total amount over 24 hours / 24 = hourly rate
- Hourly rate / 60 = minute rate
- Minute rate x drip factor = number of drops per minute
- Drops per minute / 60 = drops per second

Standard giving sets have a drip factor rate of 20 drops/ml. Paediatric (burette) giving sets have a drip factor rate of 60 drops/ml.

If administering intravenous fluids via a giving set, a fluid pump or syringe-driver must always be used to measure volumes accurately and prevent over-infusion of small patients. Regular calibration of fluid pumps and syringe-drivers is essential, as even minor inaccuracies can have significant effects when small volumes are being administered.

> **Before administration of fluids via *any* route**
>
> - Warm the fluid. Hypothermia is a huge problem in small exotic patients due to their small size and large body surface area. All fluids must therefore be warmed prior to ▶

administration and kept warm during the process. Pre-prepared maintenance fluids can be kept warm for rapid and easy administration in any patient. To keep fluids warm as they are infused, the reservoir bag can be insulated by coiling the giving set around a warmed rice bag (the bag of uncooked rice should first have been placed in a nylon stocking and heated in a microwave for 1.5–2 minutes). Alternatively, the giving set can be run through a warm water bath, allowing the fluid to be warmed by the water before it reaches the patient.

■ Ensure the correct amount and rate of administration has been calculated.
■ Ensure that the most appropriate route for administration of fluids is used in each individual patient.
■ Ensure that all equipment is ready, to minimize handling and/or anaesthetic time.
■ Prepare the patient with a topical local anaesthetic solution if necessary, at an appropriate point prior to catheter insertion.

Fluid administration rates

Mammals

The suggested maintenance rate of fluids for most healthy adult mammals varies widely between sources of information, from 50 to 150 ml/kg/day (i.e. 2–6 ml/kg/h). A general starting point in the average patient is 80–100 ml/kg/day. Rabbits and guinea pigs require approximately 100–120 ml/kg/day. To avoid fluid overload, however, it is recommended that a maximum of 70 ml/kg/day is administered intravenously. Gerbils and other desert species require lower rates (approximately 50 ml/kg/day). Most other rodents require rates in the middle of the range.

Additional requirements will depend on ongoing losses due to burns, intestinal losses, etc., and should be calculated as for dogs and cats, at approximately 4 ml/kg for each episode of vomiting or diarrhoea. The presence of palpable fluid within the large intestine of rabbits and rodents indicates significant amounts of sequestered fluid, and this should be addressed. Fluid loss via large skin deficits (e.g. fly strike) may also be significant. Surgical rates are generally two to three times maintenance, i.e. approximately 5–10 ml/kg/h. Shock rates are 80–100 ml/kg/h for up to 1 hour.

Hypertonic saline 7.5% is more effective at rapid volume expansion. It should be administered at 5 ml/kg over 5–10 minutes, and be followed by colloids.

Colloids are the preferred fluid in cases of hypovolaemia (alongside approximately 20–50% of the above crystalloid volumes, to minimize interstitial volume depletion). Boluses of hetastarch at 5 ml/kg may be given over 10–15 minutes as required, to normalize the heart rate and raise the systolic blood pressure above 90 mmHg, followed by a constant rate infusion (CRI) of hetastarch at 3–5 ml/kg/h. Colloidal solutions must be given slowly in small mammals to reduce the risk of hyperthermia, which can be seen with administration of boluses.

Oxyglobin should be given as a bolus of 2 ml/kg over 10–15 minutes until the heart rate becomes normal and the systolic blood pressure has been raised above 90 mmHg. This should be followed by a CRI of 0.2–0.4 ml/kg/h.

Blood may be given rapidly if required because of severe blood loss; however, it should initially be given at 0.5 ml/kg over 20 minutes, monitoring closely for transfusion reactions, with the remainder given over 1–4 hours, depending on circulatory health. The total amount required should be determined at the outset. In general, 20 ml/kg of whole blood (a typical dose volume) will raise the PCV by 10%. Packed red blood cells and fresh frozen plasma are administered at a dose of 10–15 ml/kg.

Blood requirement may be determined using the equation:

Blood required (ml) = (bodyweight of patient (kg) x desired PCV x 66) – (patient PCV/donor PCV)

Birds

Daily maintenance fluid requirements are 100 ml/kg/day (4 ml/kg/h) for most species (50 ml/kg/day or lower for xerophilic desert species).

For shocked birds, warmed crystalloids at doses of 10–30 ml/kg via an intravenous bolus have been widely used in a variety of species with no ill effects. Shock rates of 90 ml/kg/h are suggested. However, the use of colloids (including Oxyglobin) at 5–10 ml/kg by a slow intravenous bolus, together with 10 ml/kg of bolus crystalloids for maintenance, minimizes the risk of hypovolaemia. Blood transfusions have been used in a variety of species, in the same manner as for mammals.

Reptiles

The maintenance fluid rate for reptiles is 10–30 ml/kg/day. This is ideally given as a CRI, but may be more practically given as boluses. Frequency of administration *versus* amount given is a trade-off between efficient uptake and the stress of multiple administrations. The use of multiple routes, including the oral route, may be necessary in severely dehydrated reptiles. Fluid selection depends on the type of dehydration expected, including possible electrolyte abnormalities.

The plasma osmolality of some reptiles (in particular those from a freshwater aquatic environment) is lower than that of mammals. Solutions that are isotonic for mammals (e.g. normal saline) are therefore hypertonic in such reptiles. Dilution of solutions is advised, e.g. a 1:1 mixture of 5% dextrose and a non-lactate-containing isotonic mixed electrolyte solution. Glucose-containing solutions are helpful in reducing potassium levels in hyperkalaemic patients.

For shock rates, bolus doses of crystalloids (5–10 ml/kg) together with colloids (3–5 ml/kg) can be given intravenously or intraosseously until blood pressure is within the normal range for the species. Blood transfusions have been anecdotally reported in a number of reptile species.

Routes of administration

Enteral routes

If the mouth works, use it! Enteral fluids (water or electrolyte replacers) can be given in several ways:

- The patient drinking freely or lapping at water offered from a syringe or drinking receptacle
- Syringing fluid into the patient's mouth
- Gavage using a rigid or flexible tube passed into the crop (birds) or oesophagus
- Administration via an *in situ* feeding tube (naso-oeosophageal).

Risks and complications associated with administration of fluids via the enteral route include the following:

- It is not effective in severely dehydrated or debilitated individuals
- Some electrolyte mixtures may be unpalatable to individuals
- Mucosal burns if fluids given are too hot
- Aspiration of fluids or food due to:
  - Improper tube placement (into trachea or back of throat)
  - Regurgitation.

Damage to the oesophagus, crop, mouth or teeth, or undue stress may occur in animals that are reluctant to accept direct oral methods. In these cases, or in cases of pre-existing oral lesions, a pharyngostomy tube may be placed (Figure 6.1).

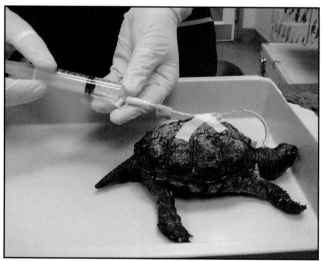

6.1 Fluid administration via a pharyngostomy tube in a 'dry-docked' pond terrapin. (© Emma Whitlock)

Administration via the oral route is only recommended where dehydration is not too severe (<5%) and where the patient is at its optimal body temperature and is able to absorb fluids via the gastrointestinal system. It is not recommended if there is vomiting or reduced gastrointestinal tract mobility, or other significant gastrointestinal pathology, although regular small feeds are important to maintain enterocyte health.

Enteral fluid administration in mammals

- Routes for enteral fluid administration in mammals include:
  - Via a syringe placed in the mouth – although aspiration is possible, especially in stressed animals or those with respiratory tract disease.
  - Via an *in situ* feeding tube (naso-oeosophageal).
- In small rodents, gavage can be achieved with the use of a crop or stomach tube; however, the patient must be scruffed and restrained sufficiently to prevent movement and to align the oesophagus with the head.
- The restraint required for gavage administration may be stressful to the patient and other methods are advised.
- **Maximum amounts** that can be delivered at any one time:
  - Rabbits: 10 ml/kg
  - Small rodents: 5–10 ml/kg
  - Guinea pigs and chinchillas: 10 ml/kg.

Enteral fluid administration in birds

- Routes for enteral fluid administration in birds include:
  - Fluid syringed into the mouth, although aspiration is very possible, especially in stressed animals, or those with respiratory tract disease
  - Gavage via a crop tube (see also Chapter 1).
    - A rigid tube is best for psittacine birds to prevent them from chewing through and ingesting the tube. Flexible tubing can be used for other species, e.g. raptors. When feeding birds without a crop (e.g. owls) it is advisable to use a longer, softer plastic tube to allow proventricular feeding.
    - A large (but not too large) blunt-ended tube should be used, to minimize the risk of accidental placement into the trachea, mucosal damage or puncture of the oesophagus.
    - Beak gags, made from plastic, metal or wood, may be used to minimize the risk of tube damage.
    - The bird can be secured in a towel and held in one hand while the crop tube is introduced into the left side of the beak, moving across so that the tube enters the oesophagus on the right-hand side and slides slowly down into the crop.
    - The tube should be directly observed passing into the pharynx. It may be seen and/or palpated passing down the oesophagus and into the crop, which is just cranial to the thoracic inlet.
- **Maximum amounts** that can be given vary depending upon the size and species of the bird and the presence or absence of the crop.

Enteral fluid administration in reptiles

- Routes for enteral fluid administration in reptiles include:
  - Via an *in situ* feeding tube
  - Via a flexible or rigid stomach tube passed through the oesophagus and into the distal oesophagus or stomach (i.e. the midpoint of the plastron in chelonians, 33–50% of the snout-to-vent length in snakes, middle to distal ribcage of lizards).
- A wooden or plastic gag (e.g. tongue depressors, syringe barrels) may be required in reptiles that have teeth (to prevent biting through the tube) or where it is difficult to hold open the mouth for gavage. Smooth metal gags may be used, with care to avoid tooth damage (Figure 6.2).
- **Maximum amounts** that can be delivered at any one time:
  - Lizards: 10–20 ml/kg
  - Snakes: 15–30 ml/kg
  - Chelonians: 5–15 ml/kg
  - In chronically anorexic reptile patients, the amount of oral fluids given should start at the lower end of the range in order to avoid re-feeding syndrome. This is a potentially fatal condition whereby rapid insulin release (a response to glucose administration in fluid or food) causes potassium to be taken into cells, resulting in hypokalaemia. This in turn can cause a fatal bradycardia. (See later for more information.)

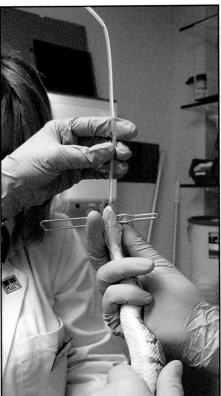

6.2 Use of a metal mouth gag to facilitate fluid administration via gavage in a snake. (Courtesy of Elisabetta Mancinelli)

Bathing reptiles

Reptiles often benefit from being placed in a warm bath (cat litter trays are ideal and may be placed on a heat mat to maintain water temperature) for up to half an hour at a time, to encourage drinking while in the water and also encourage passing of urates and faecal matter.

Chelonians (and possibly some lizards, to a much lesser extent) have the ability to exchange the contents of their bladder with that of the fluid in which they are immersed. This fluid may then be absorbed via the cloacal and bladder mucosa. It is believed that chelonians are able to absorb fluids rapidly via this route and distribute it within the systemic circulation. The bladder may be flushed with a urinary catheter and fluids administered by this route, or in a bath.

Parenteral routes

The stress of being handled and the pain caused by the various injection routes should be balanced against the need to give fluids accurately, quickly and efficiently. Whichever route is used, it is vital that fluids are injected at the correct temperature (neither too hot nor too cold) and the correct rate (not too rapidly) and, if using the intravenous or intraosseous route, that all air is removed from the syringe or giving set to avoid air embolism.

Subcutaneous administration

Subcutaneous fluids are useful for maintenance of hydration where patients do not require frequent repeated administration of fluids and in those that are <5–7% dehydrated. Due to the reduction in peripheral circulation during shock, and the slow rate of subcutaneous fluid uptake, it is not recommended that the subcutaneous route is used as the sole route of fluid administration in a shocked patient. Hyaluronidase (e.g. Wydase, Wyeth) can be added to fluids at 100–150 IU/l to increase the rate of absorption significantly.

Subcutaneous fluid administration allows for relatively large amounts to be given to mammals. The tightly adherent skin of birds and reptiles, however, limits the volumes that may be administered; larger volumes of fluid may only be given at sites with distensible skin 'pockets' (see below). The skin of birds and reptiles must never be over-distended with fluids as this may disrupt the blood supply to the area, resulting in decreased absorption from the site and potential skin necrosis.

Injection sites should be aseptically prepared to reduce the risk of infection (especially in reptiles), although care should be taken not to make the patient too wet or cold.

Subcutaneous fluids should be administered using an appropriately sized needle, gently inserted at a shallow angle under the skin to minimize the risk of puncturing air sacs or entering a body cavity. Fluids should be given slowly, to prevent leakage of fluid from the injection site and to minimize discomfort. Using a butterfly needle attached to a giving or extension set reduces the risk of the needle moving uncomfortably or in a way that will damage the patient while fluid administration is underway. In birds and reptiles with inelastic skin, a finger should be placed over the injection site when withdrawing the needle following subcutaneous fluid administration, to limit leakage of fluids through the site.

Subcutaneous administration in mammals

- Routes for subcutaneous fluid administration in mammals include:
  - Into the scruff over the dorsal scapulae
  - Into the flanks over the thoracic wall
  - Anywhere else where skin can be gently grasped and pulled away from the body wall.
- **Maximum amounts:** 10 ml/kg, divided into various sites at any one time.

Subcutaneous administration in birds

- Routes for subcutaneous fluid administration in birds include:
  - In the axillary region underneath each wing
  - In the inguinal region, where the leg meets the body
  - Over the dorsal scapulae.
- Some seabirds have subcutaneous air sac extensions, which should be avoided.
- Always draw back to check for accidental injection into an air sac.
- **Maximum amounts:** 10 ml/kg, divided into various sites at any one time.

Subcutaneous administration in reptiles

- Routes for subcutaneous fluid administration in reptiles include:
  - Lizards: The lateral thoracic areas, skin folds immediately cranial to the hindlimbs
  - Snakes: The lateral aspect of the dorsum in the caudal third of the body (Figure 6.3)
  - Chelonians: The skin folds of the neck or immediately cranial to the hindlimbs.
- Always inject between the scales.
- There is a risk of darkened pigmented skin following subcutaneous injection in some lizards (in particular chameleons).
- **Maximum amounts:** 10 ml/kg, divided into various sites at any one time.

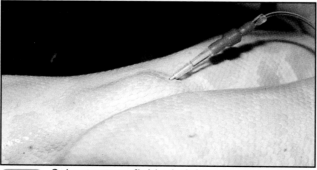

6.3 Subcutaneous fluid administration in an albino Burmese python. (Reproduced from the *BSAVA Manual of Reptiles, 2nd edition*)

Intravenous administration

Intravenous fluid administration is the most rapid and efficient method of fluid delivery but it is invasive; anaesthesia may be required to facilitate insertion of an intravenous catheter. Such catheters may not be tolerated by many exotic species, e.g. rabbits and psittacine birds.

To facilitate insertion of an intravenous catheter in mammals, topical local anaesthetic agents (e.g. EMLA cream) may be applied to the intended catheterization site following clipping, and should be left for a minimum of 30 minutes to ensure effectiveness. Other local anaesthetic agents designed for mucosal anaesthesia (e.g. Intubeaze, Dechra) may have some effect, within approximately 5 minutes.

> ⚠️ **WARNING**
> **Topical anaesthetic products should never be used on birds without extremely careful dose calculation, as their therapeutic index is lower than for mammals, and fatal central nervous system (CNS) or cardiac toxicity may result.**

Intravenous fluid administration may be achieved by off-the-needle bolus administration intermittently via an intravenous catheter or by CRI via a catheter. Catheters should be placed where either emergency intravenous access is required or repeated intravenous injections might be required, to prevent repeated damage to the veins. Intravenous catheterization minimizes the risk of repeated venepuncture; however, some problems may still be encountered.

- Veins may be difficult to access if the patient is very small, collapsed or debilitated.
- The smaller diameter of many exotic patients' veins necessitates the use of narrow-gauge catheters, with an increased risk of blockage.
- Restraint for intravenous access may be more stressful, and longer handling periods may be required than for other methods.
- Haematomas will commonly form (especially in mammals and birds). In birds, there have been fatalities where a significant amount of blood has leaked after vascular damage at venepuncture, subcutaneously around a catheter, or after removal.
- Catheters can be difficult to maintain in exotic pets; birds in particular may remove them.
- Environmental or skin bacteria may gain entry via indwelling intravenous catheters.

If an easily accessible intravenous catheter is maintained *in situ*, intravenous administration is often the least stressful method of administering fluids. Relatively large volumes of fluid can be given via this route (but should always be given slowly), and repeated intermittent boluses or CRI should be relatively painless. Where a constant infusion is to be administered, a syringe-driver or fluid pump should be used in small patients to prevent over-infusion.

Intravenous administration in mammals

- Use a 22–26 gauge hypodermic needle or catheter, depending on the patient size.
- Use a topical anaesthetic prior to inserting an intravenous catheter where appropriate.
- Suitable sites for intravenous administration include:
  - The cephalic vein (Figure 6.4)
  - The lateral saphenous veins
  - The marginal ear veins (rabbits)
  - The lateral tail vein (myomorph rodents).

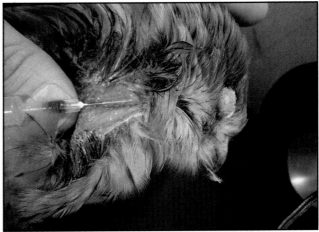

6.5 Bolus intravenous administration of the authors' suggested fluid mix via needle and syringe into the right jugular vein of a kestrel. (Courtesy of Richard Saunders)

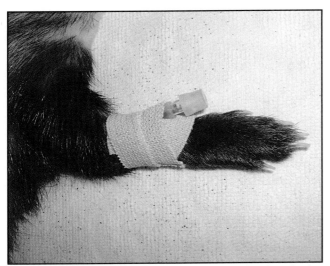

6.4 *In situ* intravenous catheter taped in place in the cephalic vein of a ferret. (Courtesy of Richard Saunders)

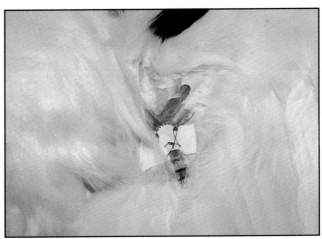

6.6 An *in situ* intravenous catheter for fluid administration via the brachial vein of a barn owl. (Courtesy of Richard Saunders)

Intravenous administration in birds

- Use a 22–26 gauge catheter, depending on the size and species of the bird.
- Do not use a topical local anaesthetic without assessing toxicity carefully.
- Suitable sites for intravenous administration include:
  - The right jugular vein (the right vein is almost always larger and therefore easier to access; Figure 6.5) – note this is not a suitable site for intravenous catheterization in most cases but may be the only accessible vein in birds weighing <150 g
  - The brachial (or cutaneous ulnar/wing) vein (Figure 6.6)
  - The medial metatarsal vein (in waterfowl and other large species).
- Transient mild bradycardia may be seen in birds given intravenous boluses of fluids.
- The small size of the catheter and its location (brachial or medial metatarsal vein) may result in kinking of the catheter. The limb should be held straight during fluid administration to avoid occlusion.

Intravenous administration in reptiles

- There are no suitable accessible peripheral vessels in reptiles.
- Intravenous catheter placement generally requires a surgical 'cut-down' technique. The most suitable vessels for this technique and catheter placement are:
  - The right jugular vein (chelonians, snakes (Figure 6.7) and small lizards)
  - The cephalic vein (in larger lizard species)
  - The ventral abdominal vein
  - The ventral tail vein.
- Crystalloid fluids may persist in the circulation for a shorter period when administered in the caudal half of the body due to the renal portal system.
- The presence of the renal portal system also means that it is not suitable to give fluids via any caudal veins, which is why only cranial sites are listed above.
- **Maximum amount:** 40 ml/kg.

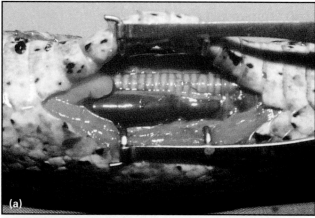

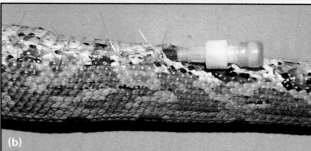

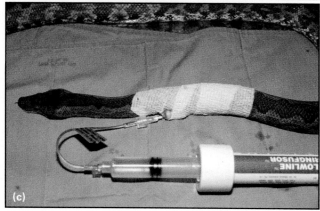

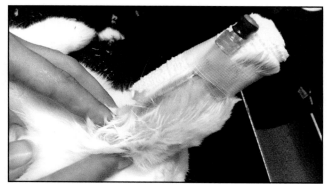

6.7 Catheterization of the jugular vein in a Solomon Island ground boa. Sedation or anaesthesia (e.g. intravenous propofol and/or isoflurane via facemask) is required; in severely debilitated reptiles a local anaesthetic may suffice. **(a)** In snakes the jugular vein is exposed by making a longitudinal incision at the junction of the lateral and ventral scales, approximately 5–8 scales cranial to the heart. (In chelonians and lizards (except chameleons) a transverse incision is made at about half the distance between the tympanum and shoulder joint.) **(b)** A small retractor aids in placement of the pre-heparinized catheter, which is then sutured to the skin. **(c)** Control of flow rate and volume requires the use of a syringe pump. (Reproduced from the *BSAVA Manual of Reptiles, 2nd edition*)

The maintenance of *in situ* catheters in exotic species is much the same as in cats and dogs.

- Patency should be ensured by regular flushing of the catheter with heparin sodium at a maximum dose of 1–10 IU/ml in saline.
- Catheter insertion sites should be protected against contamination by using suitable dressings, which must be changed at least daily.

- Rabbits commonly remove marginal ear vein catheters. This risk can be minimized by bandaging the catheter into place using a rolled-up swab within the pinna (Figure 6.8), to maintain the ear shape. An alternative method, using winged catheters, is to remove the lateral wing and glue the medial wing to the skin using veterinary surgical adhesive. Other lightweight adhesive coverings such as Opsite Flexigrid (Smith and Nephew) may be useful.
- For birds, it is not advised to bandage catheters in place in the superficial ulnar vein, as the bandage may cause feather damage or may lead to over-preening and catheter damage.
- Catheters should be removed from any one site after a maximum of 72 hours.

6.8 *In situ* intravenous catheter for fluid administration in the marginal ear vein of a rabbit. Note that the catheter has been attached to the rolled-up swab within the pinna using adhesive tape. (Courtesy of Molly Varga)

Intraosseous administration

Intraosseous fluid administration is under-utilized and is extremely useful in circumstances that may make intravenous or subcutaneous fluid therapy difficult or impossible. Intraosseous access is also recommended where an intravenous catheter is necessary but not well tolerated (e.g. in birds that interfere with the catheter). Insertion of a catheter into the medullary cavity should generally be performed under sedation or general anaesthesia but, in shocked patients, local anaesthesia by infiltration of the site may be most appropriate.

Access to the central circulation via this non-collapsible route is extremely rapid. Pain may also be felt with rapid administration of bolus fluids. Extravasation of fluids through previous catheterization attempts or fracture sites may cause local soft tissue reaction, or a build-up of fluid under the skin, leading to absence of distal limb or muscle perfusion (compartment syndrome).

The intraosseous route should be used for short-term vascular volume expansion, allowing intravenous access to be obtained if still required and if possible. Most medication or fluid that can safely and effectively be given via intravenous administration can also be given via the intraosseous route, including crystalloid and colloidal fluid products and total parenteral nutrition.

Intraosseous catheters are relatively easy to place and are tolerated well by most patients. The complications and risks relating to intraosseous catheterization and administration of therapeutics include the following:

- There is a risk of osteomyelitis, even where surgical preparation is properly maintained
- Intraosseous catheters may not be tolerated and may be removed by the patient
- Placement of an intraosseous catheter requires sedation or anaesthesia or at least local anaesthesia and analgesia
- It may not be suitable for administration of alkaline or hypertonic solutions which may cause pain upon delivery, without appropriate dilution
- The placement of intraosseous catheters may cause iatrogenic pathological fractures in patients with metabolic bone disease
- These catheters are absolutely contraindicated in cases of existing osteomyelitis or fracture of the bone to be used, due to the risks of sepsis or compartment syndrome developing
- Fluid boluses should be given more slowly than when using the intravenous route, due to the inexpansible nature of the medullary cavity
- Purpose-made intraosseous needles or spinal needles should be used, to avoid blockage of the needle lumen by bone
- Placement of the catheter close to a joint can temporarily affect limb mobility and predispose the patient to arthritis
- Ongoing analgesia is recommended as placement and maintenance cause discomfort.

Intraosseous administration in mammals

- Suitable sites include the proximal femur, cranial tibia (Figure 6.9) and proximal humerus.
- In very small patients, the medullary cavity may be too small for even a normal hypodermic needle to be inserted, making this route unsuitable.

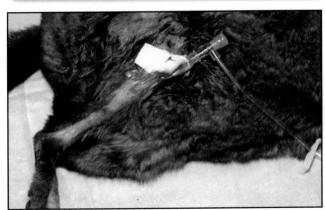

6.9 Common sites for intraosseous catheter placement in the rodent include the femur through the trochanteric fossa, or the tibia (as shown here) through the tibial crest. Placement is similar to normograde insertion of an intramedullary pin and requires strict aseptic technique during placement and maintenance. (Reproduced from the *BSAVA Manual of Rodents and Ferrets*)

Intraosseous administration in birds

- Must not be placed in pneumatized bones in birds (such as the femur or humerus typically, but anatomy of unfamiliar species must be checked).
- Suitable sites in birds include:
  - The proximal or distal ulna
  - The proximal tibiotarsus (Figure 6.10).

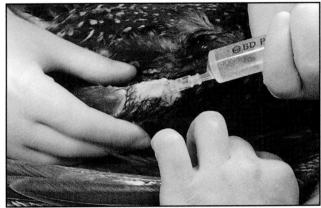

6.10 Intraosseous administration in the proximal cranial tibiotarsus of a common buzzard. (Courtesy of Elisabetta Mancinelli)

Intraosseous administration in reptiles

- Suitable sites for intraosseous administration in reptiles include:
  - Lizards and chelonians: The limb bones (typically the proximal femur)
  - Chelonians:
    - The plastrocarapacial bridge (junction of the carapace and plastron cranial to the hindlimb; Figure 6.11)
    - The costal/marginal scute junction (in softer-shelled animals).
- Some find this route unreliable and complicated in reptiles and prefer to give fluids and drugs via the intra- or epicoelomic routes, which are quick and require no specialist equipment.

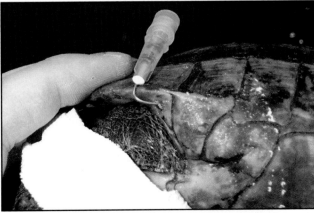

6.11 Intraosseous needle inserted into the plastrocarapacial junction. (Courtesy of Ron Rees Davis)

Nursing care of patients with *in situ* catheters

Nursing care of patients with *in situ* (intravenous or intraosseous) catheters is the same as for dogs and cats, although there may be an increased risk of infection at the insertion site due to the bacteria found on the skin of some exotic species (e.g. reptiles).

Ensure that:

■ Catheter insertion sites are aseptically prepared prior to insertion of the catheter
■ The catheter is bandaged or sutured in place effectively
■ Bandages and sutures are monitored for soiling
■ Bandages are changed every 24 hours, even if they appear clean
■ The patient does not interfere with the catheter (consider the use of bandages and collars)
■ The catheter site is checked for signs of infection; if infection is apparent, remove the catheter and inform a veterinary surgeon immediately
■ Catheters are removed and replaced in another site (if necessary) every 72 hours.

Ascertain catheter patency by:

■ Gently flushing with fluids or heparin saline. If there is resistance *do not* apply more pressure (there is a risk of clot dislodgement and embolism)
■ Monitoring for tissue swelling or wetness at the catheter site.

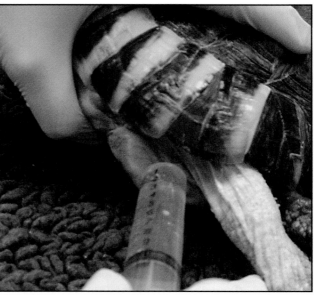

6.12 Intracoelomic fluid administration in a Horsfield's tortoise. (© Emma Whitlock)

Epicoelomic administration

The epicoelomic route allows for administration of fluids and medications close to the coelomic cavity in chelonians (Figure 6.13) but does not carry some of the risks associated with intracoelomic injection and potentially offers more efficient absorption when compared with absorption via the coelomic cavity. It is believed that this area may connect to the pericardium and other fluid storage sites, resulting in rapid effective fluid uptake and systemic distribution. The epicoelomic route is extremely useful in severely dehydrated reptiles in which intravenous access is difficult but fluids are needed urgently.

Intracoelomic administration

Reptiles (other than crocodilians) do not have separate abdominal and thoracic cavities but instead have one large space, known as the coelomic cavity, in which all visceral organs are found.

Fluids can be administered into the coelomic cavity in reptiles via an aseptically prepared site in the prefemoral fossa (Figure 6.12). There is, however, little evidence to show how effective absorption is via this route and there is anecdotal evidence to suggest that administration via the epicoelomic route is more effective. Risks and complications associated with this route include accidental puncture of the bladder, gastrointestinal tract or ovarian follicles in mature females. Where absorption is poor, overloading can occur over a longer period, with accumulation of repeated doses.

> ⚠ **WARNING**
> The intracoelomic route *must not* be used in birds. Fluid will be administered into the air sacs. This will not be absorbed effectively and may drown the bird. Even small volumes can lead to death.

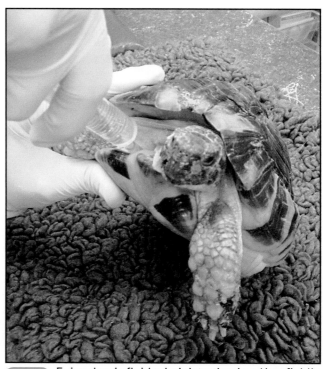

6.13 Epicoelomic fluid administration in a Horsfield's tortoise. (© Emma Whitlock)

Intracoelomic and epicoelomic administration in reptiles

- A suitable access site and method for intracoelomic administration in chelonians and lizards is the prefemoral fossa:
  1. Restrain the patient in lateral recumbency so that the viscera and reproductive organs fall away from the injection site.
  2. Insert the needle parallel to the plastron and cranially into the ventral aspect of the fossa in chelonians (see Figure 6.12), or in front of the hindlimb of a lizard.
  3. Aspirate to check for air or fluid.
     - If inserted too far dorsally, there is a risk of lung puncture.
     - If the patient urinates as the needle is inserted it may mean that the bladder has been entered. The needle should be withdrawn and the procedure repeated.
- A suitable access site and method for intracoelomic administration in snakes is the lateroventral aspect of the distal third of the body, cranial to the cloaca. Excessive volume of fluids given via this route can result in respiratory compromise. No more than 3% of bodyweight per day should be given, in divided doses.
- A suitable access site and method for epicoelomic administration in chelonians is into the epicoelomic cavity at the cranial inlet of the shell, lateroventral to the head and neck, immediately dorsal to the plastron and ventral to the pectoral musculature.
- **Maximum amounts:** 1–2% bodyweight/day in divided doses (0.5–1% recommended unless severely dehydrated).

Method for intraperitoneal administration in small mammals

1. Restrain the animal in dorsal recumbency to allow visceral organs to fall away from the injection site.
2. Insert the needle into the lower abdomen (Figure 6.14), to either side (to avoid accidental puncture of the bladder). There should be no resistance to injection.
3. Aspirate to check for accidental insertion into the bladder or intestine.

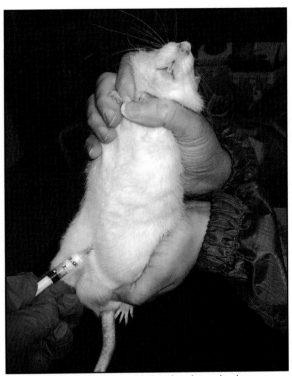

6.14 Intraperitoneal injection into the lower right quadrant of a rat. (Courtesy of Richard Saunders)

Intraperitoneal administration

This route of fluid administration is only suitable in small mammals and is not recommended in the conscious patient without excellent restraint or anaesthesia, due to the risk of visceral organ perforation and subsequent peritonitis.

Intraperitoneal administration allows rapid delivery of fluids where other administration sites are limited. Relatively large volumes of fluid can be given, with more rapid uptake than that following subcutaneous administration.

There should be minimal discomfort if appropriate volumes are administered in the correct way. Intraperitoneal administration may also warm and hydrate the gastrointestinal tract directly, with benefits in disorders such as gut stasis. There are, however, some risks associated with this method:

- Accidental organ puncture (most notably the large intestine and caecum in herbivores)
- Stressful restraint for correct positioning
- Diaphragmatic pressure may increase respiratory effort required for normal respiration
- Restraint for this route may be difficult in the conscious ferret or large rabbit.

Monitoring the effectiveness of a fluid plan

Effectiveness of the fluid plan may be assessed by monitoring the following parameters at the outset and regularly throughout the three phases (resuscitation, hydration and maintenance) of rehydration therapy:

- Clinical perfusion parameters:
  - Physical parameters: mucous membrane colour, capillary refill time, extremity and core temperatures, pulse rate and quality
  - Doppler blood pressure monitoring (note that this is unvalidated in smaller species)
  - Saturated oxygen percentage (S_pO_2) using a pulse oximeter or blood gas analysis machine, e.g. i-STAT (Abbott)
- Packed cell volume (PCV) and total protein measurement:
  - Normal PCV indicates the presence of

oxygen-carrying red blood cells but does not show whether/how well the body is utilizing that oxygen. Values must be considered alongside perfusion assessment
  – Total protein and PCV values should decrease following successful rehydration therapy. PCV values may concurrently decrease with ongoing blood losses, which may confound the picture
- Hydration status
- Bodyweight
- Frequency, concentration and approximate amounts of urine passed, based on subjective evaluation and/or laboratory analysis and measuring of fluid volumes or weights of bedding.

Detrimental effects following over-administration of fluids include:

- Serous nasal discharge
- Chemosis (conjunctival oedema)
- Restlessness
- Shivering
- Tachycardia
- Coughing
- Tachypnoea
- Dyspnoea
- Pulmonary crackles
- Ascites
- Polyuria
- Vomiting and/or diarrhoea
- Exophthalmia (abnormal protrusion of the eyeball)
- Jugular distension.

Fluid therapy should be stopped immediately if any of the above signs are observed, and the fluid and treatment plan re-evaluated. Oxygen supplementation should be considered if the patient is dyspnoeic. Diuretics may be indicated to remove some of the excess fluid.

Monitoring transfusions of natural blood products

Monitoring blood transfusion patients is vitally important, not only to ascertain whether or not the transfusion has been effective but also to identify (and manage) a transfusion reaction quickly. Acute haemolytic transfusion reactions have not been reported in exotic pets but may occur in other species following the administration of mismatched blood. Pre-treatment with antihistamines or corticosteroids has not been shown to have any effect in preventing transfusion reactions (Lichtenberger, 2004b). Signs of such reactions in small animals include:

- Vascular collapse
- Bronchospasm
- Haemorrhage associated with disseminated intravascular coagulation.

Elevation of body temperature above baseline values at any point during the transfusion requires cessation of the procedure and provision of supportive therapy with fluids, bronchodilators and corticosteroids (Lichtenberger, 2004b).

When monitoring the HBOC transfusion patient it is important to note that dose-dependent yellow-orange discoloration of the mucous membranes, sclera and urine occur, but this side effect will resolve within 3–5 days after administration. Colorimetric laboratory tests may also be invalidated for 48–72 hours after administration (Orcutt, 2000a).

Nutritional support

Nutritional support is one of the most time-consuming aspects of the nursing care of an individual patient, but is also one of the most rewarding. Provision of appropriate, effective nutrition is vitally important and cannot be ignored or underestimated.

One of the key factors when providing nutritional support to an exotic patient is an awareness of the animal's natural history and husbandry requirements; when it is understood what, how and when a particular patient would eat in its natural environment, consideration of how to provide balanced nutritional support in the hospital environment can be applied.

Providing nutritional support in the hospital environment

- Always encourage the owner to bring some of the patient's regular food in to the hospital; this reduces the need to stock every commercial diet available and minimizes the risk of the patient not eating what is offered, which is a real problem when attempting to encourage self-feeding.
- Even if the diet that is being offered at home is unsuitable, changes should be instigated gradually; it is therefore always preferable to have some of the animal's usual diet.
- For prolonged hospital stays, ensure that appropriate supplementation is provided (e.g. calcium and vitamin D for reptiles and vitamin C for guinea pigs).
- **Water should be provided for all patients at all times,** even if they live naturally in a desert environment. Ensure that water is offered in an appropriate receptacle and change it immediately if it becomes soiled. Remember that water in a hot environment (such as a vivarium) will increase the humidity considerably as it evaporates.
- In inappetent patients that normally receive their fluid maintenance requirement from their diet, it is important to ensure that those fluids are supplied via enteral or parenteral routes.

In small mammals and birds a positive energy balance must be maintained due to their high metabolic rate. Such patients should never go for more than a few hours without being fed; nutritional support should therefore be instigated immediately, alongside concurrent (rehydration) therapies. In rabbits, it is particularly important to maintain a positive energy balance in order to prevent the onset of hepatic lipidosis; this occurs when fatty acids are mobilized as a compensatory measure (usually following an anorexic episode), potentially resulting in liver failure as the body becomes overwhelmed due to the fatty acids accumulating within the hepatocytes. Regular assisted feeding of rabbits and herbivorous rodents with a high-fibre diet also maintains gastrointestinal motility and minimizes the risks associated with gastrointestinal stasis.

Re-feeding syndrome

- In (chronically anorexic) reptiles, sudden excess calories and proteins will result in rapid uptake of glucose from the bloodstream into the cells, together with potassium and phosphate ions, resulting in a potentially life-threatening hypokalaemia and hypophosphataemia (known as re-feeding syndrome).
- Monitoring of blood phosphorus and potassium is recommended in such patients but it is safe to assume that reptiles can be fed once they have passed urates (following correction of fluid deficits).

Which food to keep in stock

It is important to maintain stocks of the most commonly used diets and/or to have a local supplier so that suitable food items can be readily accessed at short notice. All food must be maintained for maximum freshness, including any diets provided by the owner. To save wastage and spoiling of food, storing small amounts is sensible and, in many cases, the shelf-life of a food item can be prolonged by freezing.

In the authors' experience, the most useful foods to keep in stock (for aiding with nutritional support) include:

- Herbivore convalescence diets such as Oxbow Critical Care Formula and Oxbow Critical Care Fine Grind (sachets can be frozen if they are not likely to be used before the use-by date)
- Avian convalescence diets such as Harrison's Recovery Formula
- Carnivore convalescence diets such as Oxbow Carnivore Care or Hills a/d
- Liquid enteral diets such as Ensure or Royal Canin Convalescence Support
- Frozen carnivore whole prey items such as day-old chicks, mice, rats and quail
- Invertebrates such as locusts, crickets and mealworms
- Herbs and salad items (a home-grown weed patch is an excellent commodity)
- Hay and/or fresh forage (good quality barn-dried grass)
- Free choice diets for the most commonly seen species.

Assisted feeding methods

Correction of fluid deficits

Before attempting assisted feeding, fluid deficits should be corrected (usually over a period of 48–72 hours). In raptors, the correction of fluid deficits will aid in the prevention of 'sour crop', caused by reduced gastrointestinal motility and food remaining and fermenting within the crop. However, in many patients provision of adequate nutrition will be a priority (and replacing fluid deficits *prior* to feeding not an option) so small amounts of food with a high fluid content should be offered regularly to ensure effective transit and digestion of nutritive material and a reduced risk of stagnation and fermentation within the crop.

The general rule when supporting hospitalized exotic species nutritionally is: 'if the mouth works use it!'. If the gastrointestinal tract cannot be utilized to provide enteral nutrition then parenteral (outside of the gastrointestinal tract) nutrition options must be considered.

Assisted feeding methods ensure that patients that are losing or failing to gain weight receive the correct calorific requirement for the day. The assisted feeding method employed will depend upon the patient and its problems, and upon the food being offered.

When instigating an assisted feeding method a nutritional plan should be made, and the patient monitored as part of this plan. Monitoring of a nutritional plan is discussed later, but *all* patients should:

- Be weighed each day at the same time on the same set of scales:
  - It is recommended that all patients are weighed at the start of the day, prior to administering any medication, food or fluids, to allow for alterations in amounts, dosing rates or frequencies where necessary
  - The patient's daily weight should be recorded and compared with that of the previous day(s)
- Be monitored for changes (positive or negative) in body condition and hydration status.

Enhancing free-choice feeding

Although not strictly 'assisted', feeding by free choice can be encouraged by:

- Offering nutritional but also highly palatable foods (e.g. for herbivores, herbs, including basil and parsley, or weeds such as dandelions)
- Offering foods that are particularly digestible, such as convalescence diets intended for syringe-feeding, which can be made to a thicker consistency and offered in a way suitable for free-choice feeding (Figure 6.15)
- Offering some of the patient's own food and/or favourite treats from the owner
- Increasing palatability of the food by crushing or heating to release the smell, or by mixing or soaking with other food items

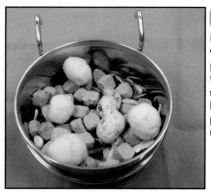

6.15 Harrison's 'Recovery Balls' mixed in with seed and pelleted diets for encouraging self-feeding in hospitalized psittacine birds. (© Emma Whitlock)

- Ensuring that food is presented appropriately for the individual patient:
  - Consider toilet areas and feeding positions, times, etc.
  - Present food in a manner appropriate to the patient (scatter-feeding rather than placing food in bowls, tearing open whole prey to look more like carrion or using naturally coloured food items such as agouti rats and mice)
- Removing food as soon as it is past its best presentation state (e.g. wilted, dried out, warm or cold) and then offering fresh food
- Abundance-feeding herbivores (Figure 6.16), where the cage floor is covered with a variety of leafy greens or forage hay or grasses (best for rabbits, guinea pigs and herbivorous chelonians).

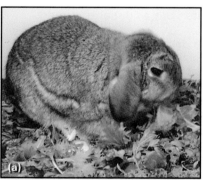

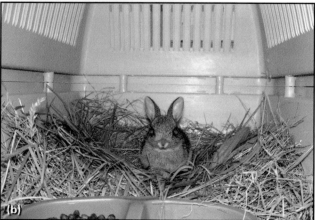

6.16 **(a)** Abundance feeding of leafy greens to a previously inappetent rabbit. (© Emma Whitlock) **(b)** Abundance feeding of good quality fresh forage to an inappetent wild rabbit. (Courtesy of Richard Saunders)

If expecting or encouraging a patient to feed by free choice, natural conditions should be simulated as closely as possible. For example, some semi-aquatic species of turtle will only eat food that is submerged in water and so food should be offered in this way. Similarly, waterfowl usually feed off or under the water, so grainy feed should be scattered in water bowls or trays.

The most important things to consider when offering free-choice foods are:

- How does the patient normally eat? Chelonians, for example, are very sight-oriented when it comes to feeding, whereas carnivores often rely on olfactory senses
- Can appetite be monitored? Cage mates may have to be separated
- Does free-choice feeding need to be supplemented with an assisted feeding method? Monitoring the patient's weight, hydration and condition gives an accurate indication as to whether or not free-choice feeding alone is adequate to maintain optimal nutritional status.

Suitable fresh greens for mammalian herbivores:

- Watercress
- Spinach
- Kale
- Carrot tops
- Herbs, including:
  - Basil
  - Parsley
  - Coriander
  - Dill
  - Oregano
  - Rosemary
- Weeds, including:
  - Dandelions
  - Clover
  - Nettle
  - Coltsfoot.

Suitable fresh greens for reptilian herbivores:

- Watercress
- Spinach
- Weeds, including:
  - Dandelions
  - Clover
  - Timothy grass
  - Nettle
  - Thistle.

Hand-feeding

Some patients that are capable of prehending and masticating food will only do so if encouraged to via hand-feeding (Figure 6.17). Likewise, such patients may only take onboard enough calories if fed regularly by hand throughout the day.

Certain species (particularly chelonians) are very sight-oriented when it comes to food selection and

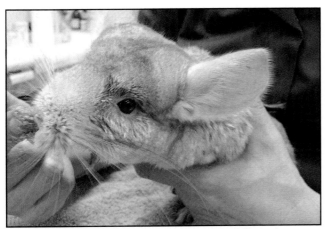

6.17 Assisted hand-feeding of a chinchilla using a herbivore convalescence formula. (Courtesy of Terri Pettis)

feeding, so will benefit from hand-feeding if they have any degree of optical impairment. The smell of fresh foods can be enhanced for sight-impaired (or inappetent) chelonians by crushing the food between the fingers before holding it just in front of the patient's face; many chelonians will then be able to find and consume the food. Smearing juices on a chelonian's beak is also helpful in encouraging self-feeding.

Where olfaction is reduced by nasal discharge or blocked nares, regular gentle cleaning of debris and/or steaming or nebulization of the environment may help to encourage the patient to feed more regularly and effectively.

Hand-feeding can also be used to encourage very lethargic or depressed patients, especially if the smell is enhanced as described above (with vegetable matter) or by heating an appropriate convalescence formula (taking great care if using a microwave, stirring well and testing for 'hot spots').

Syringe-feeding

Syringe-feeding involves syringing food into a patient's mouth for voluntary mastication and swallowing (Figure 6.18). Diets for syringe-feeding must be soft enough to pass through a syringe and into the animal's mouth. Commercially prepared diets are available, suitable for different dietary types.

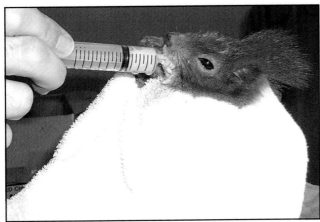

6.18 Assisted hand-feeding of a juvenile red squirrel using a syringe. (Courtesy of Richard Saunders)

Herbivores will often readily take a commercially prepared formula (e.g. Oxbow Critical Care Formula) from a syringe, although care must be taken not to over-fill the mouth before the patient has had time to swallow. To facilitate syringe-feeding with a commercially prepared convalescent formula:

- Use tepid water to make up the mixture:
  - *Always* test the temperature prior to feeding, to prevent burns
  - Avoid the use of a microwave to heat food items where possible but, if used, stir thoroughly and test for 'hot spots'
- Use a feeding syringe that has a large-bore tip (Figure 6.19), even if only feeding a small amount, to prevent food from being squirted into the patient's mouth (and possibly respiratory tract) at high pressure, especially where high-fibre foods increase the risk of nozzle blockage and sudden high pressure release of the food material
- Only syringe 1–2 ml of food into the patient's mouth at any one time
- Ensure that the syringe tip is removed from the patient's mouth to allow the patient to masticate and swallow before gently reinserting it and syringing the next 1–2 ml
- Monitor the animal following feeding for complications, including:
  - Dribbling of food
  - Abnormal respiratory signs
  - Vomiting and/or diarrhoea
  - Any signs of discomfort or deterioration in condition.

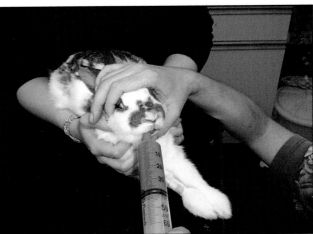

6.19 Syringe-feeding a rabbit with a convalescent herbivore formula in a wide-bore feeding syringe. (© Emma Whitlock)

Suitable fibrous diets for syringe-feeding to herbivores include:

- Oxbow Critical Care Formula.
- Oxbow Critical Care Fine Grind
- Liquidized greens made up in house
- Vetark Critical Care Formula
- Mashed pelleted diets
- Supreme Science Recovery.

Suitable diets for syringe-feeding to frugivorous and granivorous birds include:

■ Harrison's Recovery Formula or other appropriate convalescence formulas
■ Vetark Critical Care Formula
■ An appropriate juvenile-rearing diet if feeding a juvenile bird
■ Human enteral feeding products (e.g. Ensure).

Suitable diets for syringe-feeding to omnivores and carnivores include:

■ Oxbow Carnivore Care
■ Hills a/d
■ Liquivite convalescence diet
■ Home-cooked diets, including 'duck soup' for ferrets
■ Veterinary enteral feeding liquids such as Enteral Care Royal Canin Convalescence support diets
■ Human enteral feeding products (e.g. Ensure).

Specialist diet items (also suitable for syringe-feeding)

■ Nectar for nectivorous birds.
■ Dried insect food for genuine insectivores (e.g. Bogena, Prosecto Insectivorous).
■ Hand-rearing formulas.
■ Weaning formulas.
■ Liquid parenteral formulas (see later).

Gavage

Gavage is the introduction of nutritive material into the stomach by means of a tube. Feeding by insertion of a rigid or flexible tube attached to the end of a syringe is a common method for administering nutrition (and drugs and fluids) to exotic patients and is a suitable method in birds, reptiles and small rodents.

Rigid (crop) tubes tend to be used for birds to administer solutions directly into the crop, and come in a variety of sizes. It is advisable to use as large a tube as appropriate for chelonians and birds, to reduce the risk of accidental insertion of the tube into the trachea. Soft tubes can easily be made from cut-off giving set tubing, feline and canine urinary catheters and paediatric feeding tubes, and are less traumatic in animals that are likely to move when handled; however, they may be more easily passed into the trachea by accident.

To facilitate gavage in suitable patients:

■ Select a tube that is large enough to limit the risk of accidental insertion into the trachea but not so large as to damage the oesophagus or pharyngeal mucosa on insertion
■ Ensure that the tube end, whether flexible or rigid, is not sharp:

  – Manufactured feeding tubes have a smooth bulbous tip
  – Heating a cut-off plastic tube briefly over a lit flame helps to soften and round-off a sharp end
■ Ensure effective and appropriate restraint of the patient before attempting gavage
■ Ensure that all equipment is ready prior to starting and, if performing other checks or procedures on the patient, ensure gavage is performed immediately prior to returning the patient to its cage, to reduce the risk of regurgitation and accidental inhalation of solutions
■ Measure any tubes (rigid or flexible) against the patient to gauge the position of the crop or stomach and ensure that the tube does not pass further than necessary
■ Lubricate the tube lightly before use
■ Use a mouth gag (Figure 6.20) to facilitate introduction of a flexible tube if the patient is likely to bite through the tube or if it will be difficult to hold the mouth open for long enough to allow for feeding. In birds of prey, use a thumb placed in the commissure (corner) of the beak to safely hold the beak open
■ *Never* force any tube (rigid or flexible) if there is resistance
■ Ascertain the correct positioning of a crop tube in birds by gently palpating over the crop area. The tube should be felt within the crop
■ Administer solutions slowly and monitor for regurgitation constantly during feeding. If a patient does regurgitate, *do not* attempt to remove the solution but immediately place the patient back in its cage and monitor it closely. It should clear its mouth effectively itself.

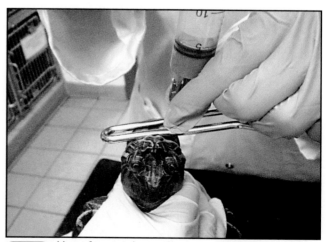

6.20 Use of a metal mouth gag to facilitate gavage for assisted nutrition in a semi-aquatic red-eared terrapin. (© Elisabetta Mancinelli)

For a full description of tube insertion in different patients see Fluid therapy, earlier.

Use of *in situ* feeding tubes

Soft feeding tubes can be inserted and then sutured or taped in position for an extended period of time to reduce the stress associated with intermittent gavage tubing. Handling a patient that has an *in situ* feeding tube is minimal and hence such tubes are recommended for patients that will require regular feeding by gavage for more than a day or two. *In situ* feeding tubes are commonly used in chelonians but are used less often in other species. However, the use of these tubes in other species is possible and in many cases they have been used successfully.

Oesophagostomy/pharyngostomy tubes

Pharyngostomy tubes are most commonly placed in anorexic chelonians (Figure 6.21). They can be left in place for an extended period of time – even for several months. Semi-aquatic species of turtle may also benefit greatly from the use of oesophagostomy tubes if they are 'dry docked', where the need for exposure to water to enable/encourage natural self-feeding can pose problems if the patient's condition prevents them from residing within an aquatic environment.

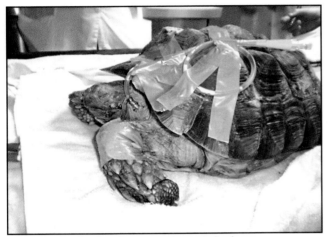

6.21 An *in situ* pharyngostomy tube in a Mediterranean tortoise. (Courtesy of Elisabetta Manicinelli)

Pharyngostomy tubes have been successfully used in ferrets in much the same way as for feline patients (Powers, 2006a) and in birds with crop lesions (Powers, 2006b).

Oesophagostomy tubes are inserted into the oesophagus via a small incision in the neck; a surgical procedure is therefore required for placement of such tubes.

Naso-oesophageal tubes

Naso-oesophageal tubes (Figure 6.22) are much the same as oesophagostomy tubes but are shorter and pass from the nasal cavity to the distal oesophagus rather than directly into the stomach, so no surgical procedure is required for placement. The nursing care required for this type of tube is therefore very much the same as that for oesophagostomy tubes, but extra care should be taken to keep the nares clean and free from debris, particularly in obligate nasal breathers such as rabbits.

Naso-oesophageal tubes tend to irritate the mucosa of the nasal cavity in small mammals, so may not be suitable in such patients, especially for long-term use. Naso-oesophageal tubes have to be narrow enough to pass through the small space of

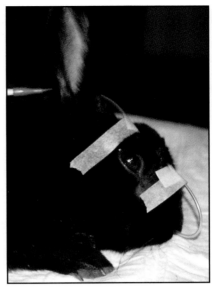

6.22 A naso-oesophageal feeding tube may be useful for delivering enteral fluid and nutritional support. (Reproduced from the *BSAVA Manual of Rabbit Medicine and Surgery*, 2nd edition)

the nasal cavity, which means that most enteral formulas (including Oxbow Critical Care Fine Grind) are too viscous to pass through and will block the tube. Vetark Critical Care Formula is less viscous and so is more suited in these cases, and can be used as a short- to medium-term solution, providing that the patient's weight, condition and clinical parameters are closely monitored.

Nursing care with *in situ* feeding tubes

- Always use a suitable tube-feeding formula appropriate to the diameter of the tube in use (Oxbow Critical Care Fine Grind or Vetark Critical Care Formula are recommended by the authors).
- When feeding the patient:
  1. Swab the hub of the feeding tube with an appropriate antiseptic solution.
  2. Draw back with an empty syringe to ascertain correct placement of the tube. If air enters the syringe, *do not feed* (the tube may be located within the respiratory tract).
  3. Flush the tube with a small amount of sterile saline before administering food to further ascertain patency and correct positioning. If the patient coughs or shows respiratory signs do not *feed*.
  4. Always flush the tube with sterile saline *after* feeding to ensure that food does not dry within the tube and block it.
- Clean around the tube placement site regularly and observe daily for any sign of infection (swelling, heat, exudate) at the insertion site.
- *Always* provide the patient with their normal diet when using an *in situ* feeding tube. Chelonians, in particular, tolerate such tubes well and will happily 'eat around' them, the idea being that the tube can be removed once the patient is no longer anorexic, so food must be offered to encourage self-feeding and establish when the patient starts to eat.

Parenteral nutrition

Although not commonly used in exotic animal medicine within the UK, parenteral nutrition offers a viable solution where appropriate and balanced enteral nutrition is impossible to achieve. Parenteral nutrition was initially described in the ferret but has now been used in small herbivores by practitioners without complication (Orcutt, 2000b).

> ### Parenteral nutrition may be considered if the following criteria can be satisfied:
>
> - Corrections have been made in electrolyte and/or acid–base abnormalities, tachycardia, volume deficits and hypotension
> - Nutritional intake is actually, or anticipated to be, less than the resting energy requirement (RER) for 3 days or more
> - An enteral nutritional route cannot be safely established or maintained, or a small intestinal disorder is confirmed or suspected
> - The patient will be hospitalized for 3 days or more.

A suitable total nutrient admixture (TNA) for parenteral nutrition in small herbivores can be made up by a specialist laboratory or a willing human hospital (compounding the mixture in-house is not viable for most practices). The primary components for a TNA suitable for use in small herbivorous mammals are dextrose, lipid and amino acids, combined with added B vitamins, trace minerals, electrolytes and crystalloid fluids to meet the patient's fluid requirement.

Delivery of parenteral nutrition is usually via a central venous catheter and the solution *must* be at room temperature. Solutions with an osmolarity of >600 mOsm/l should be used to prevent the occurrence of thrombophlebitis. If a peripheral catheter is deemed an appropriate or preferred means of providing parenteral nutrition, solutions with an osmolarity of <600 mOsm/l should be used (created by increasing the percentage of lipid within the solution). Intraosseous and intraperitoneal routes have also been used successfully (McClure *et al.*, 1992).

Using parenteral routes to deliver nutritional support to veterinary patients is a temporary method and thus nutrition need only be partial and *not* total, as it is in human medicine. Only 80% of the patient's energy requirement is necessary and this usually equates to the resting energy requirement (RER).

The most important points to consider when monitoring a patient that is receiving nutritional support via the parenteral route are those concerned with *in situ* catheter use. It is vitally important to ensure that the catheter and insertion site remain clean and free from infection and thrombi.

Nutritional plans

Nutritional plans should occur naturally as part of the nursing care plan; a specifically formulated sheet can be used to outline the plan and record administration of food and patient progress (positive or negative), or details can simply be recorded within the patient's hospital chart, but all details must be recorded for continuity of care, regardless of staff change-overs.

> ### When making a nutritional plan, veterinary staff must:
>
> - Ascertain what the patient's weight *should* be
> - Know what the patient's weight actually is at the time of making the plan
> - Assess the patient's body condition and understand what the condition should be
> - Know what daily calorific requirement the patient has
> - Understand the best method of providing adequate nutrition to each individual patient
> - Have criteria for measuring and thus monitoring the success of a nutritional plan
> - Have monitoring goals and timescales
> - Have criteria for the endpoint in the nutritional plan (e.g. once the animal is eating the correct foods by free choice and is at and maintaining optimal weight, body condition and hydration status).

In order to monitor the effectiveness of nutritional support, it is vital to know exactly what, how and when the patient is eating. In some situations, food may need to be weighed or discrete items counted before offering to the patient and this exercise repeated upon removal of uneaten food from the patient's environment, so as to assess accurately how much is being eaten. It is, however, important to consider that other losses must be accounted for. Seed- and fruit-eating birds, for example, may drop a proportion of their food on to the floor of their environment. Also, when weighing seed diets, it should be remembered that the kernel weighs a lot less then the seed shell.

In multi-animal situations, cage mates may need to be separated in order to monitor what is being eaten (and excreted) by an individual. Good record-keeping and communication is vital so that all staff members can see how the patient is being supported nutritionally. All information relating to nutritional support should be detailed on the patient's notes, including:

- A daily weight measurement for the patient (taken at the same time each day, on the same set of scales)
- Any information relating to body condition assessments and scores
- Any voluntary feeding (when and what)
- Excretion (when, what, anything unusual)
- When assisted feeding was/should be carried out (how, what, by whom and when).

Assessing body condition

The patient's body condition should be regularly assessed alongside its weight. Body condition scoring is a tool that can help to assess the overall body status of the animal in conjunction with weighing.

When assessing body condition, the following should be considered:

- Bodyweight
- Frame size
- Body condition scoring
- General health status.

Mammals

To assess body condition in mammals, palpation for fat and muscle levels over the following areas should be carried out:

- Ribs
- Backbone
- Hips.

Body condition score: Mammals

- **1/5 (Very thin):** Ribs 'visible' and spine and hips easily visible in short-coated breeds and very prominent and sharp-edged on palpation; generally poor appearance; concave rump area; no dewlap present – or dewlap with no fat deposits (rabbits only) (Figure 6.23a).
- **2/5 (Thin):** Spine likely to be visible in short-coated breeds but ribs may not be visible; both spine and ribs easily palpated; flat rump area; dewlap not present or minimal, or no fat present within it.
- **3/5 (Good):** Ribs not visible and spine not easily visible. Both palpated easily but rounded edges, not sharp; generally trim appearance. A small dewlap may be present in mature unneutered females or neutered males.
- **4/5 (Fat):** Ribs and spine not visible but palpated moderately easily; generally rounded appearance; rounded rump area; moderate dewlap in females (neutered or entire) and neutered males and smaller dewlap in entire males.
- **5/5 (Obese):** Ribs and spine not visible and palpated with difficulty; generally rotund appearance, often with large skin/fat folds; convex rump area; large dewlap present in females and males (Figure 6.23b).

Adapted from Mullan and Main (2006), with additions by Lord and Saunders.

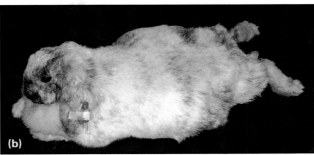

6.23 **(b)** An obese rabbit: body condition score 5/5. (Courtesy of Richard Saunders)

Birds

To assess body condition in birds, palpation for fat and muscle levels over the following areas should be carried out:

- Keel
- Ribs
- Pelvis.

Body condition score: Birds

The five-point system below uses the pectoral muscles, with a score of 1 given to a patient whose pectoral musculature is concave, 3 for a bird whose pectoral muscles is convex, and 5 when the muscles are extended beyond the keel.

- **1/5 (Very thin):** Protruding keel bone and depressed contour to breast muscles.
- **2/5 (Thin):** Prominent keel bone with poorly developed flat breast muscles.
- **3/5 (Good):** Less prominent keel bone and moderate (convex) breast muscle development.
- **4/5 (Fat):** Plump breast muscles, which provide a smooth contour with the keel.
- **5/5 (Obese):** Muscles extend beyond keel (Figure 6.24), visible fat deposits under skin (white to yellow) and partially filling the normal concavity of abdomen.

Adapted from Welle (1995).

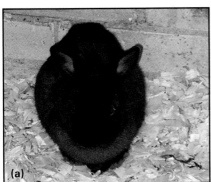

6.23 **(a)** A very thin rabbit: body condition score 0–1/5. (Courtesy of Richard Saunders)

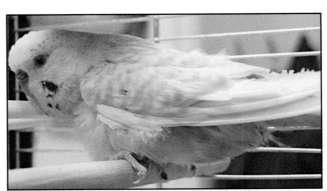

6.24 Morbid obesity in a budgerigar. It is very unusual to be able to assess body condition visually without palpation of the keel. (© John Chitty)

Reptiles

To assess body condition in reptiles, palpation over the following areas should be carried out:

- Spine
- Ribs
- Pelvis
- Tail.

Body condition score: Lizards

- **1/5 (Very thin):** Skeletal features including the spinous processes, limb bones, ribcage, pelvis and skull are easily 'visible' and prominent due to lack of fat and muscle coverage. The tail contains no fat storage and tapers sharply from the pelvis to the tip (Figure 6.25a).
- **2/5 (Thin):** The spinal processes, ribs and pelvis are still clearly visible but less prominent and sharp, with improved fat coverage along the backbone and limited muscle coverage visible in the head, limbs, shoulders and flanks. The tail contains a light amount of fat storage and tapers gradually from the pelvis to the tip.
- **3/5 (Good):** The spinal processes, ribs and pelvis are just visible or can be felt easily with light pressure, with even fat and muscle coverage along the back and flanks and good muscle coverage in the limbs. The trunk of the body has a uniform appearance from above, with the ribcage and abdomen being approximately the same width. The tail contains a moderate amount of fat storage and is slightly rounded in the middle section between the pelvis and tip (Figure 6.25b).
- **4/5 (Fat):** The spinal processes, ribs and pelvis are barely visible and can only be palpated with gentle to medium pressure. The flanks carry a moderate covering of fat over muscle and the abdomen appears slightly broader than the ribcage when viewed from above, and slightly distended when viewed from the side. The tail carries a large amount of fat storage and is notably rounded in the middle section between the pelvis and tip.
- **5/5 (Obese):** The spinal processes, ribs and pelvic bones cannot be seen from any angle and can only be palpated with moderate pressure. The back, flanks and limbs carry an excessive covering of fat masking the muscle beneath, and the abdomen appears significantly distended from the side and broader than the ribcage from above. The tail carries a very high volume of fat storage, which is significantly rounded and broad in the middle section (Figure 6.25c).

Adapted from *Practical Reptile Keeping* Dec 2009/Jan 2010.

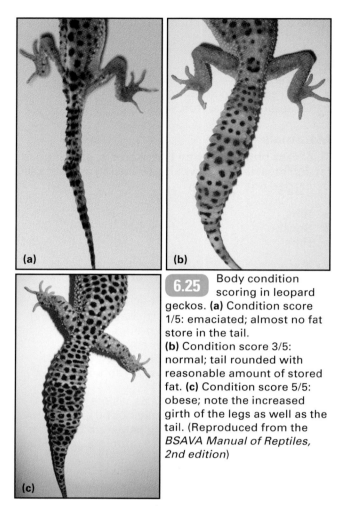

6.25 Body condition scoring in leopard geckos. **(a)** Condition score 1/5: emaciated; almost no fat store in the tail. **(b)** Condition score 3/5: normal; tail rounded with reasonable amount of stored fat. **(c)** Condition score 5/5: obese; note the increased girth of the legs as well as the tail. (Reproduced from the *BSAVA Manual of Reptiles, 2nd edition*)

In snakes, the only indicator of body condition is the concavity or convexity of the lumbar musculature; snakes appear fat or thin, dependent upon condition.

Body condition in chelonians is difficult to assess due to the anatomy of the shell and the body within it; reference can be made to published weight-to-length ratios (e.g. the Jackson's ratio), but these are species-specific, affected by other factors such as weight of reproductive tract, bladder and liver, and are often based on wild-caught animals and so must be interpreted with care. The extremities can be examined as for lizards.

Calculating calorie requirements in hospitalized patients

The patient's daily calorie requirement must be worked out on an individual basis by calculating its basal energy requirement (BER) and multiplying by a disease factor.

The basal energy requirement

The BER is the energy required by an animal at complete rest at a neutral temperature. It differs depending on the size of an animal (smaller animals require relatively more energy than larger ones) and its taxonomic group. The relative basal metabolic rate for each taxonomic group is represented by a K value.

K values

- Placental mammals: 70
- Marsupials: 49
- Passerine birds: 129
- Non-passerine birds: 78
- Reptiles: 10

The basal energy requirement is calculated using the equation:

$$\textbf{BER (kcal/day) = K x (bodyweight in kg)}^{0.75}$$

So, for each taxonomic group, the BER can be calculated as follows:

- Mammals:
  - Placental: BER (kcal/day) = 70 x (bodyweight in kg)$^{0.75}$
  - Marsupial: BER (kcal/day) = 49 x (bodyweight in kg)$^{0.75}$
- Birds:
  - Passerine: BER (kcal/day) = 129 x (bodyweight in kg)$^{0.75}$
  - Non-passerine: BER (kcal/day) = 78 x (bodyweight in kg)$^{0.75}$
- Reptiles: BER (kcal/day) = 10 x (bodyweight in kg)$^{0.75}$

It should be remembered that the correct environmental temperature for small mammals and birds should be strictly maintained to prevent energy expenditure as the patient attempts to maintain the preferred body temperature; if the environmental temperature is not optimal, calorific requirements should be adjusted accordingly.

The disease factor

In most hospital situations, patients will require more than the BER in any given day. The disease factor is used to take into account the different circumstances of individual patients:

- Growth: 1.5–2.0 x BER
- Cage rest: 1.25 x BER
- Post anorexia/starvation: 1.25 x BER
- Post surgery: 1.25 x BER
- With severe burns: 1.5–2.0 x BER
- In sepsis: 1.5–2.0 x BER
- Following trauma: 1.5 x BER
- With neoplasia: 1.5 x BER
- With hepatic disease: 1.25 x BER
- With severe renal disease: 1.25 x BER.

Recent research carried out on hospitalized dogs and cats has suggested that their energy requirements were much closer to the RER than previously thought. (RER = BER + energy required for assimilation of food and recovery from physical activity). However, experience with less common species suggests that using lower estimates of calorie requirements results in weight loss in practice. It is therefore recommended that the use of disease factors is continued until more solid research is undertaken in exotic species.

Worked example: A 1.2 kg ferret, after surgery

Using the information given above, the ferret is a placental mammal so:

$$\textbf{BER = 70 x 1.2}^{0.75}\textbf{ = 80.25 kcal/day}$$

Postsurgical energy requirement = 1.25 x 80.25 = 100 kcal/day

The ferret is being syringe-fed a diet of Hills a/d, each 156 g tin of which contains 179 kcal.

179 ÷ 156 = 1.15 kcal/g

100 ÷ 1.15 = 87 g

The ferret therefore requires approximately 87 g of Hills a/d in a 24-hour period. This should be divided into equal manageable doses.

Administering drugs

There is a common misconception among some non-specialist veterinary staff that exotic species should not be stressed by handling and medicating, and that very little should, and indeed can, be done to treat their disease problems. While such factors should be borne in mind, failing to give effective treatment is generally far more detrimental to the patient and there is now a wealth of information about treatment options, including drug dosages, available to help veterinary staff to provide gold standard care to the exotic species seen in practice and, armed with this information, to feel more comfortable prescribing and administering drugs for them.

When administering drugs for exotic species:

DO:
- Use the correct dose for each species, rather than extrapolating from the dose recommended for cats or dogs; an up-to-date exotic animal formulary (see References and further reading) should be on-hand at all times
- Administer drugs in the most appropriate site and by the most appropriate route for the exotic species concerned
- Take into account the small size of exotic patients and have the correct administration equipment available.

DO NOT:
- Extrapolate from other species and give drugs with no knowledge of their effects or toxicities in any given species (e.g. the use of avermectins in chelonians causes irreversible neurological signs, commonly leading to death)
- Administer drugs via the route you are accustomed to if there is a more effective/appropriate route in the exotic species concerned; a basic knowledge of the species' anatomy and physiology should be applied, and up-to-date texts explaining how to give drugs should be consulted.

Armed with knowledge about the species and the problems they may face, there is no need to fear the exotic species seen in practice; it is, however, important always to understand that these are non-domesticated species and to consider the stresses that this places upon the animals. The stress of handling should always be weighed against the need for a particular treatment. Therapies should be administered and the patient handled in a way that minimizes stress. Very rarely should an exotic patient be 'left' calm and quiet because of concerns about the stress of handling/treating; more commonly the patient will have a life-threatening disease or injury that will not resolve unless treated. It may, however, be appropriate to stabilize the patient by providing warmth, fluid therapy, analgesia and antimicrobials pending further examination and treatment.

Preparation

Organization and preparation are key when planning any procedure that may result in stress to exotic patients. Everything required should be out and ready before the patient is removed from its hospital housing; this will allow procedures to be carried out quickly, effectively and quietly, minimizing handling time and stress.

When preparing to dose exotic species (particularly small patients) it is vital to have a current and accurate weight prior to dosing the patient with any drug. Small species can easily be inaccurately dosed if the weight is incorrectly estimated or not current. The patient's weight should be taken every morning at the same time on the same scales *prior* to giving any therapeutics, and more frequently where necessary.

Necessary equipment

Equipment required for the administration of drugs to exotic patients is likely to be kept in the practice anyway but should include:

- Appropriately sized needles:
  - Spinal needles for intraosseous catheter placement
  - 27 gauge 5/8 inch needles
- Small dosing syringes:
  - 100 IU/ml insulin syringes for very small amounts – although the needle on an insulin syringe is often too fine for delivering through the skin of reptiles
- Short, 26–22 gauge intravenous catheters
- Syringe drivers and fluid pumps to prevent over-infusion in small patients
- Paediatric (burette) giving sets
- Rigid and flexible feeding tubes for *in situ* and intermittent use.

The mixing of different drugs in the same syringe should be avoided; the drugs may not be compatible, and dose inaccuracies due to drug contained within the needle hub may be very significant with small volumes.

Paediatric solutions

Where available, the use of human paediatric formulations should be considered, as these are easy to administer and allow more accurate dosing. Often such solutions allow for easier dosing by mouth, mixed in a small amount of food, in a favourite drink or yoghurt or given via a syringe.

Administering very small amounts

Calculating and delivering very small drug dosages is potentially prone to calamitous error. To simplify the process and to minimize delays and errors, the following should be kept to hand at all times:

- Up-to-date exotic animal drug formularies
- Calculator
- Paper and pens
- Weighing scales that are accurate to at least 0.1 g
- Pre-calculated charts or tables for commonly used or emergency medications.

Diluting drugs

When very small doses are required, it is often necessary to dilute the drug to allow the small amount of drug to be administered in a larger volume of solution (e.g. 0.001 ml of a drug is impossible to administer accurately, but the drug can be diluted 1:100 so that 0.1 ml of solution is administered and the patient receives the required dose).

When diluting drugs, a suitable substance should be used as a diluent:

- Use only sterile water or 0.9% saline if diluted drugs are to be injected
- Use tap or filtered water, or oral fluids for diluting oral drugs. To make oral dosing easier, substitute half of the water used as a diluent with petroleum jelly (e.g. K–Y), which will make the solution more viscous and easier to administer by mouth.

There are some problems with diluting drugs:

- Not all drugs can be diluted in this way, due to solubility and stability concerns
- Non-aqueous formulations do not mix evenly with water
- There is little published guidance on expiration dates for such drugs once diluted in this way. This must be taken into consideration when diluting drugs, and they should be made up freshly at regular intervals rather than kept diluted for long periods of time
- Excessive dilution may lead to larger volumes than may be safely given by intramuscular injection.

Understanding drug rates in dilution

- Drug concentration is expressed as a percentage (e.g. bupivacaine 0.25%).
- Percentage is measured in grams per ml, so that 1% = 1 g/100 ml or 1000 mg/100 ml or 10 mg/ml.
- To convert percentage to concentration (mg/ml), multiply by 10 (e.g. bupivacaine 0.25% = 2.5 mg/ml).
- If a drug is combined with a diluent, it is expressed as a dilution:

- 1:1,000 = 1 mg/ml (0.1%)
- 1:2,000 = 1 mg/2 ml (0.05%)
- 1:10,000 = 1 mg/10 ml (0.01%)
- 1:20,000 = 1 mg/20 ml (0.005%).

Worked example: Dilution

Meloxicam 5 mg/ml injectable solution, to be given to a 30 g mouse at a dose of 1 mg/kg (note that this is a considerably higher dose rate than for dogs and cats).

- Dose required = 0.03 mg = 0.006 ml. This is clearly an impractical dose to administer accurately.
- Diluting 0.1 ml of 5 mg/ml meloxicam with sterile water for injection to a total volume of 1 ml creates a solution containing 0.5 mg in 1 ml.
- This is not the same thing as adding 0.1 ml of meloxicam to 1 ml water, which would create a solution that contained 0.5 mg in 1.1 ml. The difference becomes minuscule at dilutions of 1 in 100.
- Each ingredient must be placed in turn into an appropriately sized fresh syringe (e.g. 2 ml), using a 100 IU/ml insulin syringe to draw up the drug accurately and an appropriately sized syringe (1 ml) to draw up the water, mixing well, and then withdrawing the correct amount of diluted drug with a fresh insulin syringe.
- The mixture must be very carefully mixed to avoid over- or under-dosing.
- The amount of diluted drug required is 0.06 ml.

Routes of drug administration

Slow intravenous injections (where the drug formulation is appropriate) are less painful and less irritating to tissue than are subcutaneous or intramuscular injections. Giving drugs intravenously via an indwelling catheter placed during an initial period of anaesthesia (at the time of a diagnostic work-up) and utilizing this catheter until the patient is stable and it is appropriate to give drugs orally (i.e. when the patient is eating or being fed via gavage and there are no apparent gut motility or absorption problems), reduces the stress and complications of unnecessary repeated injection and handling of the patient. It also reduces costs to the owner, as injectable drugs are often considerably more expensive than a course of oral treatment.

Oral administration

Where possible and appropriate, the gastrointestinal tract should be used. Oral dosing is suitable for most species and is often the easiest route by which to give medication. Placing oral doses on food or in drinking water is not recommended (other than for supplementary feed additives) because it is difficult to be sure that the whole dose has been taken and at the right time; it is also impossible to ascertain accurately which animal has taken a drug if there is more than one housed within the environment.

For patients that have *in situ* feeding tubes, oral medication can be given via the tube. As when feeding, care should be taken:

- Not to block the tube with the medication
- To ensure that the tube is in the correct place before administering the drug dose, by syringing a small amount of sterile saline to check for patency and position and observing for an abnormal respiratory reflex (e.g. coughing).

For administering oral drugs via gavage, it is most useful to medicate at the same time as feeding, as many oral drugs are absorbed more effectively with food. To ensure that the dose is given in full, the drug should be placed into the top of the pre-filled food syringe or into the feeding tube so that it is administered to the patient first; if the full food or fluid amount cannot be given in full (due to overfilling of the crop or regurgitation) the full drug dose will still have been given.

PRACTICAL TIP
Oral medication should not be given to birds of prey that cast the fur and feathers of their food unless the skin (with all fur/feathers) is removed from all food items before they are given to the bird.

For explanations of how best to medicate orally see Fluid therapy, earlier.

Subcutaneous administration

Many drugs can be given via subcutaneous injection, which is usually a rapid and relatively painless procedure. Repeated subcutaneous injections at the same site are not recommended, due to soft tissue damage, pain, and risk of secondary bacterial infection. Subcutaneous administration of drugs gives a relatively slow absorption rate and is not recommended in hypothermic individuals due to the further decrease in absorption time.

Complications and risks are associated with subcutaneous drug administration:

- Receiving large volumes of fluids/medication may be uncomfortable for the patient, and over-distension of the skin may disrupt the blood supply to the skin and thus decrease absorption via this route
- Tissue damage and necrosis can occur if irritant substances (e.g. enrofloxacin) are injected via this route
- Colour changes may be seen in some reptilian species, e.g. chameleons and amelanistic pythons
- Care must be taken not to puncture the body wall, which can easily happen accidentally in very small patients.

For suitable sites and explanations of subcutaneous administration in different species see Fluid therapy, earlier.

Intramuscular administration

Intramuscular administration of drugs is commonly used in exotic animal medicine. It is no more difficult in exotic patients than in dogs and cats, other than the often considerably smaller muscle mass at the injection site. Because of the vascular nature of the musculature, drug delivery is more rapid and reliable than via the subcutaneous route. Restraint time for intramuscular injection is usually minimal, so it may be a less stressful route than slow intravenous infusion.

Complications and risks of intramuscular injection include the following.

- Injection may be painful.
- There is a risk of blood loss due to the vascular nature of the musculature.
- It is not feasible in patients with too little musculature (very small or cachexic patients).
- Significant tissue damage and necrosis can occur due to volume, dosage frequency and drug formulation (e.g. high or low pH extremes). This may lead to self-trauma and, in extreme cases, distal limbs may be chewed off.
- The higher doses of drug required according to metabolic scaling principles (see later) may lead to relatively higher volumes, which may be too large to administer safely to a single site by this route. Multiple sites or alternative routes may be required.
- Colour changes may be seen in some reptilian species, e.g. chameleons and amelanistic pythons.

To minimize pain on intramuscular injection, the least sensitive sites (where the muscle fascia is not too tight) should be used. Injection sites should be alternated or rotated between doses (e.g. left pectoral and right pectoral) to minimize trauma to one particular site. Clear notes must be made on the patient's hospital chart to show which sites have been used.

Intramuscular administration in mammals

- Suitable sites include:
  - Lumbodorsal epaxial musculature (muscles either side of the spinal column just cranial to the hip)
  - The neck (cervical muscles) if enough musculature is available to inject into
  - The shoulder area (in larger animals only, such as rabbits and some guinea pigs)
  - The quadriceps muscle (never along the medial aspect due to the possibility of damaging the sciatic nerve).
- The biceps femoris muscle group is *not advised* due to the proximity to the sciatic nerve.
- **Maximum amounts:** entirely dependent upon patient size, muscle size, and formulation and concentration, but could be as little as 0.05 ml into the quadriceps muscle of a mouse.

Intramuscular administration in birds

- Suitable sites include:
  - The pectoral muscles (large 'breast' muscles either side of the sternum)
  - The thigh muscles at the top of the leg in larger birds or predominantly ground-dwelling birds with proportionally larger hindlimb muscles.
- Avoid the posterior aspect of the femur in birds, to reduce the risk of damage to the sciatic nerve.
- Avoid (or take extreme care and use a very shallow injection technique) pectoral muscle injection in fledgling birds that still have a cartilaginous sternum; these are more at risk of accidental penetration into the liver or air sac.
- Note that some owners of birds of prey or racing pigeons may not wish for intramuscular injections to be given into the pectoral muscles due to the perceived effect on the flight musculature; this should be discussed with the owner and consent sought before medication is administered.
- **Maximum amounts:** 1–2 ml/kg amounts that are >2 ml/kg should be given across multiple sites (Chitty, 2008).

Intramuscular administration in reptiles

- Suitable sites in lizards:
  - Caudal muscle groups of the front legs
  - Epaxial muscles along the back, neck and lumbar region (the muscles of the tail may be used, but should be avoided in species that autotomize their tails)
  - Cranial thigh muscles.
- Suitable site in snakes:
  - Midway between the dorsal midline and the lateral aspect, approximately 33–50% of the snout to vent length.
- Suitable sites in chelonians:
  - Caudal muscle groups of the front legs
  - Cranial thigh muscles.
- **Maximum amounts:** entirely dependent upon patient size, muscle size, drug formulation and concentration.

Intravenous administration

Relatively high volumes of drug can be given via this route (but should always be given slowly) (Figure 6.26), and repeated injection (intermittent infusion) is relatively painless. Where a CRI is administered to a small patient, a syringe driver or fluid pump should be used to ensure accuracy.

For intravenous administration sites, volumes and methods see Fluid therapy, earlier.

Intraosseous administration

Most drug preparations that may be given intravenously may also be given via intraosseous administration. Extravasation through any holes or fracture

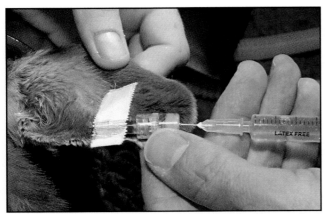

6.26 Intravenous drug administration in the marginal ear vein of a rabbit. (Courtesy of the University of Bristol)

sites in the bone may allow drugs to leak locally, which may cause soft tissue damage with irritant drugs.

Intracoelomic and epicoelomic administration

The intracoelomic and epicoelomic routes are suitable for reptiles that possess a coelomic cavity, and are widely used to administer drugs where other routes are impractical or impossible. Irritant drugs should be diluted with appropriate fluids.

For intracoelomic and epicoelomic administration sites, volumes and methods see Fluid therapy, earlier.

Intraperitoneal administration

The intraperitoneal route is recommended for small mammals where access to other suitable sites is limited or impractical, and allows for relatively large volumes to be administered. However, uptake is not as reliable as intravenous or intramuscular administration; needle damage to abdominal organs and gut perforation are possible, and irritant drugs may provoke peritoneal inflammation and adhesion formation. Its use is usually restricted to large-volume injections of non-irritant drugs where intravenous access is not practical.

For intraperitoneal administration site, volumes and methods see Fluid therapy, earlier.

Allometric or metabolic scaling

Allometric, physiological or metabolic scaling is based on the concept that the metabolic rate, and therefore the drug or nutrient requirement per unit bodyweight of an animal, is dependent on its size. This has implications for drug doses and dose frequency, with smaller animals requiring higher doses, and more frequent dose intervals. (See also Nutritional support, earlier.)

Nursing care plans

Nursing care plans are becoming more popular within the veterinary nursing profession. Originating from human nursing models, care plans provide a way for nurses to practise a patient-oriented approach rather

than the more common and popular disease-oriented approach used by many veterinary staff. Nursing care plans provide a way of ensuring individualized, organized care to each patient; in particular, they allow less experienced nurses, or those branching out into a new area of the profession, to consider all of the needs of the patient – known as a holistic approach – rather than focusing only on the obvious clinical needs. Holistic nursing is a philosophy of nursing practice that considers the physical, emotional and social needs of the patient and, although relatively recently applied to veterinary nursing care, it is widely agreed that a holistic approach and the use of nursing care plans greatly improves patient care. The nursing model is the original theoretical idea upon which the nursing care plan is based, and is usually described as a set of ideas, beliefs and values about the nature and purpose of nursing.

The nursing process

In order to understand the ability of a nursing model, and for a nursing care plan to be effective, one must first have an understanding of the nursing process. The nursing process is a problem-solving framework that enables the nurse to plan and implement individualized patient care. It helps to ensure good quality nursing care to each patient. The nursing process is:

- **Systematic:** Doing things in a specific order to reach the best outcome
- **Dynamic:** Understanding that it is a process and that there is frequently regression to earlier stages before moving forward
- **Interpersonal:** Understanding that not all patients, as with humans, are the same and so avoiding generalization and assumption about an individual case
- **Outcome-focused:** Implementing gold standard care must involve monitoring how effective the care is, and allowing for changes to the process (see Dynamic, above) and to any plan that would provide more effective care and/or treatment
- **Universally applicable:** Providing the versatility that is so well recognized in nursing care models and plans, nurses (and indeed other clinical staff) can apply the process to a wide range of species with a variety of problems in many different environments.

The nursing process is a dynamic and interactive process that is never stagnant or still but is continually evolving and changing; it must therefore allow for updating and improvement. There are five important steps.

The five important steps of the nursing process

1. Assessment.
2. Nursing diagnosis (different from a veterinary diagnosis).
3. Planning.
4. Implementation.
5. Evaluation.

The nurse is required to use these five steps during each interaction with a patient. Experienced nurses are likely to follow these steps subconsciously, whereas inexperienced nurses (or those entering a new area of the profession, such as exotic pets) may have to think about each stage. A nursing care plan can help to steer nurses who are inexperienced in a particular area down the right paths, so that they do not have to think consciously about each of the five steps.

Understanding the stages of the nursing process

This section does not provide guidance regarding how to make a plan but instead focuses on developing an understanding of how to use the nursing process effectively. Once understood, ideas will automatically be implemented as a plan is worked through.

Assessment

This stage can be thought of as data collection, or gathering information. It is almost certainly the most important stage and should not be rushed – otherwise the process and any nursing care plans created could be ineffective.

Assessment should be holistic, rather than 'what is the animal doing and thus what is wrong?'. The bigger picture must be looked at. Owners are often only too happy to explain more about their pet; however, in practice this is constrained by time limits (appointment slots, planned surgeries, etc.). Sometimes a nurse does not have the opportunity to speak directly with the owner (e.g. nurses that work at referral centres may have little contact with the owners); however, good communication between colleagues should help in such cases. A telephone conversation with the client at a later time is also always an option.

Gathering information about a patient usually involves:

- Observation
- Interviewing the owner or carer
- Physical assessment of the patient
- Discussion with the clinical team (often between an individual veterinary surgeon and nurse, sometimes with externs, interns, residents, care staff, etc.). A thorough discussion often occurs during 'rounds' at the start of the day or during handover to specialized night staff; a nurse should therefore be prepared to make changes to plans during these times.

When gathering information, there are several different sources:

- The patient (objective data)
- The owners (subjective and some objective data)
- Current and previous nursing (and medical) records (subjective and objective data)
- Records from other veterinary professionals
- Statements and information from paraprofessionals, witnesses to accidents, police and RSPCA officers, etc.

As many of these sources as possible should be utilized to continue with the holistic approach.

The importance of understanding natural requirements

When implementing the nursing process for exotic species, it is vital that the animal's natural requirements are understood in order to minimize stress and provide the correct husbandry during the patient's hospital stay (and on discharge, to allow the owner to continue appropriate care).

If unsure, the natural requirements of the animal should be investigated. Information can be found using the Internet, or by contacting an exotic species specialist or even a good quality exotic animal breeder or pet shop. The animal's natural situation should never be ignored. Without effective husbandry, all other treatment will be pointless (at least in the long term).

Nursing diagnosis

Totally different from veterinary diagnosis, where a causal explanation for a range of signs and symptoms is sought, a nursing diagnosis is a judgement of priority and care needs that fall within the scope of nursing practice (e.g. assistance with nutrition, restoration of fluid balance, pain management and mobility). The registered veterinary nurse (RVN) is now accountable for his/her own actions; the nursing diagnosis is used to implement care for which the nurse is accountable.

Planning

Planning allows nursing and other clinical staff to establish realistic outcomes and time-frames, ready for the implementing care and evaluation stages of the nursing process. Three types of planning should take place:

- Initial planning
- Ongoing planning
- Discharge planning.

Planning allows the nursing team to establish goals, which may be short-term, long-term or intermediate. The key to planning and achieving goals is to set the criteria for success from the outset. An individual cannot assess the effectiveness of any care that has been given if they do not know what they are looking for (positive or negative).

KEY POINTS

- Remember that the nursing process is **dynamic**; any plan, even if not progressed to a full scale nursing care plan, should be fluid and readily adapted.
- Planning should *not* be a one-off exercise. Re-evaluation will allow the effectiveness of any treatment and care given to be monitored, but planning can be re-instigated and implemented at any point during the process if deemed appropriate.

Implementing care

Once the plan has been established and the goals set, with criteria in place to monitor the effectiveness of care, the nurse should be able to carry out the practical care of the patient successfully. The key to caring for a patient in line with the nursing process is that there should be regular monitoring of the effectiveness of care, and interventions should be prompt where necessary. It must be remembered that the point of nursing models and nursing care plans is to provide a holistic approach, with gold standard care.

Excellent nursing care:

- Is based upon evidence-based practice, relevant research and professional standards of care
- Understands the nursing process described and the rationale for the actions implemented and, most importantly, questions any actions that are not readily understood
- Can be adapted to each individual patient
- Is safe and takes account of risk
- Respects the dignity of the patient and owner
- Adopts a holistic approach, taking into account the physical, psychological and social needs of the patient
- Is a continuous assessment of the patient.

Evaluation of care

If goals are not being met, or if other problems are arising, the nurse can adapt the plan and increase effectiveness. Evaluating also allows the nursing team to gain valuable feedback on procedures and protocols in the species seen in exotic practice, which, in turn, can help to provide better care for other patients. Evaluation can be performed in several ways, the three most common of which are:

- **Ongoing** – dependent upon patient response and need
- **Intermittent** – occurring at set intervals
- **Summative** – ascertaining the patient's condition at the end of care (summarizing its condition at that time).

It is important to understand what is being evaluated, and when such outcomes are appropriate for each individual patient. Possible outcomes of evaluation include:

- Reaching the nursing goals (e.g. restoration of hydration status, as may be ascertained via a packed cell volume (PCV) examination)
- Making progress towards the nursing goals (e.g. an improved but not yet normal PCV result)
- Not making any progress towards the nursing goals (e.g. no improvement in PCV result over the desired time period)
- Moving further away from the nursing goals (e.g. a deterioration in the PCV result).

If the outcome is a movement further away from the nursing goals, one of the following actions should take place:

- The nursing goals should be adapted
- The nursing action should be adapted
- The evaluation dates should be revised.

Specific nursing models

There are numerous named nursing models, all of which evolved within the human nursing profession. Several of these models have been applied to veterinary nursing, the most popular being the Roper, Logan and Tierney model. More detail on nursing models can be found in the *BSAVA Textbook of Veterinary Nursing*.

The Roper, Logan and Tierney model of nursing

The only model to have been developed in the UK, the Roper, Logan and Tierney model is utilized widely within the veterinary nursing profession and can be applied easily and effectively to exotic patients that are hospitalized, regardless of the hospital setting. This model is more popular and appropriate to veterinary nursing than other models; although it may have different ideas and 'systems' to other models, all are aiming towards the same goal, which is **to provide the best possible care to each individual patient using a holistic approach**.

Roper, Logan and Tierney based their model of nursing on their cited 'activities of living', the idea being that these activities define what 'living' means and promote maximum independence. The model has five components.

The five components of the Roper, Logan and Tierney model

- The activities of living (ALs).
- The patient's lifespan.
- Dependence–independence continuum.
- Factors influencing the activities of living.
- Individuality in living.

The activities of living

- Maintaining a safe environment.
- Communication.
- Breathing.
- Eating and drinking.
- Eliminating (defecating and urinating).
- Personal cleansing and dressing (grooming).
- Thermoregulation.
- Mobilization.
- Working and playing.
- Expressing sexuality.
- Sleeping.
- Dying.

Lifespan

The patient's lifespan runs from birth to death, and is closely related to other parts of the model, in particular the dependence–independence continuum. Some patients may not fulfil the entire potential lifespan – i.e. they may die before they reach old age. The lifespan can be plotted early on in the plan and throughout the patient's nursing care records so that it is visible at a glance. Lifespan is presented on paper as shown below. A point should be marked on the line to indicate how old the animal is.

Neonate ⟶ Geriatric

Dependence–independence continuum

The continuum acknowledges that an individual may not yet, or may no longer, be capable of performing some of the activities of living independently. The continuum is presented on paper in the same way as lifespan, as shown below. A point should be marked on the line to indicate how independent the animal is.

Total ⟶ Total
dependence (D)   independence (I)

The idea is that the patient's dependence–independence continuum should be plotted for each activity of living and should also be plotted throughout the provision of care. As the patient's problems (resulting in a lack of ability to perform activities of living independently) resolve, their dependence–independence continuum will be plotted at a different place, giving an impression of the patient's overall dependence in an easy-to-read form.

Factors influencing the activities of living

There are five key factors that are known to influence the activities of living:

- Biological – The impact on overall health
- Psychological – The impact of emotion and cognition (and, in humans, spiritual beliefs and the ability to understand)
- Sociocultural – The impact of society and culture
- Environmental – Consideration of the environmental impact on the individual
- Politocoeconomic – This factor is irrelevant in the non-human patient and so will not be discussed within this context.

Consideration of these factors enables a holistic approach to the patient, which is integral to the nursing care plan.

Individuality in living

Individuality simply means acknowledging that each patient is different and may respond differently in any given scenario. A holistic view looks at the patient as a whole, on an individual basis.

> **KEY POINT**
> It is important to understand that the Roper, Logan and Tierney model of nursing is intended to be a 'cognitive approach to the assessment and care of the patient, not on paper as a list of boxes but in the nurse's approach to and organization of the care provided', as the authors intended.

Figure 6.27 highlights the relationship between each of the components of the Roper, Logan and Tierney model of nursing, and shows how the model for living is adapted as a model for nursing.

Initially, the model may seem complicated, but it is actually a representation of the theories and ideas that comprise the definition of independence. By using diagrams to represent the patient's position along its lifespan, and its ability to perform its

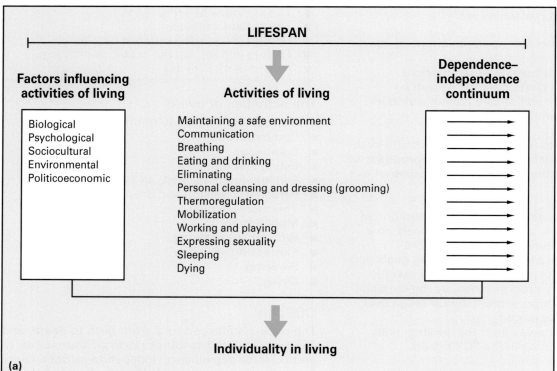

6.27

(a) The Roper, Logan and Tierney Model for living. (b) The Roper, Logan and Tierney Model for nursing. (Reproduced from the *BSAVA Manual of Practical Veterinary Nursing*) (continues) ▶

LIFESPAN

Factors influencing activities of living

Biological
Psychological
Sociocultural
Environmental
Politicoeconomic

Activities of living

Maintaining a safe environment
Communication
Breathing
Eating and drinking
Eliminating
Personal cleansing and dressing (grooming)
Thermoregulation
Mobilization
Working and playing
Expressing sexuality
Sleeping
Dying

Dependence–independence continuum

Individuality in living

(a)

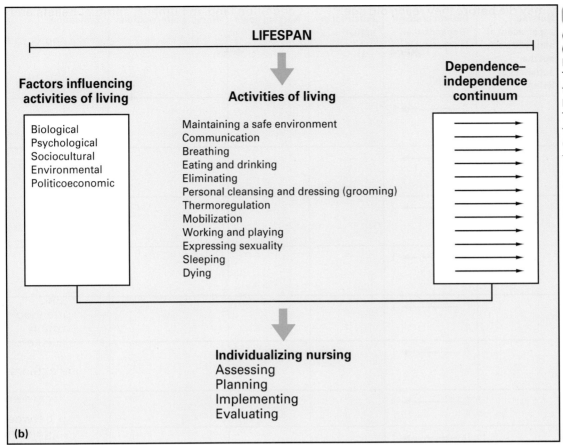

(continued) **(a)** The Roper, Logan and Tierney Model for living. **(b)** The Roper, Logan and Tierney Model for nursing. (Reproduced from the *BSAVA Manual of Practical Veterinary Nursing*)

activities of living in an independent manner (or not), the plan is readily available for nurses to utilize in an endless variety of patients and situations.

Recently, a model specifically based on veterinary nursing requirements has been proposed that is a synthesis of both the Roper, Logan and Tierney model and Orem's 'Self-Care' model. Orem's model is based upon the concept of patients as self-caring individuals, with consideration given to self-care requisites including universal (activities integral to health), developmental (according to lifespan) and health deviation (situations demanding healthcare). In contrast to the Roper, Logan and Tierney model, Orem considers interuterine life and birth as part of a patient's lifespan and it has the ultimate desire to enable patients to meet their self-care needs through appropriate nursing interventions, empowerment, education and support.

The new combined model differs slightly in that it focuses on the abilities of the animal during the initial assessment stage, allowing care to be tailored to the individual animal throughout. It should be noted that this model, while very suitable for cats and dogs, is more difficult to apply to many exotic species due to the lack of knowledge of the normal behaviours expected.

Putting the nursing model into practice

Once understood, the processes of nursing care and the theories of the nursing model can be utilized practically in the form of the nursing care plan. By using a template (Figure 6.28) and adapting it for individuals (Figure 6.29), the nursing care plan can be used for an endless number of patients and nursing situations.

It is vital to seek advice where there are areas of knowledge lacking that might inhibit the full process from being carried out or that might reduce the efficacy of the plan. In order to ensure the process is dynamic, a plan can be added to or changed as frequently as necessary, or new plans can be created throughout the care of an individual patient as its condition changes.

The most important properties of a nursing care plan

- The process should be **dynamic** (never stagnant or still); care must incorporate a holistic approach throughout
- **Evaluation** must be fulfilled at appropriate points and necessary changes to the plan or goals implemented as required
- There must be a **team approach** to the use of a care plan; this is one of the most valued advantages of a plan
- It should create a **common goal** for all care staff within a realistic and known time-frame.

Activity of living	Nursing assessment of ability to carry out the activities of living	Patient problem (Dependent or Independent)	Potential or actual	Nursing goals	Nursing interventions	Evaluation
Maintaining a safe environment		D ———► I				
Communicating		D ———► I				
Breathing		D ———► I				
Eating and drinking		D ———► I				
Eliminating		D ———► I				
Personal grooming		D ———► I				
Thermoregulation		D ———► I				
Mobilization		D ———► I				
Working and playing		D ———► I				
Expressing sexuality		D ———► I				
Sleeping		D ———► I				
Dying		D ———► I				

Patient details:

Lifespan position: Neonate ————————————————————► Geriatric

Date/time:

6.28 An example of a nursing care plan template (Roper, Logan and Tierney Model).

Activity of living	Nursing assessment of ability to carry out activities of living	Patient problem (Dependent or Independent)	Potential or actual	Nursing goals	Nursing interventions	Evaluation
Maintaining a safe environment	Needs a secure cage to prevent flight/danger	D ←——— I	Actual	Avoid free flight	Place in cage within avian ward and catch up in a towel before leaving the ward	A safe environment was maintained throughout Louis' stay
	Cannot balance on a high perch due to weakness			Avoid the need for climbing/elevated perching	Give low perches with food and water easily accessible to prevent the need to climb	
	Risk of pathogenic disease from other psittacine patients			Keep away from other inpatients and outpatients	Place in avian ward with own ventilation and ensure handled prior to, or avoid handling after, dealing with other potentially infective patients	
	Is in danger of becoming very stressed if placed near predators			Avoid contact or sight-line to likely predators, and ensure nurses' behaviour is not too threatening	Housed in avian ward away from predators. Staff not to peer into cage or talk at Louis while in cage unless interacting for a reason (i.e. asking to 'step up' prior to handling)	
Communicating	Is unable to communicate through vocalization. Is able to communicate through body language	D ←——— I	Potential	Ensure all nurses recognize behavioural signs displayed by Louis	Assess behaviour during any interventions with handling	Nurses built up a good relationship with Louis and avoided getting bitten – he stepped up well when asked to throughout his stay
Breathing	Louis has an abnormal respiratory rate and pattern due to the large syringeal aspergilloma	D ←——— I	Potential	Improve patient's respiratory function and monitor throughout treatment	Provide oxygen therapy and nebulization (F10 in water 1:250 ml) q6h. Monitor respiratory rate and pattern for improvement/deterioration and maintain air sac tube *in situ*. Monitor respiratory signs hourly and record	Louis' respiratory effort deteriorated; assessment showed an infected air sac tube insertion site and blocked tube. General anaesthetic used to insert new tube, and nebulization increased to q4h
Eating and drinking	Louis is not drinking/feeding consistently on his own and is not maintaining weight	D ←——— I	Potential	Supplement patient's free-choice feeding and monitor weight for changes. Ensure hydration status is maintained. Encourage self-feeding	Feed by gavage q6h and give intravenous fluids q6h. Weigh q24h at 8 am and compare with previous weights. Give food-oriented toys, placed low around cage, and favourite treats mixed in with parrot mix and pelleted diet	Louis' weight was maintained with gavage feeding but hydration status was hard to maintain and Louis removed his intravenous catheter. Subcutaneous fluid therapy was instigated but Louis became sore

6.29 An example of a nursing care plan (Roper, Logan and Tierney Model). (continues)

Activity of living	Nursing assessment of ability to carry out activities of living	Patient problem (Dependent or Independent)	Potential or actual	Nursing goals	Nursing interventions	Evaluation
Eliminating	Louis is able to eliminate naturally and has no diarrhoea	D ——|—→ I	Potential	Monitor faecal/urinary output and ensure normal elimination	Assess and record faecal/urinary output daily and alert veterinary surgeon of any changes	Louis had no problems with elimination but urinary output decreased when hydration status subnormal. Improved once subcutaneous fluids instigated
Personal grooming	Louis is feather-plucking at times due to stress and is not preening as normal	D —|——→ I	Potential	Monitor feather-plucking and encourage/instigate grooming. Keep stress to a minimum/allow time to preen	Record feather-plucking activities and feather loss daily (compare with previous records). Mist cage daily to increase humidity and instigate/improve preening. Delay handling/medicating if Louis is preening when ward entered	Louis continued to feather-pluck but began preening more frequently and effectively
Thermoregulation	Louis is showing signs of feeling cold but must not be allowed to overheat	D —|—→ I	Potential	Maintain temperature but ensure Louis does not overheat	Monitor temperature and provide supplementary heat if required – but check regularly to prevent overheating (use time checks on patient hospital chart)	Louis required supplementary heat at night but not during the day. When provided, Louis maintained his correct temperature
Mobilization	Louis can move around normally but is too weak to climb safely or perch in an elevated position	D —|——→ I	Potential	Ensure Louis mobilizes but prevent danger from unnecessary climbing	Use low perching and place food and water low to remove the need to climb	Louis used the low perches and was able to reach his food and water bowls
Working and playing	Louis cannot climb about his cage or come out for free flight in the normal way	D —|——→ I	Potential	Stimulate Louis and prevent boredom. Allow some movement when not too weak	Use low food-oriented toys around the cage to stimulate limited movement and allow out of the cage q12h to climb around a parrot tree	Louis did not play with the toys but self-fed his favourite treats and utilized his time out on the parrot tree
Expressing sexuality	Louis has not got a mate and usually expresses his sexuality via interaction with his owner	D —|——→ I	Actual	Prevent loneliness and separation anxiety (from owner)	Instigate regular interaction with Louis and organize owner visits	Louis improved following visits from his owner and began to interact better with the nurses and interns

6.29 (continued) An example of a nursing care plan (Roper, Logan and Tierney Model). (continues)

Activity of living	Nursing assessment of ability to carry out activities of living	Patient problem (Dependent or Independent)	Potential or actual	Nursing goals	Nursing interventions	Evaluation
Sleeping	Louis may not be able to sleep in an unfamiliar hospital environment	D ——— I	Potential	Provide distinct day/night periods	Minimize disturbance and light at night, cover Louis' cage and reduce the need for handling at night with thoughtful and appropriate medication timing	Louis often 'nodded off' during the day, indicating that he had not had enough sleep at night
Dying	The final act of living; veterinary intervention would be required if Louis entered this point of his lifespan	D ——— I	Potential	Maintain life and prevent death. Maintain analgesia	Monitor closely, provide adequate analgesia and treat as prescribed to maintain life and improve condition. Humane euthanasia with the owner's consent may be carried out by the veterinary surgeon if death becomes imminent and Louis' quality of life is further reduced	Louis' condition deteriorated rapidly as the aspergilloma did not reduce in size and systemic infection took hold. He was euthanased with his owner's consent 10 days after admission

Patient details: Louis, 2-year-old Amazon parrot

Lifespan position: Neonate ——|————————————▶ Geriatric

Date/time: 10/10/10 10:00am

6.29 (continued) An example of a nursing care plan (Roper, Logan and Tierney Model).

When using a nursing model, it helps to have an initial idea of the actual and potential problems that exist in an individual (Figure 6.30) before drawing up a full plan.

Activity of living	Actual problems	Potential problems
Maintaining a safe environment		
Communicating		
Breathing		
Eating and drinking		
Eliminating		
Personal grooming		
Thermoregulation		
Mobilization		
Working and playing		
Expressing sexuality		
Sleeping		
Dying		

6.30   It is helpful to have an initial idea of the actual and potential problems that a patient has before drawing up a full nursing care plan.

References and further reading

Ballard B and Cheek R (2010) *Exotic Animal Medicine for the Veterinary Technician, 2nd edn*. Wiley-Blackwell, Oxford

Best D and Mullineaux E (2003) Basic principles of treating wildlife casualties. In: *BSAVA Manual of Wildlife Casualties*, ed. E Mullineaux *et al.*, pp. 6–28. BSAVA Publications, Gloucester

Carpenter JW (2005) *Exotic Animal Formulary, 3rd edn*. Saunders Elsevier, Missouri

Chitty J (2008) Basic techniques. In: *BSAVA Manual of Raptors, Pigeons and Passerine Birds*, ed. J Chitty and M Lierz, pp. 62–72. BSAVA Publications, Gloucester

Davis C (2007) The nursing process and nursing models. In: *BSAVA Manual of Practical Veterinary Nursing*, ed. E Mullineaux and M Jones, pp. 95–104. BSAVA Publications, Gloucester

Dorrestein GM (2000) Nursing the sick bird. In: *Avian Medicine*, ed. TN Tully *et al.*, 74–111. Butterworth Heinemann, Oxford

Gajanayake I, Lumbis R, Greet G and Girling S (2011) Nutrition and feeding. In: *BSAVA Textbook of Veterinary Nursing, 5th edn*, ed. B Cooper *et al.*, pp. 305–345 BSAVA Publications, Gloucester

Girling S (2003) *Veterinary Nursing of Exotic Pets*. Blackwell Publishing, Oxford

Gosden C (2004) *Exotics and Wildlife*. Butterworth Heinemann, London

Graham J (2006) Common procedures in rabbits. *Veterinary Clinics of North America: Exotic Animal Practice* **9**, 367–388

Harcourt-Brown N and Chitty J (2005) *BSAVA Manual of Psittacine Birds, 2nd edn*. BSAVA Publications, Gloucester

Highfield AC (1996) *The Tortoise and Turtle Feeding Manual*. Carapace Press, London

Holland K, Jenkins J, Solomon J and Whittham S (2008) *Applying the Roper, Logan and Tierney Model in Practice, 2nd edn*. Churchill Livingstone Elsevier, Philadelphia

Hotston Moore P (2007) Practical fluid therapy. In: *BSAVA Manual of Practical Veterinary Nursing*, ed. E Mullineaux and M Jones, pp. 127–139. BSAVA Publications, Gloucester

Jeffrey A and Ford-Fennah S (2011) The nursing process, nursing models and care plans. In: *BSAVA Textbook of Veterinary Nursing, 5th edn*, ed. B Cooper *et al.*, pp. 346–364. BSAVA Publications, Gloucester

Joiner T (2000) An holistic approach to nursing. *Veterinary Nursing* **15**, 142–148

Lichtenberger M (2004a) Principles of shock and fluid therapy in special species. *Seminars in Avian and Exotic Pet Medicine* **13**, 142–153

Lichtenberger M (2004b) Transfusion medicine in exotic pets. *Clinical Techniques in Small Animal Practice* **19**, 88–95

Lichtenberger M (2007) Shock and cardiopulmonary-cerebral resuscitation in small mammals and birds. *Veterinary Clinics of North America: Exotic Animal Practice* **10**, 275–291

Lichtenberger M and Hawkins MG (2009) Rodents: physical examination and emergency care. In: *BSAVA Manual of Rodents and Ferrets*, ed. E Keeble and A Meredith, pp. 18–31. BSAVA Publications, Gloucester

Lichtenberger M and Lennox A (2004) Emergency and critical care of small mammals. In: *Ferrets, Rabbits and Rodents Clinical Medicine and Surgery, 3rd edn*, ed. KE Quesenberry and JW Carpenter, pp. 532–544. Saunders, St. Louis

Longley L (2008) Anaesthesia and analgesia in rabbits and rodents. *In Practice* **30**, 92–97

Longley L (2010) *Saunders' Solutions in Veterinary Practice: Small Animal Exotic Pet Medicine*. Saunders Elsevier, St. Louis

Maclean B and Raiti P (2004) Emergency care. In: *BSAVA Manual of Reptiles, 2nd edn*, ed. S Girling and P Raiti, pp. 63–70. BSAVA Publications, Gloucester

Mader DR and Rudloff E (2006) Emergency and critical care. In: *Reptile Medicine and Surgery, 2nd edn*, ed. DM Mader, pp. 533–548. Saunders Elsevier, St. Louis

Marshall KL (2008) Rabbit haematology. *Veterinary Clinics of North America: Exotic Animal Practice* **11**, 551–567

Martini ME (2008) Laboratory animal medicine. In: *Mosby's Comprehensive Review for Veterinary Technicians. 3rd edn*, ed. M Tighe and M Brown, pp. 287–310. Mosby Elsevier, Philadelphia

Martinez-Jiminez D and Hernandez-Divers SJ (2007) Emergency care of reptiles. *Veterinary Clinics of North America: Exotic Animal Practice* **10**, 557–585

McArthur S (2004) Feeding techniques and fluids. In: *Medicine and Surgery of Tortoises and Turtles*, ed. S McArthur *et al.*, pp. 257–271. Blackwell, Oxford

McClure SR, Welch RD and Johnson TL (1992) Use of an implant for intraosseous infusion as supportive therapy for a Vietnamese pot-bellied pig with urethral obstruction caused by a polyp. *Journal of the American Veterinary Medical Association* **201**, 1587–1590

Meredith A and Johnson-Delaney C (2010) *BSAVA Manual of Exotic Pets, 5th edn*. BSAVA Publications, Gloucester

Mitchell MA (2006) Therapeutics. In: *Reptile Medicine and Surgery, 2nd edn*, ed. DM Mader, pp. 631–664. Saunders Elsevier, St. Louis

Mitchell MA and Tully TN Jr (2009) *Manual of Exotic Pet Practice*. Saunders Elsevier, St. Louis

Moon-Massat PF (2007) Fluid therapy and blood transfusion. In: *BSAVA Manual of Canine and Feline Anaesthesia and Analgesia*. ed. C Seymour and T Duke-Novakovski, pp. 166–182. BSAVA Publications, Gloucester

Mullan SM and Main DCJ (2006) Survey of the husbandry, health and welfare of 102 pet rabbits. *Veterinary Record* **159**, 103–109

Best D and Mullineaux E (2003) Basic principles of treating wildlife casualties In: *BSAVA Manual of Wildlife Casualties*. ed. E Mullineaux *et al.*, pp. 6–28. BSAVA Publications, Gloucester

Orcutt C (2000a) Oxyglobin administration for the treatment of anaemia in ferrets. *ICE2000 Proceedings* **2.3**, 44–46

Orcutt C (2000b) Parenteral nutrition for small exotic herbivores. *ICE2000 Proceedings* **2.3**, 39–43

Orcutt C (2000c) Use of vascular access ports in exotic animals. *ICE2000 Proceedings* **2.3**, 34–38

Orcutt C (2001) Update on oxyglobin use in ferrets. *ICE2001 Proceedings* **3.3**, 29–30

Pizzi R (2008) Examination, triage and hospitalization. In: *BSAVA Manual of Raptors, Pigeons and Passerine Birds. 2nd edn*, ed. J Chitty and M Lierz, pp. 48–61. BSAVA Publications, Gloucester

Powers LV (2006a) Techniques for drug delivery in psittacine birds. *Journal of Exotic Pet Medicine* **15**(3), 193–200

Powers LV (2006b) Techniques for drug delivery in small mammals. *Journal of Exotic Pet Medicine*, **15**(3), 201–209

Ramsey I (2011) *BSAVA Small Animal Formulary, 7th edn.* BSAVA Publications, Gloucester

Redig PT (1996) Avian emergencies. In: *BSAVA Manual of Raptors, Pigeons and Waterfowl*, ed. N Forbes and N Harcourt-Brown. BSAVA Publications, Gloucester

Redig TP (1996) Nursing avian patients. In: *BSAVA Manual of Raptors, Pigeons and Waterfowl*, ed. N Forbes and N Harcourt-Brown. BSAVA Publications, Gloucester

Rees Davies R and Klingenberg RJ (2004) Therapeutics and medication. In: *BSAVA Manual of Reptiles. 2nd edn*, ed. S Girling and P Raiti, pp. 115–130. BSAVA Publications, Gloucester

Samour J (2008) Medical procedures. In: *Avian Medicine, 2nd edn*, pp. 98–118. Mosby Elsevier, Philadelphia

Schumacher J (2008) Chapter 20: Fluid therapy in reptiles. In: *Zoo and wild Animal Medicine: Current Therapy, volume 6*, ed. M Fowler and E Miller, pp. 160–164. Saunders Elsevier, St. Louis

Stocker L (2005) *Practical Wildlife Care, 2nd edn.* Blackwell Publishing, Oxford

Thorson TB (1968) Body fluid partitioning in Reptilia. *Copeia* **3**, 592–601

Timmins F and Horan P (2007) A critical analysis of the potential contribution of Orem's (2001) self-care deficit nursing theory to contemporary coronary care nursing practice. *European Journal of Cardiovascular Nursing* **6**, 32–39

Ward M (2008) Pet rodents: what every vet should know. *Irish Veterinary Journal* **61**, 176–181

Welle KR (1995) Body condition scoring in companion birds. *Proceedings of the Annual Conference of the Association of Avian Veterinarians*, pp. 487–489

Self-assessment questions

1. Definite skin turgor, anorexia, increased capillary refill time and sunken eyes within orbits (not always obvious) indicates what percentage dehydration?
   a. <5%
   b. 7–9%
   c. 10–12%
   d. 13–15%
2. Which of these sites is unsuitable for intraosseous fluid therapy provision in a bird?
   a. The proximal ulna
   b. The proximal tibiotarsus
   c. The distal ulna
   d. The humerus
3. Why should no more than 3% of bodyweight be given per day as fluids via the intra- or epicoelomic routes in chelonians?
   a. Because excessive volumes of fluids via this route can result in respiratory compromise
   b. Because excessive volumes of fluids via this route can result in renal washout
   c. Because chelonians can rehydrate themselves without the need for fluid therapy
   d. Because chelonians will not eat if they are hydrated
4. Free-choice feeding can be enhanced by
   a. Offering favoured food items
   b. Offering an abundance of fresh green forage or dried forage
   c. Removing food as soon as it is past its best presentation state
   d. All of the above
5. When feeding an avian patient via gavage with a rigid crop tube, why should you choose as large a tube as is appropriate?
   a. Because it encourages swallowing
   b. Because it keeps the bird's neck rigid whilst you feed it
   c. Because it allows large volumes to be given at once, saving time later on in the day
   d. So that the risk of accidental insertion into the respiratory tract is minimized
6. When syringe feeding small mammals, which of the following statements is correct?
   a. You should syringe as much food into the mouth as possible to minimize the stress associated with handling and to speed up feeding time
   b. You should use a narrow bore feeding tube so that the food is syringed at high pressure
   c. You should administer 1–2 ml at a time with a wide bore syringe and remove the tip to allow for mastication and swallowing, before introducing the tip into the mouth again
   d. You should leave any dribbled food to dry around the mouth to encourage self-feeding by the patient later on
7. Which of the following would **not** help in administering very small amounts of drug to exotic patients
   a. A calculator
   b. Weighting scales that are accurate to at least 0.1 g
   c. Up-to-date exotic animal drug formularies
   d. Wide bore syringes
8. Which of the following is a known problem when diluting drugs?
   a. Not all drugs can be diluted due to solubility and stability concerns
   b. There is little published guidance on expiration dates for such drugs once diluted
   c. Excessive dilution may lead to larger volumes than may be safely given by intramuscular injection
   d. All of the above
9. Why should oral administration of medication be utilized where appropriate/possible?
   a. Because in most situations it is the least stressful method of administering a medication
   b. Because it encourages the patient to eat afterwards
   c. Because it allows the nurse to see if the patient can swallow
   d. Because it encourages urination and defecation
10. The fundamental reason for using nursing care plans with hospitalized in-patients is
    a. To provide documentary evidence in case of litigation
    b. To give the owner something to look at when the patient is discharged
    c. To encourage staff to practice a patient-oriented approach
    d. To encourage staff to follow a disease-oriented approach

7

Anaesthesia and analgesia

Lesa Thompson and Wendy Bament

This chapter is designed to give information on:

- Recognition of pain and provision of analgesia
- Commonly used sedative, analgesic and anaesthetic drugs and their potential effects on patient physiology
- Anaesthesia protocols
- Intubation, including specific anatomical differences among species and intubation techniques
- Anaesthetic monitoring and the use of monitoring equipment
- Pre- and post-anaesthetic care
- Recognizing problems, their underlying causes and strategies to correct them

Anaesthesia and analgesia of exotic pets can be daunting for veterinary nurses because of a fear of the unfamiliar. However, veterinary nurses already possess foundation knowledge and skills, based on other species, which can be drawn upon and adapted for various exotic and wildlife species. This chapter promotes the use of existing veterinary nursing skills and assumes a willingness to learn species-specific requirements. Veterinary nurses can bring an important contribution to the overall planning and conducting of the anaesthesia and analgesia regimes of exotic patients.

Several reasons for administering an anaesthetic exist:

- To restrain an animal that is fearful
- To provide muscle relaxation
- To provide adequate analgesia.

In order to make a full assessment and apply appropriate treatment in exotic and wildlife species, the above reasons often demand more rapid intervention than for other species. There may therefore be less opportunity for pre-anaesthetic stabilization.

Recognition of pain and provision of analgesia

Relief from pain should be considered for exotic and wild animals as for dogs and cats. The benefits of analgesia in relation to anaesthesia are two-fold:

- Provision of relief from pain will speed recovery after anaesthesia, e.g. will enable a more rapid return to normal appetite
- Some analgesics also have sedative properties, reducing the dose requirement of other agents in the anaesthetic regime.

Recognition of signs of pain

Exotic species and wild animals typically hide signs of pain (usually as a protective mechanism in prey species), and this makes recognition of the need for analgesia, and the monitoring of response to analgesics, extremely difficult. While some reasons for pain will be obvious, e.g. lameness in a fractured limb, the signs of pain are frequently subtle and may be specific to a species – or even to an individual. Pain is often demonstrated more by an absence of normal behaviour; veterinary staff should therefore be aware of the normal behavioural characteristics of species in their care.

Clinical signs of pain that are not species-specific may include vocalization or 'guarding' a painful area. Vague signs of pain may include inactivity, reduced appetite and lack of grooming.

Mammals

The gastrointestinal tracts of herbivores such as rabbits and hystricomorph rodents (guinea pigs, chinchillas and degus) are exquisitely susceptible to stress, including that associated with pain. In these animals pain may present as altered faecal output, e.g. small faecal pellets and/or reduced faeces production.

Birds

Any change in behaviour noted by owners in the home environment should not be dismissed, even if it is imperceptible in the veterinary practice. Animals (particularly birds) will mask signs of illness and pain more in a strange environment.

Environmental stressors may increase pain in birds, e.g. housing them in the presence of predator species such as dogs and cats, or excessive handling and restraint. Reduction of such stressors will reduce pain (Paul-Murphy, 2006).

Reptiles

Indications of pain in an anaesthetized reptile may include voluntary movement or elevated heart or respiratory rate. Note that cold narcosis does *not* provide analgesia (Bennett, 1998).

Pathophysiology and mechanism of action of analgesics

Local anaesthesia

Local anaesthesia is useful in exotic patients. Regional anaesthesia and analgesia is produced. However, care should be taken in small patients to avoid fatal overdosage, by weighing the animal and calculating the maximum safe dose before administration. Dilution of the drug may be required. Signs of possible toxicity include ataxia, stupor, seizures and cardiac arrest. The toxic dose of lidocaine in birds is around 4 mg/kg (Huckabee, 2000). In birds, local anaesthetic ointments are best avoided as dose calculation is difficult and they may damage plumage.

Lidocaine and bupivacaine can be utilized in combination. Lidocaine is more rapid-acting, but bupivacaine is longer-acting.

The simplest form of applying local anaesthetic is as a splash block (i.e. it is dripped on or into a subcutaneous space just before closing a surgical incision). In reptiles, intercostal nerve blocks and interpleural anaesthesia have been reported. Dental nerve blocks can be performed in larger species such as rabbits. Epidural analgesia is another option in larger animals such as rabbits and ferrets.

Systemic analgesics

In mammals, pain relief is predominantly associated with mu and kappa opioid receptors. Opioid receptor distribution and function vary between species. For example, pigeons have high proportions of kappa receptors in their forebrain. While buprenorphine may be effective in several bird species, butorphanol is thought to have limited effectiveness as an analgesic in birds. One study showed butorphanol (a kappa agonist) to be effective in cockatoos and African grey parrots but not in Amazon parrots (Curro, 1993; Curro *et al.*, 1994). Opioids may result in cardiorespiratory depression.

The mechanism of action of non-steroidal anti-inflammatory drugs (NSAIDs) is via inhibition of cyclo-oxygenase-1 (COX-1) and COX-2 enzymes, both of which are involved in inflammation. NSAIDs may be associated with renal or gastrointestinal side effects in many species.

Some anaesthetic agents have analgesic properties, e.g. the alpha-agonists medetomidine and ketamine. Reversal of the alpha-agonist at the end of the anaesthetic protocol will result in loss of the analgesia provided.

Using analgesics

Where possible, analgesia should be administered pre-emptively before 'wind-up' (physiological changes in the nervous system leading to increased sensitization to further pain) occurs. This is paramount where surgery will be performed, ideally including analgesic(s) in the anaesthetic protocol. After anaesthesia many conditions will require continued analgesia, although the agent and route of administration may vary (Figure 7.1). For many species there are gaps in current knowledge regarding which analgesics are effective, what dose is required and the dose frequency; most published doses are empirical and the clinician has to use his/her own judgement.

Species	Drug	Dose (mg/kg)	Route		Comment
Mammals					
Rabbits	Buprenorphine	0.01–0.05	Subcutaneous/intramuscular/intravenous		
	Butorphanol	0.1–0.5	Intramuscular/subcutaneous/intravenous		
	Carprofen	4	Subcutaneous		
	Ketoprofen	1–3	Subcutaneous		
	Meloxicam	0.2–0.6	Oral/subcutaneous		
Rodents	Buprenorphine	0.05–0.10	Subcutaneous		

7.1 Suggested analgesic doses in various species groups. (continues) ▶

Species	Drug	Dose (mg/kg)	Route	Comment
Mammals (continued)				
Mice	Carprofen	5	Subcutaneous	
	Meloxicam	1–2	Subcutaneous/oral	
Rats	Carprofen	5	Subcutaneous	
	Ketoprofen	5	Subcutaneous	
	Meloxicam	1–2	Subcutaneous/oral	
Hamsters	Carprofen	5	Subcutaneous	
	Ketoprofen	5	Subcutaneous	
Gerbils	Carprofen	5	Subcutaneous	
	Ketoprofen	5	Subcutaneous	
Guinea pigs	Carprofen	4	Subcutaneous	
	Ketoprofen	1	Subcutaneous/intramuscular	
Chinchillas	Carprofen	4	Subcutaneous	
	Ketoprofen	1	Subcutaneous/intramuscular	
Ferrets	Butorphanol	0.1–0.5	Intramuscular/subcutaneous/intravenous	
	Carprofen	1	Oral/subcutaneous	
	Meloxicam	0.1–0.2	Oral	
	Ketoprofen	1	Subcutaneous/intramuscular	
Birds				
Most species (no species-specific doses published)	Bupivacaine	1–2	Local, e.g. intra-articular/ subcutaneous/intramuscular	
	Carprofen	2–4	Oral/subcutaneous/intramuscular/intravenous	
	Ketoprofen	2–5	Oral/subcutaneous/intramuscular	
	Lidocaine	1–3	Local	Toxic >4 mg/kg
	Meloxicam	0.1–0.2	Oral/intramuscular/subcutaneous	q24h
Reptiles				
Most species (no species-specific doses published)	Butorphanol	0.4–2.0	Subcutaneous/intramuscular/intravenous	
	Carprofen	1–4	Oral/subcutaneous/intramuscular/intravenous	Half dose if repeat after 24h
	Ketoprofen	2	Subcutaneous/intramuscular	
	Lidocaine	1–5	Local	Toxic >10 mg/kg
	Meloxicam	0.1–0.2	Oral/intramuscular/subcutaneous	q24h

7.1 (continued) Suggested analgesic doses in various species groups.

Example: Analgesic protocol for a 3-year-old sugar glider undergoing castration

Case presentation
The anaesthetic protocol involved induction in a chamber with isoflurane, with maintenance via a facemask. Pre-emptive analgesia was provided by meloxicam at 0.2 mg/kg s.c. before commencement of surgery. A closed castration was performed and the skin closed using an intradermal suture pattern.

After recovery from the anaesthetic, the patient was seen to be traumatizing its surgical wound. This species has relatively long lower incisors, used in the wild to gouge bark to release sap (a constituent of their diet); these teeth would make short work of most suture materials. In this case, the self-trauma was suspected to be due to a combination of discomfort and rapid alertness postoperatively. Further analgesia was required.

Considerations
Consideration was given to the analgesics already provided (NSAIDs) and to the animal's demeanour. It was thought likely that the sugar glider would persistently chew at the wound if not prevented from doing so. Due to the animal's small size and its flexibility, it would be difficult to employ methods to prevent it reaching the wound. It was decided to provide additional analgesia (from a drug group other than NSAIDs) as well as administering a sedative.

Protocol
A combination of butorphanol (1.7 mg/kg) and acepromazine (1.7 mg/kg) was administered. ▶

(continued)

To reduce stress for the patient, the drugs were given orally.

Outcome
Mild sedation resulted and the animal ceased to traumatize the wound. A second dose of the combination butorphanol and acepromazine was not deemed necessary, but analgesia was continued using meloxicam daily for a period of 5 days after the surgery. The animal made an uneventful recovery.

Pre-anaesthetic care

For each individual patient it is essential to perform a thorough clinical examination and compile baseline parameters of normal biological data in the first instance. These include accurate weight (Figure 7.2), respiratory rate, heart rate and rhythm, temperature, blood pressure and blood measurements. Despite the usefulness of referring to species-specific data, it is ideal to refer any observations to the individual's normal baseline parameters.

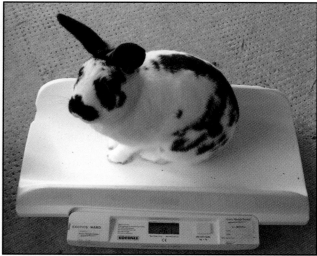

7.2 Acquiring an accurate bodyweight is essential in pre-anaesthetic assessments and when preparing anaesthetic and emergency drugs and making fluid therapy calculations.

The effects of stress

Handling, travelling and spending time in waiting rooms will dramatically elevate baseline parameters, particularly in mammals and birds, and can provoke cardiac arrhythmias. Respiratory rate should be measured either before approaching the animal or after it has become calmer in a less stressful environment. Wildlife species are usually in a state of heightened vigilance for a 'flight or fight response' from a potential threat as soon as they are seen and approached by a human; this makes baseline data collection challenging until the animal is sedated or anaesthetized. Once the patient has been admitted

it should be transferred to a low-stress environment such as a darkened, quiet room. Prey species (e.g. most birds and small mammals) and predator species (e.g. ferrets, foxes, birds of prey and snakes) should be housed in separate rooms where possible (see Chapter 5).

Careful planning with efficient administration of treatments will minimize required handling.

Warming reptiles

Reptiles may become cold during transport. It is advisable to warm the patient gently, using a bath (Figure 7.3) or heated vivarium, prior to the full clinical examination.

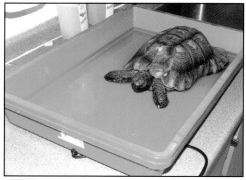

7.3 Shallow warm water baths (e.g. using seed propagators) can be useful prior to anaesthesia of reptiles, such as this marginated tortoise, to allow full clinical assessment and rehydration. Care should be exercised in patients that should be receiving nil by mouth.

Blood tests

Blood tests may be useful. Commonly used parameters include:

- Packed cell volume (PCV) and total protein – to assess hydration and circulating blood volume
- Blood urea (mammals) or uric acid (reptiles and birds) – to assess waste product metabolism
- Glucose – to assess nutritional status, particularly in ferrets and other carnivorous mammals and birds.

For further details on blood collection sites (Figure 7.4) and techniques see Chapter 10.

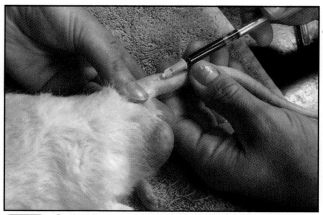

7.4 Collecting a pre-anaesthetic blood sample from a rat using the lateral tail vein.

Analgesia

Analgesia should be considered early, while the patient is being assessed. During anaesthesia, a patient's sensation of pain can be interpreted by sudden changes in heart and respiratory rates. Pre-empting the occurrence of postsurgical pain will allow reduced concentrations of anaesthetic agents to be used and will contribute towards an uneventful anaesthesia and recovery.

Nutritional and hydration support

This may be required before anaesthesia can commence, especially in collapsed or nutritionally compromised individuals. See Chapters 1 and 6.

Fasting

This encompasses the period of time in which food is withheld from the patient (Figure 7.5). Fasting should be minimized and only undertaken if the patient is stable and not already nutritionally compromised. Fasting times should be shorter for immature animals that will be more susceptible to hypoglycaemia. Smaller animals and those that are immature should be monitored closely and glucose should be administered if required.

Species	Can this species vomit/regurgitate?	Maximum fasting times prior to anaesthesia (withhold food from all species once patient is premedicated)	Recovery re-feeding timing (to prevent hypoglycaemia and/or ileus)
Mammals			
Rabbits	No	1 hour of no vegetables, to ensure no food in the mouth at the time of intubation	Within 1–2 hours to prevent ileus. Suggest assisted feeding if not observed to eat within 1–2 hours of recovery
Mice and rats	No	Not usually required	Within 2 hours to prevent hypoglycaemia
Hamsters	No, but can store food in their cheek pouches	Not usually needed, but cheek pouches may need to be gently emptied at induction	Within 2 hours
Guinea pigs and chinchillas	No	1 hour to ensure no food present in the oropharynx	Within 1–2 hours to prevent hypoglycaemia and ileus
Chipmunks and squirrels	Yes	2 hours	Within 1–2 hours
Ferrets and skunks	Yes	2–4 hours	Within 4 hours
Foxes	Yes	8–10 hours	Within 4–6 hours
Badgers	Yes	4–6 hours	Within 4–6 hours
Hedgehogs	Yes	1–1.5 hours of no vegetables, to ensure no food in the mouth at the time of intubation	Within 6–8 hours
Bats	Yes	1.5 hours	Within 4 hours
Seals <6 months old	Yes	4–6 hours	2–3 hours
Seals >6 months old	Yes	8–10 hours	4–6 hours
Birds			
Birds <100 g	Yes	Remove food for 30 minutes to empty crop	10 minutes to 1 hour post perching; feed via crop tube with recovery/support food
Birds 100–300 g	Yes	Remove food for 1 hour to empty crop	30 minutes to 1 hour post perching; feed via crop tube with recovery/support food
Birds >300 g	Yes	8–10 hours	30 minutes to 1 hour post perching; feed via crop tube with recovery/support food
Birds of prey	Yes	12 hours and a cast (indigestible food, e.g. bones, fur or feathers) produced	30 minutes to 1 hour post perching; feed via crop tube with recovery/support food
Waterfowl	Yes	Remove food for 1 hour to empty crop	30 minutes to 1 hour; feed via crop tube with recovery/support food, e.g. ground waterfowl pellets
Reptiles			
Lizards	Yes	Insectivores: 24 hours for live prey to be fully digested	30 minutes to 1 hour; tube-feed carnivore/herbivore recovery/support food
Snakes	Yes	2 days to reduce any pressure on heart and lungs	30 minutes to 1 hour; tube-feed carnivore recovery/support food
Chelonians	Yes	30 minutes to 1 hour may be beneficial relative to procedure	30 minutes to 1 hour; tube-feed carnivore/herbivore recovery/support food

7.5 Pre-anaesthetic fasting and suggested re-feeding times on recovery. (Data from Lawton, 1996; Flecknell, 2000; Girling, 2003; Longley, 2008; Chitty, 2010)

Pre-anaesthetic problems

It is well recognized that many exotic and wildlife species conceal their true suffering as a survival tactic, and during pre-anaesthetic examination it is vital to address any concerns regarding suitability to undergo anaesthesia and possible surgery.

- Some underlying illnesses are acute and can be stabilized satisfactorily preceding an anaesthetic. However, acute illness may require postponement of anaesthesia or careful anaesthetic planning and monitoring. The owner must be made aware of any heightened risks.
- Wildlife species are often compromised physically by parasitic load, injury, poor nutritional or seasonal condition and/or acute stress, but it may be difficult to assess the patient fully without first sedating it. The stress of implementing sedation can put both patient and handler at great risk, and preparation is vital in minimizing this risk.
- Other stressors observed are due to handling, travelling, unfamiliar or unsuitable environmental conditions, and close proximity to potential predators. These conditions can lead to predisposed species-specific problems such as congenital epilepsy in gerbils (Hollamby, 2009) and extreme tonic immobilization, which can be difficult to avoid, in rabbits.

Premedicants, sedatives and anaesthetic agents

Premedicants and sedatives

Agents used to premedicate animals before anaesthesia have several uses:

- They may provide sedation and/or analgesia before anaesthesia is induced
- They may reduce handling stress
- They usually lower the doses of other agents required in an anaesthetic protocol.

In some instances, these agents may prolong the recovery time (particularly after short procedures). This can be an advantage in some cases where a smooth recovery is optimal, e.g. following an orthopaedic repair.

Phenothiazine derivatives

This group includes acepromazine. Sedation is produced by central blockade of dopamine. Acepromazine is frequently used in combination with other agents to reduce doses required to produce surgical anaesthesia.

Butyrophenones

These include fluanisone and droperidol and are similar to phenothiazines. Combinations are commonly used, such as fluanisone with fentanyl (Hypnorm, Janssen Pharmaceuticals).

Alpha-2 agonists

These include medetomidine (stereoisomer: dexmedetomidine) and xylazine. Alpha-2 adrenoceptor stimulation inhibits presynaptic calcium influx and neurotransmitter release. These potent sedatives result in muscle relaxation, anxiolysis and variable analgesia. They potentiate most anaesthetic drugs. Cardiopulmonary effects may be significant, e.g. resulting in increased sensitivity to catecholamine-induced cardiac arrhythmias. (Note that the drug doses given in this chapter pertain to the racemic mixture containing two stereoisomers of medetomidine, rather than the preparation containing solely dexmedetomidine.)

Anticholinergic drugs

These drugs include atropine and glycopyrrolate. They may be given as a premedicant to reduce hypersalivation and respiratory secretions occurring in response to gaseous anaesthetic agents. Although they reduce bronchial and salivary secretion volume, this may result in more viscous secretions that can obstruct the airways (Flecknell, 1996). Atropine can be given to reptiles prior to induction to help prevent intracardiac shunting (Jepson, 2009). Atropine may also be used to protect the heart from vagal inhibition or in cases of bradycardia. Overdosage may result in seizures (Hedenqvist and Hellebrekers, 2003). Most rabbits and some rats possess hepatic atropinesterase, and glycopyrrolate should therefore be used in preference to atropine.

Benzodiazepines

These drugs include diazepam, midazolam and zolazepam. Benzodiazepines potentiate GABA (gamma-amminobutyric acid), resulting in sedation and skeletal muscle relaxation; they are also anticonvulsants. Midazolam is shorter-acting but is more potent. Flumazenil specifically antagonizes these agents. These sedatives result in anterograde amnesia.

Opioids

This group includes butorphanol, buprenorphine, morphine and fentanyl. Many narcotic analgesics cause moderate sedation. Butorphanol is an analgesic with some sedative properties, and is frequently used in combination with other drugs such as alpha-2 agonists and the dissociative agent ketamine.

Anaesthetic agents

Physiological effects of agents can be found in Figure 7.6, along with factors that must be considered when using them.

Injectable agents

Due to the risks of overdosage, small patients should always be weighed accurately and drug doses calculated carefully before administration of injectable agents. For very small specimens, drugs may need to be diluted in order to measure the dose accurately (see Chapter 6).

Drug	Effects	Cautions
Acepromazine	Sedation	No analgesia. Long duration of action, response variable, moderate hypotension, reduced thermoregulation, lowered CNS seizure threshold (Short, 1987; Hedenqvist and Hellebrekers, 2003). Avoid in dehydrated patients
Alfaxalone	Anaesthesia	
Atipamezole	Antagonist of alpha-2 agonists, specific for medetomidine (less effective for xylazine)	Shorter-acting than medetomidine. Repeat if re-sedation seen
Anticholinergic drugs, e.g. atropine, glycopyrrolate	Reduce bronchial and salivary secretion volume. Protect heart from vagal inhibition or in cases of bradycardia	Respiratory secretions may become thicker. Ineffective in many rabbits and rats
Diazepam	Sedation, skeletal muscle relaxation	Possible liver toxicity (Strombeck and Guildford, 1991)
Gaseous agents, e.g. halothane, isoflurane, sevoflurane	Anaesthesia via enhancement of GABA receptors. Some analgesia	Smell and airway irritation may lead to breath-holding (especially in rabbits). Poor analgesia. Require use of anaesthetic machine/circuit
Fluanisone	Sedation	Hypotension (less than acepromazine), bradycardia, respiratory depression, hypoxia, hypercapnia, acidosis (Hedenqvist and Hellebrekers, 2003). Long duration of action. Paradoxical excitement and aggression in some animals (Heard, 1993)
Halothane	Potent anaesthetic	Moderate respiratory depression, reduced myocardial contractility, risk of arrhythmias (Brunson, 1997). Ease of overdosage in birds – cardiac and respiratory arrest are simultaneous. Risks to veterinary staff (hepatotoxicity, possible teratogenicity)
Isoflurane	Rapid induction of anaesthesia and recovery. Moderate analgesia and muscle relaxation	Respiratory depression similar to halothane, but cardiac effects less pronounced
Ketamine	Anaesthesia	Possible discomfort on injection. Tremors and muscular rigidity if used as sole anaesthetic agent. Moderate respiratory depression (but also bronchodilation). Usually loss of corneal reflex, so need to protect eyes using ocular lubricant
Medetomidine	Sedation	Cardiorespiratory depression (species- and dose-dependent). Analgesic properties weak in rabbits, guinea pigs and hamsters (Hedenqvist and Hellebrekers, 2003). Hypoglycaemia (Lukasik, 1999)
Midazolam	Sedation, skeletal muscle relaxation	Prolonged recovery time with higher doses
Naloxone	Reversal of opioid	Loss of analgesia
Opioids, e.g. buprenorphine, butorphanol, fentanyl	Analgesia, sedation	Respiratory depression, some affect gastrointestinal motility (Flecknell, 1996)
Propofol	Anaesthesia	Apnoea common
Sevoflurane	Rapid induction of anaesthesia and recovery	
Xylazine	Sedation	More side effects than medetomidine. Cardiac arrhythmias in some species (Flecknell, 1996). Avoid in pregnant animals (increases uterine tone in some species) (Hedenqvist and Hellebrekers, 2003). Hypoglycaemia (Feldberg and Symonds, 1980)
Yohimbine	Antagonist of alpha-2 agonists, specific for xylazine	

7.6 Physiological effects of agents used in anaesthesia.

Dissociative agents

Agents such as ketamine and tiletamine are lipophilic cyclohexamines. They work by antagonizing NMDA (N-methyl-D-aspartate) receptors, resulting in a 'dissociative state'. These drugs are often used in combination with other agents to produce more balanced anaesthesia.

Although various injectable anaesthetic regimes involving ketamine are published for several species of bird, care should be taken to weigh the patient accurately, to reduce the risk of fatal overdose. Birds should also be given oxygen during anaesthesia with ketamine when possible.

Ketamine is a relatively safe agent in reptiles. Effects (including recovery time) are dose-dependent. Several routes of administration are viable.

Propofol

This alkyl phenol is administered intravenously and induces anaesthesia rapidly by enhancing GABA receptor function. Hepatic metabolism and therefore recovery are rapid. Apnoea is frequently seen after administration of this agent, and intubation should be performed (or at least preparations made to intubate) in cases of apnoea. Cardiovascular depression and respiratory depression are dose-dependent.

Alfaxalone

This steroid is usually administered intravenously to induce anaesthesia and is frequently used in reptiles. Top-ups can be given to prolong anaesthesia.

Inhalational agents

The immense benefit of gaseous anaesthetic agents is the rapid recovery time. Induction of anaesthesia with gaseous agents in small rodents is usually rapid (due to their high respiratory rate). These drugs enhance the inhibitory neurotransmitters GABA and glycine. Rapid recovery is seen after anaesthesia with gaseous agents as they do not require a great deal of metabolism.

Although several texts discuss the sole use of gaseous agents to induce anaesthesia in rabbits, breath-holding is common (Gonzalez-Gil *et al.*, 2006; Jepson, 2009). This may lead to hypoxia, hypercapnia and bradycardia, and potentially death.

Chloroform derivatives

Halothane is an example of a chloroform derivative agent. Induction of anaesthesia in birds using high concentrations of halothane is dangerous, with fatal levels building up in posterior air sacs (Jepson, 2009).

Halogenated ethers

Overdoses of halogenated ethers such as isoflurane and sevoflurane cause apnoea before cardiac arrest, allowing intervention in carefully monitored patients.

Most isoflurane is expired, with only 0.2% metabolized in the liver. Hystricomorph rodents (e.g. guinea pigs and chinchillas) often hypersalivate in response to isoflurane. Administration of an anticholinergic agent such as atropine (see earlier) will reduce this. Sevoflurane has negligible airway irritant effects.

Both isoflurane and sevoflurane are protective against myocardial infarction. In most species, both induction and recovery are rapid with these agents.

Reversal agents

Alpha-2 adrenergic antagonists

These agents include atipamezole and yohimbine. Atipamezole is used to reverse alpha-2 agonist agents such as medetomidine. Yohimbine is a more specific reversal agent for xylazine. Note that after administration of the reversal agent, any beneficial effects of the alpha-2 agonist (such as analgesia) are also lost.

Benzodiazepine reversal agents

Flumazenil is a benzodiazepine antagonist. Sarmazenil is a partial agonist of benzodiazepine receptors.

Naloxone

This agent reverses the action of opioids, including full opioid agonists such as fentanyl and partial agonists such as buprenorphine. Sedative and analgesic effects of the opioid are both lost after reversal.

Anaesthesia protocols

Commonly used anaesthetic protocols for species seen frequently in small animal practice are given in Figure 7.7.

Species–specific considerations

Species–specific considerations must be borne in mind when anaesthetizing the exotic patient (Figure 7.8).

Species	Drug	Dose	Route	Comment
Most species				
Any	Atipamezole	<5 times medetomidine dose	Intramuscular	Reversal of medetomidine
Most species	Atropine	0.01–0.04 mg/kg	Intramuscular/subcutaneous	Anticholinergic premedicant. Ineffective in most rabbits and many rats
	Benzodiazepines, e.g. diazepam	0.5–1.0 mg/kg	Intramuscular/intravenous	Sedation
Mammals				
Rabbits	Fentanyl/fluanisone	0.2–0.5 ml/kg	Intramuscular	Results in sedation
	Fentanyl/fluanisone, followed by midazolam	0.2–0.3 ml/kg, then 0.5–2 mg/kg	Intramuscular, then intravenous (10 minutes later)	
	Glycopyrrolate	0.01–0.02 mg/kg	Subcutaneous/intravenous/intramuscular	Anticholinergic premedicant
	Medetomidine	0.1 mg/kg	Intramuscular	Results in sedation

7.7 Commonly used anaesthetic protocols for commonly seen species. (continues) ▶

Species	Drug	Dose	Route	Comment
Mammals (continued)				
Rabbits (continued)	Medetomidine + ketamine + butorphanol	0.1 mg/kg + 5 mg/kg + 0.5 mg/kg	Intramuscular	
	Midazolam	0.5–2.0 mg/kg	Intramuscular/subcutaneous	Results in sedation
	Naloxone	0.01–0.10 mg/kg	Intramuscular/intravenous/intraperitoneal	Reversal of opioids
	Propofol	3–6 mg/kg	Intravenous	Induces anaesthesia after premedication
	Sevoflurane	To effect	Intubate or use facemask to maintain anaesthesia	
Rodents	Medetomidine	0.1 mg/kg	Intramuscular	Results in sedation
	Midazolam	1–2 mg/kg	Intramuscular/subcutaneous	Results in sedation
Small rodents in general	Isoflurane	To effect (usually induce 3–5%, maintain 0.25–4%)	Induction chambers to induce, then use facemask to maintain	Intubate if possible
	Sevoflurane	To effect	Induction chamber to induce, then use facemask to maintain	Intubate if possible
Mice	Medetomidine + ketamine	1 mg/kg + 50–75 mg/kg	Intramuscular	
Rats	Glycopyrrolate	0.01–0.02 mg/kg	Subcutaneous/intravenous/intramuscular	Anticholinergic premedicant
	Medetomidine + ketamine	0.5 mg/kg + 75 mg/kg	Intramuscular	
Gerbils	Fentanyl/fluanisone	0.5–1.0 ml/kg	Intramuscular	Results in sedation
Guinea pigs	Medetomidine + ketamine	0.5 mg/kg + 40 mg/kg	Intramuscular	
Chinchillas	Acepromazine + ketamine	0.4–0.5 mg/kg + 40–50 mg/kg	Intramuscular	
	Medetomidine + ketamine	0.06 mg/kg + 5 mg/kg	Intramuscular	
	Naloxone	0.05 mg/kg	Subcutaneous/intraperitoneal	Reversal of opioids
Ferrets	Fentanyl/fluanisone	0.3 ml/kg	Intramuscular	Results in sedation
	Halothane	To effect	Induction chamber or facemask to induce, then intubate or use facemask to maintain	
	Isoflurane	To effect (usually induce 3–5%, maintain 0.25–4%)	Induction chamber to induce, then intubate or use facemask to maintain	
	Medetomidine	0.1 mg/kg	Intramuscular	Results in sedation
	Medetomidine + ketamine	0.08 + 5 mg/kg	Intramuscular	
	Medetomidine + ketamine + butorphanol	0.08 mg/kg + 5 mg/kg + 0.1 mg/kg	Intramuscular	
	Midazolam	0.3–1.0 mg/kg	Intramuscular/subcutaneous	Results in sedation
	Naloxone	0.01–0.03 mg/kg	Intramuscular/intravenous	Reversal of opioids
	Propofol	1–3 mg/kg	Intravenous	Induces anaesthesia after premedication
		8 mg/kg	Intravenous	Induces anaesthesia if un-premedicated
	Sevoflurane	To effect	Induction chamber to induce, then intubate or use facemask to maintain	

7.7 (continued) Commonly used anaesthetic protocols for commonly seen species. (continues) ▶

Species	Drug	Dose	Route	Comment
Mammals (continued)				
Small non-human primates	Medetomidine + ketamine	0.1 mg/kg + 10–15 mg/kg	Intramuscular	
	Sevoflurane	To effect	Induction chamber to induce, then intubate or use facemask to maintain	
Wild mammals				
Foxes	Medetomidine + ketamine + butorphanol	0.02 mg/kg + 4 mg/kg + 0.4 mg/kg	Intramuscular	
	Sevoflurane	To effect	Intubate or use facemask to maintain anaesthesia	
Badgers	Medetomidine + ketamine	0.04 mg/kg + 5.0–7.5 mg/kg	Intramuscular	
	Medetomidine + ketamine + butorphanol	0.02 mg/kg + 4 mg/kg + 0.4 mg/kg	Intramuscular	
	Sevoflurane	To effect	Intubate or use facemask to maintain anaesthesia	
Hedgehogs	Isoflurane	To effect (usually induce 3–5%, maintain 0.25–4%)	Induction chamber to induce, then use facemask to maintain	Intubate if possible
	Naloxone	0.16 mg/kg	Intramuscular	Reversal of opioids
	Sevoflurane	To effect	Induction chamber to induce, then use facemask to maintain	
Bats	Isoflurane	To effect (usually induce 3–5%, maintain 0.25–4%)	Induction chamber to induce, then use facemask to maintain	
	Sevoflurane	To effect	Induction chamber to induce, then use facemask to maintain	
Birds				
Most species	Isoflurane	To effect (usually induce 3–5%, maintain 0.25–4%)	Use facemask to induce	Intubate if possible
	Ketamine + midazolam	10–40 mg/kg + 0.2–2.0 mg/kg	Subcutaneous/intramuscular	Sedation (depth varies depending on dose and species)
	Propofol	<14 mg/kg (dose to effect)	Intravenous	Induction of anaesthesia
Waterfowl	Ketamine + xylazine	5 mg/kg + 1–4 mg/kg	Intramuscular/intravenous	
	Medetomidine + ketamine	0.15–0.3 mg/kg + 3–5 mg/kg	Intravenous/intramuscular	
Reptiles				
Most reptile species	Medetomidine + ketamine	0.05–0.10 mg/kg + 5 mg/kg	Intramuscular/intravenous	Species variation in response
	Alfaxalone	10–15 mg/kg (dose to effect)	Intravenous	Some effect after intramuscular administration
	Ketamine	<60 mg/kg (usually 5–20)	Intramuscular/lower dose required if intravenous	Sedation
		60–90 mg/kg	Intramuscular/lower dose required if intravenous	Anaesthesia
	Propofol	<10 mg/kg	Intravenous	Induction of anaesthesia; lower dose if premedicated
	Tiletamine/ zolazepam	4–10 mg/kg	Intramuscular	Results in sedation

7.7 (continued) Commonly used anaesthetic protocols for commonly seen species. (continues) ▶

Species	Drug	Dose	Route	Comment
Reptiles (continued)				
Lizards	Medetomidine/ ketamine	0.1–0.15 mg/kg + 5–10 mg/kg	Intramuscular/intravenous + intramuscular	
Snakes	Tiletamine/ zolazepam	10–40 mg/kg	Intramuscular	Induction of anaesthesia; recovery variable

7.7 (continued) Commonly used anaesthetic protocols for commonly seen species.

Mammals

- Rabbits and rodents are nasal breathers – the soft palate is locked around the epiglottis when the mouth is closed. This could potentially lead to suffocation if the nares are blocked in any way. When conscious, nasal breathers will panic if the nares are forced closed, and care should be taken not to block or cover nares in unintubated anaesthetized animals.
- Mammals with large abdomens/hindguts (e.g. rabbits, rodents and ferrets) should be positioned in sternal recumbency where possible, with the chest elevated slightly more than the abdomen.
- Hypothermia is a risk factor due to their reduced size/mass to high body surface area ratio.
- Iatrogenic bloat or the filling of the stomach with air may occur, caused by intubating the oesophagus instead of the trachea.
- Rabbits require glycopyrrolate rather than atropine to treat bradycardia, due to the high chance they possess atropinesterases.
- Rodents will often require atropine or glycopyrrolate to compensate for/appease the excessive production of saliva and porphyrin secretions.
- Gerbils can suffer from congenital epilepsy, which becomes apparent when they are stressed.
- Ferrets can develop a massive fall in blood pressure following an apparently successful recovery, especially where there has been blood loss.

Birds

- Complete tracheal cartilaginous rings; therefore cuffed tubes should not be used, to prevent 'pressure necrosis' of the tracheal lining (Girling, 2003; Degernes, 2008).
- Lungs are rigid and attached to thoracic vertebrae.
- Air sacs and pneumonized bones are intrinsic to the respiratory system; air is cycled through the air sacs and lungs over two respiratory cycles (Girling, 2003; Longley, 2008).
- No diaphragm.
- The 'dive response' of waterfowl means that apnoea and bradycardia are common in mask induction of these species, thought to be caused by stimulation to the beak and nares. Positioning helps to reduce the risks associated with this; lateral recumbency is preferred.
- Birds should be intubated for procedures >5 minutes in duration to prevent mucus movement/respiratory secretions in the upper airway.
- If IPPV is not available, movement of the wings, keel and legs may simulate normal respiration movements by causing the air sacs to act as bellows, circulating the air through the lungs.
- Care should be taken to avoid ocular damage when testing for the corneal reflex.
- Air sacs can accumulate gases, which may prolong recoveries.

Reptiles

- Snake and lizard tracheas have incomplete (C-shaped) rings.
- The trachea is particularly long in snakes.
- Chelonians have complete tracheal rings and therefore should not have a cuffed ETT.
- Chelonians have a very short trachea (sometimes branching into two bronchi within the neck); it is therefore possible to intubate only one bronchus if the tube is advanced too far, resulting in inadequate ventilation and damage.
- Lizards and snakes have intercostal muscles to move the ribcage.
- The rib cage of chelonians is fixed; they must move their limbs and neck in order for air to enter and leave the lungs.
- No diaphragm.
- Chelonians can hold their breath for extended periods of time (>24 hours in some species), and some lizards can also hold their breath for up to 5 hours; intubation is therefore required to ensure adequate respiration throughout anaesthesia and recovery.
- Apnoea is most common during recovery, and chelonians can survive for long periods without drawing breath by converting to anaerobic respiration. Therefore, care must be taken not to over-ventilate using IPPV and 100% oxygen, as this will depress the respiration.
- Many lizards shed their tails (autotomize) with careless handling.

7.8 A summary of species-specific considerations for anaesthesia.

Mammals

In general, small rodents are not premedicated, as inhalational agents are typically used for induction and maintenance of anaesthesia. In some species, premedication may be used to reduce stress and side effects of gaseous agents (such as hypersalivation), for example in guinea pigs and chinchillas. Isoflurane and sevoflurane result in rapid recovery. Sevoflurane is preferred for induction as it is less irritant to respiratory passages. Induction may be performed in a chamber, although larger species such as ferrets may be restrained while a facemask is applied. Intubation is feasible in larger species such as ferrets and rabbits but is challenging in smaller species including rodents. Please refer to the section on intubation later in this chapter.

Injectable agents are rarely used on their own in small species, but are useful for prolonged and/or painful procedures. Injectable anaesthetics are useful for oral or neck procedures, although oxygen should be routinely supplemented to all patients during anaesthesia. However, species such as rabbits frequently hold their breath if anaesthetic induction is attempted using only inhalational anaesthetics. Injectable combinations are more routinely used in this species. In some cases, injectable premedication (e.g. with a benzodiazepine, or butorphanol and medetomidine) may be utilized. This will sedate the rabbit and may help to reduce breath-holding before induction using an inhalational agent. Rabbits should always be pre-oxygenated before use of gaseous agents to induce anaesthesia.

Birds

Birds do not have a diaphragm; movements of the keel accomplish respiratory movements. Air is passed unidirectionally, enabling very efficient gas exchange, through the lungs by use of air sacs that act as bellows. Some bones are also connected to the airways, for example the humerus in most species.

Premedication may be used to sedate a stressed bird and/or to provide analgesia before a painful procedure is performed. Common options (sometimes used in combination) include butorphanol, benzodiazepines and low doses of ketamine.

For most species encountered in general practice, including psittacine and passerine birds, anaesthesia is induced and maintained using solely inhalational agents; the bird is restrained and induced via a facemask. Induction in a chamber may be slightly less stressful for small birds. Birds are pre-oxygenated for a short period before addition of gaseous anaesthetics.

Diving species such as ducks may breath-hold with gaseous agents, and so injectable anaesthetics are often used in these species. Benzodiazepines, in combination with ketamine or propofol, are frequently employed.

Reptiles

Reptiles (apart from crocodilians) do not have a diaphragm.

For non-invasive, non-painful procedures such as conscious radiographs, the vasovagal reflex can be used, as discussed in Chapter 1, but should never be used for painful procedures.

Premedicants such as butorphanol or ketamine may be used in reptiles. These may precede induction using gaseous agents (either in a chamber or after intubation, see below) or intravenous anaesthetics.

Ketamine is a safe anaesthetic in reptiles. Effects are dose-dependent, and the clinician can use this agent as a sedative or full anaesthetic. However, high doses are associated with a prolonged recovery (possibly days) (Lawton, 1992).

In large or particularly defensive chelonians such as *Geochelone* species (e.g. leopard and African spurred tortoises) the animal may pull its limbs inside the shell, prohibiting intravenous access (Figure 7.9). Intramuscular premedicants and/or anaesthetics are required in these patients. Ketamine may be used alone or in combination with alpha-2 agonists.

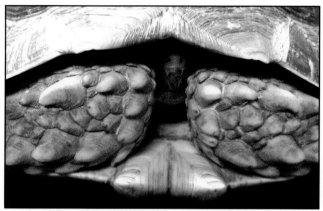

7.9 Some species of tortoise, such as this African spurred tortoise, will resist examination of the head, making jugular access challenging in the conscious animal.

Anaesthesia is usually induced in lizards and chelonians using injectable agents. Drugs of choice include the short-acting agents propofol and alfaxalone. In most chelonian species, the jugular vein is relatively easy to access, while the ventral coccygeal vein is used in lizards. Care should be taken with species of lizard that autotomize their tail, such as leopard geckos; unless the individual is very calm or weak, the intramuscular route is preferred. The ventral coccygeal vein is often more difficult to access in the short tail of snakes, and anaesthetic agents are more commonly injected intramuscularly in these animals. Anaesthesia of small snakes may be induced in an airtight container using gaseous agents. In larger non-venomous snakes, conscious intubation may be performed for induction using intermittent positive pressure ventilation (IPPV) of gaseous anaesthetics.

Wildlife

Anaesthesia of wildlife patients is usually the best (and sometimes only) means of allowing the patient to be handled by veterinary staff. For example, anaesthesia is usually required before a hedgehog can be unrolled and examined. Preparations should include consideration of any procedures that may need to be performed. For example, the animal should be examined in detail, samples (e.g. blood) obtained, medications and fluids administered, and imaging or surgery performed. As with other species discussed in this chapter, time given to preparation before the anaesthetic is well spent and will minimize the animal's anaesthetic time.

Wild animals generally carry zoonotic disease, often asymptomatically (see Chapter 6); staff should therefore take care to wear personal protective equipment (PPE) when handling these patients. This is paramount when working closely with anaesthetized patients. Equipment should be thoroughly disinfected between patients to reduce transfer of pathogens.

Sedation or tranquillization is very useful to reduce stress in hospitalized wildlife. Premedicants may be helpful to calm birds of prey.

Smaller wildlife species (including garden birds, hedgehogs and bats) and medium-sized birds (such as seabirds and birds of prey) are usually induced with gaseous anaesthetics as for most pet birds, usually in a chamber to minimize stress in small species, or using a facemask for medium-sized birds restrained manually.

Delicate species, such as bats, require careful handling during induction and a non-traumatic facemask when maintaining anaesthetic gas delivery, such as a soft plastic Spigot connector for an Ayre's T-piece circuit (Figure 7.10).

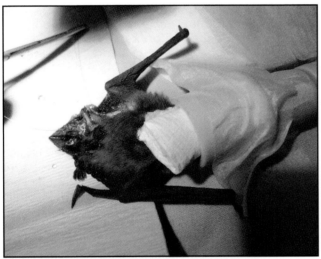

7.10 A common pipistrelle bat induced and maintained using sevoflurane and a Spigot connector for an Ayre's T-piece breathing circuit.

An examination glove stretched over the facemask can be used to provide a good seal around thin beaks, e.g. for seabirds such as gannets. These techniques can also be used for small mammals such as hedgehogs. The use of gaseous anaesthetic agents alone permits rapid post-anaesthetic recovery.

The dive response in some birds (particularly waterfowl) may occur in response to induction of anaesthesia. This stress response results in episodes of apnoea and bradycardia. Injectable protocols are therefore preferred in waterfowl, for example ketamine with xylazine administered intravenously in swans.

Larger mammalian species such as foxes and badgers pose a safety risk to staff involved in their treatment. Injectable anaesthetics, such as ketamine with medetomidine, are usually used to induce anaesthesia in such animals. Use of such a protocol minimizes restraint time during gaseous induction, reducing stress for the animal and reducing the risk of staff being bitten.

For all species, anaesthesia is maintained or topped-up using gaseous anaesthetics. Intubation is possible in larger species.

Intubation

Intubation protects the patient's airway from aspiration of fluids (either from the oral cavity or regurgitated), permits oxygen and anaesthetic gas provision, and allows IPPV. The ability to intubate exotic and wildlife species should be viewed as an essential element of a veterinary nurse's skill set and as part of their responsibility to preserve life.

When to intubate

In general, it is preferable to intubate anaesthetized patients. However, for many exotic species this is frequently not straightforward due to their small size and anatomical considerations, and unsuccessful attempts can extend the period of anaesthesia or potentially damage the patient. While the authors recommend intubation for species whenever practical, this should be balanced against detrimental effects.

For many short procedures, e.g. phlebotomy and radiography, the simplest and quickest method of anaesthesia would be an inhalation anaesthetic via a facemask. This reduces time waiting for intramuscular injectables to take effect and allows for a much faster reversal of effects once anaesthetic gases are turned off. In these instances, the anaesthetist should have intubation equipment on-hand, in case the situation is prolonged or deteriorates. Intubation should always be performed for longer procedures, for patients with respiratory disease or for anaesthetic combinations likely to result in apnoea.

Anatomical considerations

Mammals

Diminutive size is the main issue affecting intubation of exotic mammals. If orotracheal intubation is not possible, performing a tracheostomy should be considered in an emergency.

Birds

In general, intubation of birds is relatively straightforward, with the glottis located midline at the base of the tongue. However, anatomical variations in some species can make the procedure trickier, e.g. the fleshy tongue of parrots and the tracheal crests of certain bird species, including some waterfowl (Figure 7.11). The tracheal rings of birds are complete and use of a cuffed endotracheal tube could damage the trachea, which may result in stricture formation. Use of a cuffless endotracheal tube (ETT) is preferred (see Equipment, later).

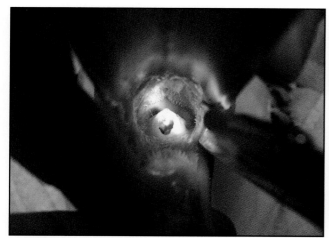

7.11 The glottis of a swan. Note the surrounding tracheal crests.

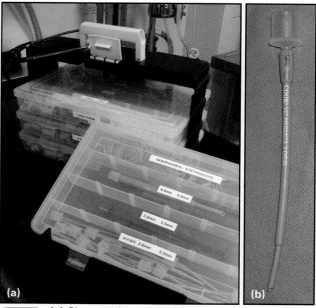

7.13 (a) Clean and protected storage of a variety of ETTs for exotic patients. (b) A Cook ETT.

Reptiles

The glottis of reptiles is located at the base of the tongue. In snakes it is very obvious, as they have a thin tongue (Figure 7.12); in chelonians and lizards (with fleshier tongues) the glottis may be more difficult to see but is still relatively rostral.

In tortoises there is only a short length of trachea before it bifurcates, often within the neck. A short ETT should be used in these species to avoid intubating a single bronchus.

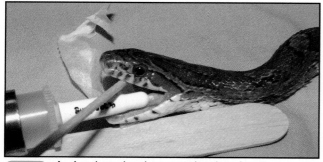

7.12 An intubated red cornsnake showing the rostrally positioned glottis.

Equipment

The veterinary practice should stock a variety of ETTs, including various sizes and shapes (Figure 7.13a). As a guide, a 2.5 kg rabbit will probably require a 2.5–3 mm ETT, while a 300 g parrot also requires a 3 mm ETT. Tubes may be made of rubber or latex; the latter may be transparent and provide advantages for monitoring breathing (using the presence of condensation).

Many exotic and wildlife species do not require cuffed ETTs; this is particularly true for species with complete tracheal rings, such as birds and tortoises. Cook ETTs (Figure 7.13b) have a step or shoulder, so the narrow end sits within the trachea but a seal is created at the glottis by the thicker portion.

Whichever ETT is used, attention should be paid to minimizing dead space within the anaesthetic circuit by reducing the length of ETT outside the animal's body. This often requires ETTs to be shortened before use.

For very small patients, ETTs can be fashioned from intravenous catheters. Obstruction by respiratory secretions is common with such small tubes; this is reduced if IPPV is performed throughout the procedure. If obstruction occurs, the tube should be extracted and cleaned before replacing.

A laryngoscope is used to depress the tongue and visualize the glottis (Figure 7.14). A suitably sized laryngoscope blade should be used, such as a Wisconsin size 0 or 1 for rabbit or larger mammal species intubation.

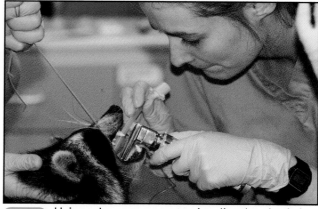

7.14 Using a laryngoscope to visualize the glottis in a raccoon. (Courtesy of Job Stumpel)

Procedures for common species

Mammals

Ferrets are intubated as for small cats. Orotracheal and nasotracheal intubation are both possible in rabbits, and nasotracheal intubation is also possible in rodents. However, nasotracheal intubation may introduce pathogens from the upper airways into the lower airways.

The main challenges of rabbit intubation are the long and narrow buccal cavity, and the tendency for laryngospasm and oedema. Despite these anatomical challenges, various successful protocols/techniques have been developed, ranging from using endoscopy to visualize the epiglottis, to the 'blind' technique, which merely requires the ETT and a keen sense of hearing. The procedure described below uses direct visualization of the rabbit's epiglottis with an auriscope (otoscope), and is the technique used routinely by the author (WB). It cannot be stressed enough that before attempting to perform this procedure, and even before a sedative/anaesthetic is administered, the required equipment should be assembled and everyone involved must be briefed regarding the intubation procedure.

Rabbit intubation procedure

Equipment (Figure 7.15a (overleaf))

- Small forceps to hold out the tongue.
- An auriscope with a long enclosed cone (or laryngoscope with size 0 or 1 Wisconsin blade) to visualize the trachea/glottis.
- Local anaesthetic to minimize laryngospasm.
- A selection of uncuffed ETTs (2–3.5 mm) of good length (50–70 mm).
- An 'introducer' such as a 6Fr dog catheter with the port removed (does not always fit down the lumen of 2 mm ETTs).
- A tie to secure the ETT in place, e.g. a length of open weave bandage.
- A breathing circuit with bag, oxygen and anaesthetic gas.
- Capnography to assess successful intubation if available, including ETT connectors with a side-sampling port.

Technique

1. The selected ETTs are measured against the patient and the point of exit from the mouth identified on the tube (Figure 7.15b).
2. The rabbit is positioned in sternal recumbency, ideally with oxygen supplied. The author (WB) prefers this position, although some texts (e.g. Flecknell, 1996) describe positioning in dorsal recumbency. The handler holds the rabbit behind its head with their hand palm-side up, placing their fingers under the jaw and gently hyperextending the head so that the larynx is in a straight vertical position (Figure 7.15c). The person intubating may find it easier to hold the head until the glottis is visualized. If the head is overextended the airway will be blocked.
3. Forceps are used to grasp and extend the tongue gently, to ensure it is not obscuring the field of view. The auriscope is carefully inserted into the mouth, if the jaw tone is relaxed, and over the tongue until the glottis is visualized (Figure 7.15d). Care must be taken in smaller rabbits to ensure that delicate orophayngeal membranes are not damaged upon insertion of the auriscope cone. Repeated probing of the glottis can result in oedema and inflammation that may jeopardize intubation attempts or airway patency. There should be no more than three intubation attempts.
4. Local anaesthetic is sprayed on to the end of the introducer (Figure 7.15e) or down the cone or blade. The rabbit can then be put back into normal sternal recumbency and given 100% oxygen by facemask for about 30 seconds (to allow the local anaesthetic to take effect). After this time, assuming the rabbit is still stable, the patient is repositioned for intubation as in steps 1 and 2. Once the opening and closing of the epiglottis is visualized, the introducer is then inserted approximately 1 cm past the epiglottis (Figure 7.15f).
5. The auriscope is carefully removed while the introducer is held in place
6. The ETT is threaded on to the introducer and inserted until the pre-marked point on the ETT is reached (Figure 7.15g). The introducer is removed and the ETT secured in place with a tie (e.g. bandage material), behind the ears and head (Figure 7.15h). The ETT is connected to a circuit supplying oxygen and anaesthetic gas as soon as possible.
7. **Placement confirmation**: There may not be a cough response in rabbits. The tube's placement is checked by: attaching the tube to a circuit and using IPPV; observing condensation in clear tube connectors or on a glass slide held to the tip of the ETT; or placing a small tuft of hair in front of the tube and observing its movement with each breath. **On no account should the chest be compressed; this could easily damage the rabbit or displace the tube.** If capnography is available, this can be used to show CO_2 emissions if the trachea has been intubated correctly.

Birds

Birds are easily intubated, and this should be done for all but very short procedures (see When to intubate, earlier). The glottis is typically easy to visualize in the midline at the base of the tongue (Figure 7.16). Cartilage rings in the avian trachea are complete and ETTs should be uncuffed (ideally cuffless). The lumen is relatively large (e.g. a 3 mm ETT is required for a 300 g parrot).

After induction using a facemask, an assistant holds the bird's head (including the upper beak) towards the anaesthetist. The anaesthetist pulls the lower beak down to reveal the glottis. In species with a fleshy tongue this may need to be depressed to visualize the glottis. The ETT is inserted without force into the trachea and secured in place. ETTs are usually attached to the lower beak using adhesive paper tape.

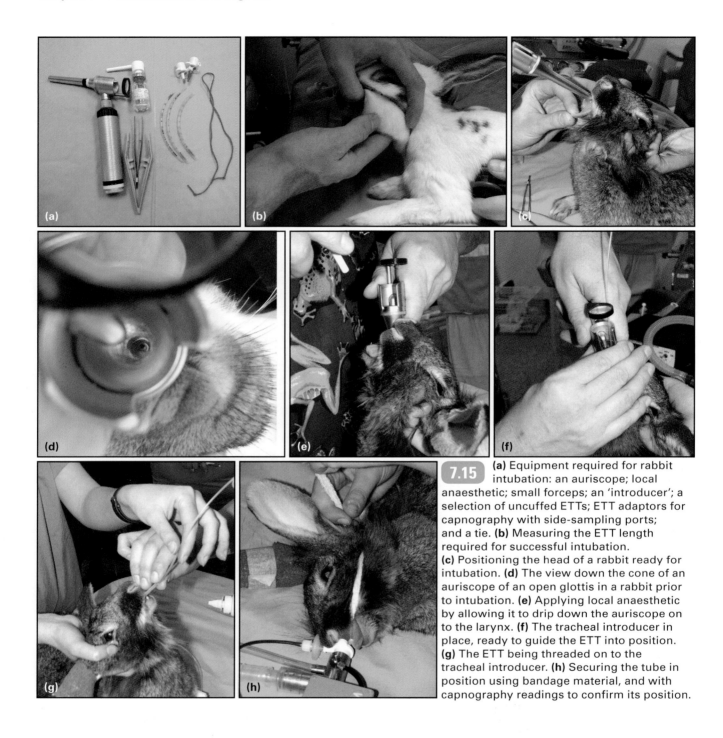

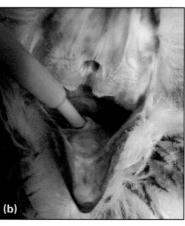

7.15 (a) Equipment required for rabbit intubation: an auriscope; local anaesthetic; small forceps; an 'introducer'; a selection of uncuffed ETTs; ETT adaptors for capnography with side-sampling ports; and a tie. (b) Measuring the ETT length required for successful intubation. (c) Positioning the head of a rabbit ready for intubation. (d) The view down the cone of an auriscope of an open glottis in a rabbit prior to intubation. (e) Applying local anaesthetic by allowing it to drip down the auriscope on to the larynx. (f) The tracheal introducer in place, ready to guide the ETT into position. (g) The ETT being threaded on to the tracheal introducer. (h) Securing the tube in position using bandage material, and with capnography readings to confirm its position.

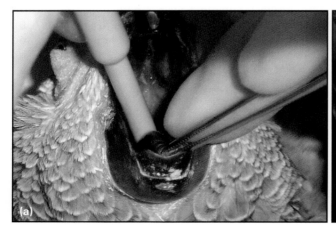

7.16 Intubation using an ETT in (a) an African grey parrot (Courtesy of Kevin Eatwell) and (b) an eagle owl.

Air sac cannulation

Air sac cannulation is an extremely useful technique. For dyspnoeic patients with upper airway disease, it provides access to the respiratory tract for provision of air/oxygen (and also inhalational anaesthetic agents as required). For patients requiring surgical intervention on the head or neck, utilization of an air sac cannula in the caudal part of the bird permits better access for the surgeon.

The cannula is inserted into either the abdominal or caudal thoracic air sacs (see Chapter 3). The cannula should be soft with lateral fenestrations, and of a size proportional to the bird (e.g. 4 mm for a 350 g parrot). Proprietary tubes are available, but cut-down ETTs can be used in an emergency.

The patient is restrained in right lateral recumbency (usually under inhalational anaesthesia induced using a facemask), permitting access to the left lateral body wall. The hindlimb is pulled either cranially or caudally, enabling the clinician to make a skin incision just caudal to the last rib, halfway down the body wall (ventral to the flexor cruris medialis muscle if the leg is drawn cranially). Small haemostats are used to puncture the musculature of the body wall and enter the air sac. Sutures can be used to keep the cannula in place.

Reptiles

Intubation is also relatively straightforward in reptiles. The glottis is situated in the midline at the base of the tongue; it is more rostral in carnivorous species such as monitor lizards. In snakes, the glottis is fairly rostral and very easy to see when the oral cavity is opened. As previously discussed, a short ETT should be used in chelonians to ensure a single bronchus is not entered. In reptiles the resting position is closed, with the glottis opening during inspiration/expiration, at which time the ETT can be gently inserted. The ETT is then secured in place with tape to the lower jaw.

Anaesthetic monitoring

Sensitive monitoring and management skills, and clear communication between the anaesthetist and surgeon, are vital for identifying and rectifying early signs of problems. When monitoring an animal, it is ideal to acquire and refer to its baseline parameters and consistently maintain data collection methods to avoid variation in values. Throughout the anaesthesia and recovery period, the anaesthetist should be vigilant for trends and changes in the patient's biological parameters, e.g. heart rate, respiratory rate and temperature.

The role of the nurse or anaesthetist cannot be fulfilled by machines. Monitoring and/or maintenance devices should be used in conjunction with observation by the veterinary team, to enhance the monitoring process and therefore optimize sensitive and successful anaesthesia. Despite the comfort of using machines, it is vital to look at the patient rather than to focus on digital displays.

Figure 7.17 provides an example of an anaesthetic and recovery record.

Preparing the patient

Setting up equipment before anaesthesia will reduce time spent preparing the patient and minimize anaesthetic time. This also includes pre-prepared emergency drugs (see Figure 7.27). Attachment of monitoring devices such as a temperature probe, capnograph, Doppler ultrasound probe and blood pressure cuff should be done as soon as the patient is stable under anaesthetic. Thoughtful preparation of the surgical site will ensure temperature loss is minimized, e.g. reducing the clipped/plucked and scrubbed surgical area and applying warm surgical preparations rather than cold could delay a drop in body temperature.

Positioning

Inappropriate positioning of the patient can significantly compromise respiratory and anaesthetic efficiency, and positioning should be carefully considered throughout the procedure. Rabbits and other hindgut fermenters should be positioned in sternal recumbency where possible, with the chest slightly elevated (see Figure 7.20). Birds should be kept in lateral recumbency to minimize the restrictions posed to the expansion of their air sacs. Reptiles can generally be kept in sternal recumbency, although chameleons will lie better in lateral recumbency.

It is advisable to release dental gags every 10–15 minutes to relax facial muscles, particularly in rodents. For further information see Anaesthetic problems, later.

Ocular desiccation

Mammals in particular suffer from desiccation of the cornea when they are heavily sedated or anaesthetized, as the intermittent blink reflex to rehydrate the corneal surface is lost. The eyelids can be taped closed, or ocular lubricants can be used (with repeated application during long procedures). A small amount of lubricant can also be applied to the eyes of birds, taking care not to interfere with the corneal reflex checks. Snakes and some lizard species do not require lubricant owing to the presence of fused, transparent eyelids (spectacles).

Heart rate

Heart rates in some anaesthetized exotic species, particularly small mammals and birds, can reach >350 beats per minute, and consequently many mechanical devices struggle to achieve a consistent reading. For observers, the heart rate will be too fast to count, resulting in a reliance upon sensitive hearing to detect any changes in rhythm and rate. It is, however, possible to count beats over a shorter time period, e.g. 5 or 10 seconds, and then multiply appropriately to convert to beats per minute.

EXOTIC AND WILDLIFE ANAESTHESIA RECORD

Date: / / Case number:......................... Species:............................... Procedure:...

Animal's name: .... Owner's name: .... Bodyweight:................................

Sex: *M / F / N / E* Age: *(years)*........ *(months)*............ Vet & VN:...

Pharmaceuticals (Induction, Analgesia, Maintenance & Recovery)

Drug name	Dose rate mg/kg or %	Total dose (ml)	Route (i.v., i.m., s.c., i.o., i.p.)	Time given	Time of effect and comments

Emergency drugs (pre-calculate maximum safe dose for individual patient)

Drug name	Dose rate mg/kg or %	Total dose (ml)	Route (i.v., i.m., s.c., i.o., i.p.)	Time given	Time of effect and comments
Adrenaline (1 mg/ml)					
Atropine (0.6 mg/ml)					
Diazepam (5 mg/ml)					
Doxapram (20 mg/ml)					
Glycopyrrolate (0.2 mg/ml)					
Naloxone (0.04 mg/ml)					

Fluid therapy – .... *ml/kg/h. Total/h:* .... *Bolus amount (* .... *ml) and frequency (* .... *)*

RECOVERY MONITORING (Commence when gas turned off and/or reversible drugs administered)

Min	0	15	30	45	60	75	90	105	120	135	150	165	180	195	210
Actual time															
Heart rate															
Respiratory rate															
Temperature															
Head lift															
Coordinated movement (actual time)															
Fluid therapy															
Other events or treatments															

7.17 An example of an anaesthetic and recovery record for exotic and wildlife patients. (continues) ▶

Time (min) + Actual time	Pre-anaesthetic parameters	0	5	10	15	20	25	30	35	40	45	50	55	60	65	70	75	80	85	90	95	100	105	110	115	120
Iso %																										
Sevo %																										
O_2																										
IPPV (√)																										
>350																										
350																										
300																										
280																										
260																										
240																										
220																										
200																										
180																										
160																										
140																										
120																										
100																										
90																										
80																										
70																										
60																										
55																										
50																										
45																										
40																										
35																										
30																										
25																										
20																										
15																										
10																										
05																										
00																										
Temp																										
Fluids																										
Event																										

Key: Heart rate = **X** Respiratory rate = ◯ Blood pressure = ● End tidal CO_2 = ∧ O_2 saturation = ∨

* = Anaesthetic event 1:.. # = Anaesthetic event 2:..

Notes: ....
....
....

7.17 (continued) An example of an anaesthetic and recovery record for exotic and wildlife patients.

Electrocardiography

Electrocardiography (ECG) can be useful in providing instantaneous data that will clearly determine any maintenance and emergency treatments. For many exotic pets, blunted crocodile clips can be used or, for lizard species, clips can be attached to needles inserted into the skin. For normal rabbit ECG values, see Fraser and Girling (2009) and Lord *et al.* (2010). For ECG probe placement in exotic species, see Bailey and Pablo (1998).

Doppler ultrasonography

Doppler ultrasonography provides audio monitoring of the heart and, once in place, allows hands-free constant monitoring. When using a Doppler ultrasound probe it is possible to connect non-invasive blood pressure monitoring equipment to mammals, including small rabbit breeds. Placement of the probe in a small mammal is most easily done over the cephalic vein (or lateral tail veil in rats). The fur must be clipped or plenty of contact gel applied.

The most accessible pulse points in birds are over the ulnar vein (Figure 7.18) in most species, or the tarsometatarsal vein in waterfowl.

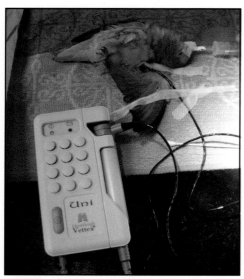

7.18 An anaesthetized peach-faced lovebird having its heart rate monitored by a flexible transducer Doppler probe. Note the position of the bird in dorsal recumbency, as opposed to the preferred lateral recumbency, owing to the nature of the surgical site over the keel.

Rigid Doppler probes are more useful in reptiles, where chelonians' and lizards' heart rates can be measured at the thoracic inlet (between the forelimb and jaw) (Figure 7.19), and snakes' (and also lizards') pulses can be found directly over the heart.

Respiration

For most veterinary nurses, the extent of respiratory monitoring involves observing the rate, rhythm and, rather subjectively, the volume of the patient's breaths. Some affordable and practical machines can facilitate respiratory monitoring, but those basic monitoring techniques should never be discarded.

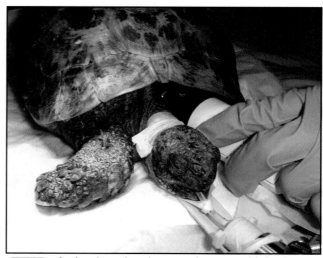

7.19 An intubated and recovering spur-thighed tortoise having its heart rate monitored using a rigid Doppler probe placed at the thoracic inlet. (Courtesy of Kevin Eatwell)

Respiratory monitors such as capnographs and pulse oximeters are particularly useful in small exotic species. Mucous membrane colour and capillary refill time are also useful indicators of oxygen saturation and circulation efficiency (being more reliable in species with pink mucous membranes than those with pigmented membranes).

Capnography

Non-invasive capnography monitors are useful indicators of respiratory physiology and cardiovascular changes. They measure the percentage of CO_2 exhaled by the patient. Stanford (2004) provides a useful review of their use and interpretations in exotic animal anaesthesia. Special ETT adaptors can be employed to reduce the dead space and improve the capnograph's sampling capabilities in 'side-stream' sampling machines. In side-stream machines, the analyser is not directly next to the expired gases of the patient but is positioned a distance away and a small amount of the expired gases is continually pumped to the analyser for measurement of CO_2 (Figure 7.20); even if the patient is not intubated but is being maintained via a facemask, the side-stream connector can extract adequate samples when attached to a tight-fitting facemask. From this sample, a graph and percentage values are displayed for interpretation, e.g. inspired values should be 0 mmHg and end-tidal values should read between 35 and 45 mmHg (Stanford, 2004).

Pulse oximetry

Pulse oximetry measures the degree of oxygenation in the blood; this measurement can be used to indicate ventilation efficiency. The pulse oximeters used in many practices are useful for dogs and cats, but for the high metabolic and pulse rates of exotic species a more sensitive pulse oximeter will be required (Figure 7.21), such as one that records up to 350 beats per minute. Locations for the probes will depend on the species; they may be placed either on the skin or in the oesophagus, rectum or cloaca.

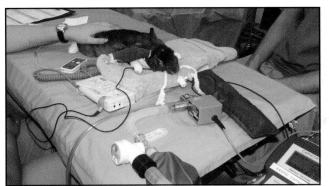

7.20 Monitoring biological parameters during the initial recovery stages in a rabbit immediately following surgery. The rabbit is still intubated, is in sternal recumbency and the chest has been slightly raised. This photo shows the continued use of capnography, thermometer probes and heart rate monitor (Doppler), with the option of IPPV (via ventilator or breathing circuit) should the rabbit become apnoeic. Rapid/sudden recoveries are not uncommon and an anaesthetist/assistant should place a hand on the rabbit until it is extubated and has been secured in an incubator or cage.

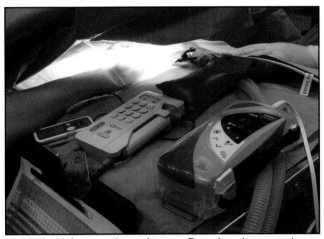

7.21 Using a pulse oximeter, Doppler ultrasound probe and long thermometer probe during endoscopy of a lovebird where access to the patient is limited.

Mechanical and manual ventilation

Mechanical or manually controlled IPPV should commence when successful intubation of patients is achieved, to facilitate optimal ventilation. When setting the rate and depth of pressure-cycled ventilators, this should start on the lowest setting and be gradually increased to mimic the patient's normal respiratory depth and pattern.

Ambu-bags, which are easy to use, are particularly useful during bird and reptile recovery. Reptile respiration needs to be stimulated by the presence of carbon dioxide in room air.

Body temperature

Owing to the large surface area to body mass ratio of small animals, many exotic and wildlife species are predisposed to a significant increase in body heat loss per gram. Conversely, many species possess no sweat glands, making hyperthermia a risk without careful consideration. Care should be taken when using cloacal or oesophageal thermometer probes for reptiles and birds, as it can be easy to damage these structures. Resistance may occur on insertion into the cloaca, or infection can be provoked if the probe enters the urinary tract.

Equipment that can be used to increase temperature includes water circulating blankets, forced warm air blankets, sterile clear plastic drapes, portable heaters to warm room air, microwavable heat packs, heated surgical tables, temporary warm water-filled surgical gloves, and hot water bottles (see Chapter 9).

Blood pressure

Data gathered from blood pressure readings will inform the anaesthetist of the animal's current blood volume and circulating pressure. It will help to have baseline levels from the conscious animal or at the sedation phase to compare; for example:

- **No variation:** Suggests that the patient is stable and so should be maintained and supported with appropriate fluid therapy, i.e. to replace fluids lost due to the drying effects of anaesthetic gases, continuing insensible losses and to replace loss due to any periods of not eating pre- and postoperatively
- **Increase:** Suggests inadequate anaesthesia and analgesia
- **Decrease:** Suggests a possible overdose of anaesthetic, or surgery which has led to blood and fluid loss.

Equipment required for blood pressure assessment includes a Doppler ultrasound probe and contact gel, placed over a pulse point (e.g. the carpal artery in most small mammals), and a blood pressure cuff attached to a sphygmomanometer (pressure gauge and pump). The cuff's width should be 30–40% of the patient's limb circumference, and should be placed proximal to the Doppler probe. This is useful in most mammal and bird species (Figure 7.22), but cannot be used in animals smaller than rats or canaries, respectively.

Invasive arterial blood pressure monitoring is possible in birds, mammals and medium to large (>300 g) reptiles. It is the gold standard of accurate arterial blood pressure monitoring but is not considered practical, particularly for reptiles, for several reasons. These include the requirement for costly sophisticated equipment, a surgical procedure to access the artery (as there are limited superficial vessels available) and considerable skill in placement of an intra-arterial catheter, which creates a high risk of thrombosis formation (Chinnadurai *et al.,* 2009).

The non-invasive technique, using the Doppler, cuff and sphygmomanometer as used in mammals and birds, is more practical than invasive techniques and this equipment can be positioned around a limb in lizards and chelonians, or at the base of the tail distal to the cloaca in snakes and lizards. In reptiles it can, however, be a challenge to isolate and maintain the location of the Doppler and cuff depending on the species (e.g. body size may be too small for

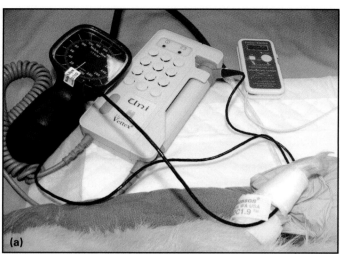
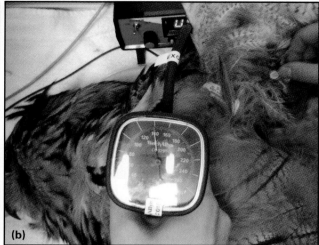

7.22 **(a)** Blood pressure monitoring of an anaesthetized ferret using the forelimb. **(b)** Measuring the blood pressure of an eagle owl using a Doppler ultrasound probe and sphygmomanometer.

the smallest available cuffs) and procedure (some procedures will limit the accessibility to certain body regions). Reptiles will also be more sensitive to environmental temperatures; a warm environment will generally increase blood pressure (Hernandez-Divers, 2008).

Reflexes

Nevarez (2005) identifies assessment of diverse reflexes as 'the most basic form of monitoring an anaesthetized animal'. Responses to various stimulations provide an indication of the depth and reactivity of anaesthesia. Reflexes that are useful in small mammals include pinch withdrawal, muscle relaxation (jaw tone, anal/cloacal tone), righting reflex, and palpebral and corneal reflexes. Some exotic species require specific reflex assessments. Suggestions of reflexes of exotic species associated with the different anaesthetic planes are given in Figure 7.23.

Reflexes observed	Stage/plane of anaesthesia			
	1	**2**	**3**	**4**
Mammals				
Righting reflex	P	A	A	A
Jaw tone	P	SR	A	A
Tail (care in gerbils and degus) or toe pinch	P	SR	A (SR – sometimes in rabbits)	A
Response to noxious stimuli (e.g. movement away from inhalant gas, apnoea or nose-rubbing in rodents)	P	A	A	A
Swallow reflex (easier to assess this in larger species, e.g. foxes and badgers)	P	A	A	A
Palpebral (can be lost in early or late stages in rabbits)	P	A	A	A
Anal tone	P	P	SR	A
Birds				
Corneal reflex (involuntary)	P	P	SR	A
Voluntary movement of nictitating membrane	P	A	A	A
Righting reflex	P	A	A	A
Palpebral	P	A (SR – mainly in birds of prey)	A	A
Pedal and wing muscle pinch/withdrawal	P	SR	A	A
Cere pinch/poke	P	SR	A	A

7.23 Anaesthetic planes and associated motor responses/reflexes in exotic species. Stages are identified as follows: Stage 1 (voluntary excitement); Stage 2 (involuntary excitement); Stage 3 (surgical anaesthesia); Stage 4 (medullary paralysis prior to death). Responses and reflexes are categorized as: P = present and rapid response to stimuli; SR = slower response to stimuli; A = absent. (Data from Smith and Swindle, 1994; Girling, 2003; Nevarez, 2005; Longley, 2008; Flecknell, 2009; Lierz and Korbel, 2012; Sladky and Mans, 2012) (continues) ▶

Reflexes observed	Stage/plane of anaesthesia			
	1	**2**	**3**	**4**
Birds (continued)				
Jaw tone	P	SR	A	A
Eyelids droop	P	A	A	A
Response to noxious stimuli (e.g. movement away from inhalant gas)	P	A	A	A
Muscle relaxation (head lowered)	P	A	A	A
Cloacal tone	P	P	SR	A
Reptiles: snakes and lizards [a]				
Righting reflex	P	SR	A	A
Jaw tone	P	SR	?SR	?SR
Tail (take care in geckos) or toe pinch	P	P–SR	SR	?SR
Bauchstreich reflex (particularly in snakes)	P	SR	A	A
Response to noxious stimuli (e.g. writhing)	P	A	A	A
Vent tone	P	SR	SR	?SR
Tongue withdrawal	P	A	A	A
Limb extension	P	SR	A	A
Corneal (not in snakes and some species of lizard)	P	SR	A	A
Reptiles: chelonians [a]				
Jaw tone	P	SR	SR	A
Limb or neck extension	P	SR	A	A
Tongue withdrawal	P	A	A	A
Vent tone	P	A	SR	A
Response to noxious stimuli (e.g. apnoea)	P	A	A	A
Palpebral	P	SR	A	A
Corneal	P	P	P	Lost just before death
Tail pinch	P	A	A	A

7.23 (continued) Anaesthetic planes and associated motor responses/reflexes in exotic species. Stages are identified as follows: Stage 1 (voluntary excitement); Stage 2 (involuntary excitement); Stage 3 (surgical anaesthesia); Stage 4 (medullary paralysis prior to death). Responses and reflexes are categorized as: P = present and rapid response to stimuli; SR = slower response to stimuli; A = absent. [a] Stages are difficult to identify in reptiles and their anaesthetic monitoring may produce different results from those given here. (Data from Smith and Swindle, 1994; Girling, 2003; Nevarez, 2005; Longley, 2008; Flecknell, 2009; Lierz and Korbel, 2012; Sladky and Mans, 2012)

Small mammals

Palpebral reflex and jaw tone may be retained through a deep surgical plane of anaesthesia; these are therefore misleading reflexes to interpret and anesthetists should refer to more reliable responses such as the deep pain withdrawal reflex (e.g. toe pinches) and the effect on biological parameters such as heart rate and respiration (Bailey and Pablo, 1998; Flecknell, 2000).

Birds

The corneal reflex (Figure 7.24) is arguably the most useful reflex to use in birds and involves the sweeping movement of the nictitating membrane across the cornea when gently touched with a damp cotton bud. If checks are repeated too often, however, this may impede responsiveness. The speed of the nictitating membrane moving across the cornea and returning to its hidden position can be relative to the depth of

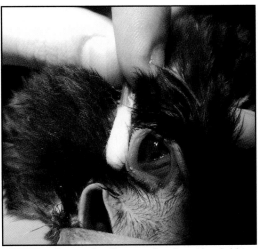

7.24 Corneal reflex testing in a Harris' hawk, using a wet cotton bud.

anaesthesia, whereby the slower the action the deeper the plane of anaesthesia; in contrast, a faster sweeping action of the membrane would indicate a lighter plane of anaesthesia.

Birds are also very sensitive to having their wing muscles gently squeezed, which will often cause increased inspiration; this is useful in recovering birds to stimulate breathing.

Reptiles

During anaesthetic induction, reptiles (particularly snakes) demonstrate muscle relaxation from the head to the tail; recovery proceeds in the opposite direction. These reflexes are therefore important for assessing the desired plane of anaesthesia (Bailey and Pablo, 1998). Tail pinches are useful as they indicate pain sensation and a withdrawal reflex (as with toe pinches in mammals); however, some lizard species, such as geckos, have fracture planes along their tail for autotomy and so tail pinches should be avoided. In snakes, the Bauchstreich reflex is observed when the underside of the snake is stroked, triggering movement away from the stimulus (Lawton, 1992; Girling, 2003).

Post-anaesthetic monitoring and care

Rabbits and rodents

Monitoring these patients requires vigilance, as apnoea, hypothermia and hypoglycaemia are often encountered. Initial recovery from the anaesthetic will be relatively rapid when gases and reversible agents are implemented. It is important to keep the patient warm and in sternal recumbency, with the chest slightly elevated above the hindgut. Small rodents will often become mobile and eat within 30 minutes of regaining consciousness and can be tempted with recovery formulas, baby food, or vegetables. Rabbits can take much longer (see Figure 7.5). Incubators provide warmth and security, but the temperature must be regularly monitored. Fluid therapy should be maintained followed by supplemental feeding until the rabbit is eating and maintaining its weight. Gut motility stimulants (e.g. ranitidine, metoclopramide) and appropriate pre-emptive analgesia (e.g. meloxicam, buprenorphine) should be administered to prevent gut stasis/ileus occurring and to encourage voluntary feeding.

Birds

As soon as the anaesthetic gases have been turned off, the still-intubated birds should be supported with 100% oxygen and IPPV until they are breathing voluntarily. Room air and a resuscitator bag (e.g. Ambu-bag) should be used when the corneal reflex returns and the bird begins to shiver or show muscular tension. The body should be supported in an upright position to ensure that air sacs are not compromised, lightly wrapping it in a towel (Figure 7.25) to prevent the wings flapping and potentially damaging the bird. Recovering birds may shake their heads and require rapid extubation, but they are prone to becoming

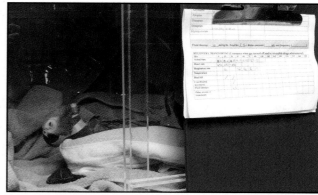

7.25 Sick birds can have extended recoveries, such as this African grey parrot, which is recovering from an anaesthetic in an incubator, supported in a towel in a doughnut shape. Note the jugular catheter and recovery monitoring sheet.

apnoeic and requiring re-intubation. Continued ventilation and positional support is required until the bird is able to perch and support its weight.

Reptiles

Reptiles tend to show the most prolonged recoveries owing to the need to use injectable anaesthetics, which need to be metabolized and excreted. Reptiles must be kept at their optimal temperature. Following anaesthesia, the patient should remain intubated and room air should be administered using a resuscitator bag, until coordinated movement and jaw tone return.

Nutritional and hydration support

Nutritional and hydration support are necessary for most exotic and wildlife patients recovering from anaesthesia.

- High metabolic rates predispose animals to the rapid onset of hypoglycaemia, particularly those with a short gut transit time such as ferrets and small birds.
- Rabbits and rodents are prone to developing ileus rapidly if dehydrated.
- Prolonged recovery times may occur where injectable anaesthetics are used or an animal becomes hypothermic.

Nutritional imbalances will be specific for individual dietary and metabolic requirements. It is best practice to support the patient's requirements until it is able to eat and/or drink voluntarily. Food should be offered as soon as it is safe to do so. Assisted feeding (Figure 7.26) is routinely carried out in patients not showing interest in food or at high risk of hypoglycaemia and gut stasis problems (see Chapter 6 for more information about assisted feeding). Some exotic pets are not fed optimal diets, and a recovery formula will improve recovery. A number of proprietary recovery or supplemental formulas are available for feeding a variety of animals (e.g. Oxbow Critical Care Formula, Vetark Critical Care Formula and Supreme's Recovery Formula). It may be useful in some instances to assess blood glucose during the initial stages of recovery.

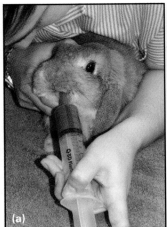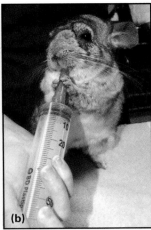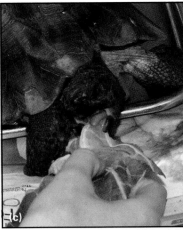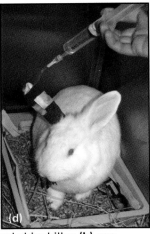

7.26 Supportive nutritional and hydration therapy in various exotic species. Rabbits **(a)** and chinchillas **(b)** can be syringe-fed recovery formulas. **(c)** Hand-feeding, such as with this marginated tortoise, can also be an effective, yet simple, technique. **(d)** The flexibility and reasonably non-invasive extension adaptors that can be attached to intravenous catheters allow fluid therapy to be administered with relatively little disturbance to the patient, even while it is being tempted to eat some parsley.

Case study: Snake anaesthetic recovery

All species show some variation between individual responses to stimuli and medications. Snakes can be slow to show voluntary movement and it is difficult to assess their analgesia requirement. Recent literature and studies provide practical tips to improve the understanding and success of snake recovery (Lawton, 1992; Longley, 2008; Eatwell, 2010).

Key considerations
- Fluid therapy.
- Nutritional support.
- Heat.
- Analgesia.
- Quiet environment (snakes are sensitive to noise vibrations).

In anticipation of a prolonged recovery, basic equipment should be assembled during pre-anaesthetic preparations, and a vivarium should be heated to the snake's preferred optimum temperature range (POTR, see Chapter 4).

Equipment checklist
- Heat sources:
  - Pre-warmed vivarium to POTR
  - Water-circulating heat mat
  - Microwavable heat packs
  - Hairdryer
  - Overhead lights/lamps.
- Thermometer probe.
- Ambu-bag or resuscitator unit.
- Doppler ultrasound probe and lubricating gel.
- Force-feeding:
  - Mouth gag (tongue depressor or soft plastic implement)
  - Dosing catheter or soft tubing
  - Recovery formula (e.g. Vetark, Oxbow, Supreme, Lectade).

Reflexes
Various reflexes are used in reptiles to determine stages of recovery, as well as stimulating the patient to commence voluntary ventilation. The most useful in snakes include:

- The tail pinch reflex
- The righting reflex, where the snake responds to being put on its back by 'righting' itself back on to its ventral surface
- Jaw tone
- Cloacal tone
- The stroking or Bauchstreich reflex, whereby the ventrum or lateral aspect of the snake is gently stroked in the direction of the scales. A mildly sedated or non-sedated snake will instantly move its body away from the stimulus.

When snakes are anaesthetized using gas, these reflexes are important to assess the desired plane of anaesthesia and recovery; Heard (2001) observed that 'snakes relax from the head to the tail and recover in the opposite direction'.

Fluid therapy
Dehydration will lead to visceral gout due to the insolubility of uric acid in the blood, resulting in microcrystals forming within the reptile's tissues (see Chapter 4). Subcutaneous or intraperitoneal fluid therapy is beneficial for most reptile recoveries (see Chapter 6). When the snake has demonstrated voluntary ventilation and movement it can be offered water, but this should be supervised.

Nutritional support
It is advisable for snakes to be gavage-fed a recovery formula within 1 hour of showing coordinated voluntary movement during recovery, to help rehydrate and support gastric motion.

▶

(continued)

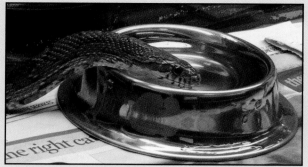

A cornsnake drinking water from a bowl while recovering from an anaesthetic.

Temperature regulation

Heat support is required. A thermometer can be carefully placed either into the cloaca or oesophagus or alongside the snake's body. During anaesthesia and recovery the snake can be placed on a water-circulating heat mat or similar and/or a hairdryer used by targetting the warm air flow along the snake's body, ensuring a low setting is selected and constant monitoring of temperature applied to avoid burning the skin. A hypothermic snake will have a prolonged recovery, and the resulting slow metabolic rate may reduce the benefits of fluid therapy, antibiotics and analgesia.

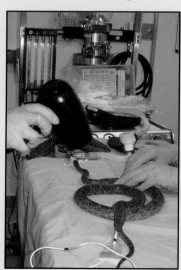

A cornsnake in the initial stages of recovery following an anaesthetic. Snakes can be gently heated up using a hairdryer, but a hand should be placed in the line of the airflow to ensure overheating or burns do not occur.

Analgesia

Signs of discomfort in snakes include restlessness, increased respiration, unnatural posture, sensitive withdrawal from contact and even attempts to bite the handler or location of pain (see Bays *et al.*, 2006 for more detailed discussion). It should be assumed that snakes will require analgesia after surgery. When a snake is recovering it may be experiencing pain but also anxiety, due to constant movements and noise vibrations in its environment. It is therefore considerate to cover the vivarium between recovery checks and ensure that noise levels are kept to a minimum.

Respiration

A recovering snake's respiration is stimulated or increased in response to low levels of oxygen (hypoxia) and high levels of carbon dioxide (hypercapnia). Providing the reptile with 100% oxygen would lengthen its recovery. Maintenance of IPPV and the airway should be achieved using room air and a resuscitator bag until the snake's muscle and/or jaw tone returns.

Heart rate and rhythm

A Doppler ultrasound probe is best placed directly over the heart. This is positioned at one-third of the snake's length from its head. Movement of the heart can be seen when the snake is turned on its back and the position marked with a piece of tape for rapid repeat assessments. Lubricating gel should be used to create good contact with the skin and to minimize interference from the snake's scales.

Anaesthetic considerations

Preparation and keen observation are key to preventing or minimizing problems. Preparation requires consideration of the potential problems that could arise from anaesthesia and should involve the following:

- Preparation of emergency and maintenance drugs, fluids and equipment, specific to the individual patient (Figure 7.27)
- Intravenous or intraosseous and tracheal access, to ensure efficient emergency and maintenance responses
- Planning the anaesthetic protocol.

The observational skills of veterinary nurses will demand heightened sensitivity with exotic pet anaesthesia, to discern subtle changes in behaviour and to pick up on physiological cues. Observation should involve the following:

- Constant awareness of a patient's status through continuous cycles of reflex and physiological assessments
- Regular, clear communication with other staff involved with managing a patient's status, and immediately sharing any concerns.

For veterinary nurses, an 'emergency kit' (Figure 7.28), containing all emergency drugs (see Figure 7.27) and equipment, will already be a familiar part of anaesthesia.

Commonly encountered problems

Figures 7.29 to 7.31 show the commonly encountered anaesthetic problems in mammals, birds and reptile species, respectively, along with their signs, potential causes and methods to correct them. If any problems do occur, it is important to review actions to improve responses for future procedures.

Species	Emergency drug dosages (mg/kg)						
	Adrenaline for cardiac resuscitation (1 mg/ml)	**Atropine** prevents/ corrects bradycardia. Reduction of mucus production (0.6 mg/ml)	**Diazepam** anticonvulsant, muscle relaxant, epileptic seizures (5 mg/ml)	**Doxapram** to stimulate respiration (20 mg/ml)	**Glycopyrrolate** to reduce oral and bronchial secretions (0.2 mg/ml)	**Naloxone** to reverse the effects of opioid agonists (0.4 mg/ml or 0.02 mg/ml)	**Lidocaine** for local anaesthesia (20 mg/ml)
Mammals							
Rabbits	0.1–0.2 mg/kg i.v.	0.02–0.04 mg/kg Possible repeat injections q10–15 min. (Not always effective in some rabbits due to atropinesterase)	1 mg/kg i.v.	5–10 mg/kg i.v., i.m., s.c., i.p. (sublingual once only)	0.011 mg/kg i.v., i.m.	0.04 mg/kg	Epidural: 0.3 ml/kg Cardiac arrhythmias: 1–2 mg/ml i.v. or 2–4 mg intratracheal (NB no more than 4 mg/kg)
Mice	0.003 mg/kg i.v.	0.04–0.1 mg/kg i.m., s.c.	2.5–5 mg/kg i.m., i.p.	5–10 mg/kg i.v., i.m., s.c., i.p. (sublingual once only)	0.01–0.02 mg/kg i.v., i.m.	0.01–0.1 mg/kg s.c., i.v., i.p.	1–3 mg/kg (NB no more than 4 mg/kg)
Rats	0.003 mg/kg i.v.	0.04–0.1 mg/kg i.m., s.c.	2.5–5 mg/kg i.m., i.p.	5–10 mg/kg i.v., i.m., s.c., i.p. (sublingual once only)	0.01–0.02 mg/kg i.v., i.m.	0.01–0.1 mg/kg s.c., i.v., i.p.	1–3 mg/kg (NB no more than 4 mg/kg)
Hamsters	0.003 mg/kg i.v.	0.04–0.1 mg/kg i.m., s.c.	2.5–5 mg/kg i.m., i.p.	5–10 mg/kg i.v., i.m., s.c., i.p. (sublingual once only)	0.01–0.02 mg/kg i.v., i.m.	0.01–0.1 mg/kg s.c., i.v., i.p.	1–3 mg/kg (NB no more than 4 mg/kg)
Gerbils	0.003 mg/kg i.v.	0.04–0.1 mg/kg i.m., s.c.	2.5–5 mg/kg i.m., i.p.	5–10 mg/kg i.v., i.m., s.c., i.p. (sublingual once only)	0.01–0.02 mg/kg i.v., i.m.	0.01–0.1 mg/kg s.c., i.v., i.p.	1–3 mg/kg (NB no more than 4 mg/kg)
Guinea pigs	0.003 mg/kg i.v.	0.04–0.1 mg/kg i.m., s.c.	0.5–5.0 mg/kg i.m.	2–5 mg/kg i.v., s.c., i.p.	0.01–0.02 mg/kg i.v., i.m.	0.01–0.1 mg/kg s.c., i.v., i.p.	1–3 mg/kg (NB no more than 4 mg/kg)
Chinchillas	0.003 mg/kg i.v.	0.04–0.1 mg/kg i.m., s.c.	2.5–5 mg/kg i.m., i.p.	5–10 mg/kg i.v., i.m., s.c., i.p. (sublingual once only)	0.01–0.02 mg/kg i.v., i.m.	0.01–0.1 mg/kg s.c., i.v., i.p.	1–3 mg/kg (NB no more than 4 mg/kg)
Ferrets	0.02 mg/kg s.c., i.m., i.v., intratracheal	0.04–0.1 mg/kg s.c., i.m., i.v.	2–5 mg/kg i.m.	5–10 mg/kg i.v., i.m., s.c., i.p. (sublingual once only)		0.01–0.04 mg/kg i.v., i.m., s.c.	1–3 mg/kg (NB no more than 4 mg/kg)
Birds							
	0.1–1.0 mg/kg i.v., i.o., intracardiac, intratracheal	Organophosphorus poisoning: 0.04–0.5 mg/kg i.v., i.m., q4h Bradycardia:0.01–0.02 mg/kg i.v.	Seizures: 0.1–1 mg/kg i.v., i.m. Raptor appetite stimulant: 0.2 mg/kg q24h	5–20 mg/kg i.m., i.v., i.o., intratracheal	As a premedicant 0.01–0.03 mg/kg i.m., i.v.	No information available	Local anaesthesia: <4 mg/kg (NB not with adrenaline)
Reptiles							
	0.5 mg/kg i.v., i.o. or 1 mg/ kg intratracheal dilute 1 ml/100 g of bodyweight	0.01–0.04 mg/kg i.m., i.v.	Seizures: 2.5 mg/kg i.m., i.v.	4–12 mg/kg i.m., i.v., orally	0.01 mg/kg i.m., i.v.	No information available	Given to effect s.c., dilute 1:1 with sterile water <5 mg/kg in total

7.27 Emergency drug dosages for the main exotic species/groups encountered in practice.

- **Drugs:**
  - Adrenaline
  - Atropine
  - Glycopyrrolate
  - Doxapram: injectable and drops (stored in fridge)
  - Atipamezole
  - Diazepam
  - Naloxone
- **Intubation equipment:**
  - Portable auriscope with appropriate-sized cones/laryngoscope with Wisconsin blade size 1 or 0
  - Pen torch
  - Spare batteries for the above listed equipment
  - Small atraumatic dressing forceps and plastic forceps
  - Local anaesthetic spray
  - ETT introducer/stylet selection: 6Fr dog catheter for >2.5 mm diameter tubes, guide wire for tubes <2.5 mm diameter
  - Selection of uncuffed and avian ETTs: 1 mm diameter/ intravenous catheter adapted to 4 mm in most exotic species, larger sizes for some wildlife species
  - Bandage or tying-in material for securing ETTs
- **Intravenous or intraosseous access:**
  - Selection of intravenous catheters (26 to 20 gauge)
  - Selection of spinal needles for intraosseous catheterization
  - T-connectors/extension sets
  - Injection ports/bungs
  - Heparin/saline flush (dilution = 1000 units heparin: 5000 units saline 0.9%)
- **Consumables:**
  - Non-traumatic tape, e.g. thin and wide
  - Selection of syringes (0.3 ml insulin syringes to 20 ml syringes)
  - Selection of needles (27 gauge 5/8 inch to 21 gauge 5/8 inch and 1 inch)
  - Tongue depressors (securing ETTs or used as a gag)
  - Sterile lubricating gel
  - Cotton buds
  - Swabs
- Ocular lubricant
- Ambu-bag

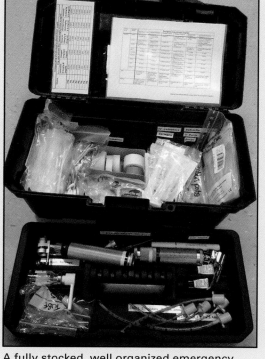

A fully stocked, well organized emergency kit. Note the inclusion of an emergency drugs doses chart.

7.28 The emergency kit should contain all emergency drugs and equipment required for anaesthesia.

Problem	Signs	Main causes	Corrective strategies
Pre-anaesthesia (in all cases patients should be stabilized and fully assessed for suitability prior to anaesthetizing)			
Anorexia and hypoglycaemia	Poor body condition, no gut sounds in rabbits and rodents, weakness/lethargy, ataxia	Lack of suitable diet, pain/ discomfort, disease, stress	Give supportive nutrition and investigate underlying cause
Dehydration	Tenting of the skin, sunken eyes, dry/tacky mucous membranes	Lack of access to fluid, disease, heat stress	Stabilize and treat underlying issues. Intraosseous, intraperitoneal, subcutaneous, intravenous or oral fluid administration. Diagnostic tests required prior to anaesthesia
Ileus	No gut sounds, no recent faecal material	Chronic/acute stress or poor husbandry	Stabilize and treat underlying issues. Supportive feeding, gut stimulants, etc. Diagnostic tests required prior to anaesthesia
Dyspnoea	Respiratory movements become shallower and/or irregular, open mouth breathing or collapse	Airway obstruction or lungs compressed, heat stress	Administer oxygen. Quiet, stress-free environment
Stress and fear	Trying to hide, aggression, shaking and increased respiratory rate, regurgitation	Travel effects, handling, pain or physically compromised, unaccustomed to close human contact	Allow to calm down in a warm, darkened and quiet enclosure. Minimize handling. Avoid contact or close proximity to predator species. Investigate causes of pain or discomfort. Consider sedation

7.29 The most common problems encountered before, during and after anaesthesia of mammal patients. (continues)

Problem	Signs	Main causes	Corrective strategies
During anaesthesia (anaesthetic equipment and heart rate should be checked first)			
Reduced respiration	Respiratory movements become shallower and/or irregular	Airway obstruction or lungs compressed, reduced cardiac output, anaesthetic gases or drugs	Reduction, cessation or reversal of anaesthetic drugs. Oxygen provision and IPPV/occasional chest compressions and reflex stimulation, e.g. toe pinch. Check positioning of patient, e.g. rabbits and rodents should have thorax slightly elevated. Ensure correct placement of ETT and check the lumen is clear. Mucolytics if excessive oral secretions (atropine or glycopyrrolate)
Apnoea/ respiratory arrest	Respiratory movements cease, pale mucous membranes or cyanosis, poor or low reading on pulse oximeter	Airway obstruction, lungs compromised, ETT in too far (entered a single bronchus) or blocked by secretions, hypercapnia, anaesthetic overdose	1. Create a stimulus, e.g. toe pinch or reposition. 2. Turn off anaesthetic gases and/or give reversible drugs. 3. Attempt quick intubation or replace blocked ETTs. 4. Apply IPPV via ETT or tight-fitting mask, and gentle chest compressions or cranial-caudal rocking motion. 5. Apply doxapram injection/drops. 6. Check monitoring equipment and verify the situation by evaluating the patient
Dysrhythmia	Irregular heart rate (tachycardia/bradycardia) and rhythm	Disease, inappropriate or overdose of anaesthetic, pain or too close to consciousness. Severe blood loss (bradycardia)	If other reflexes and signs are stable it may be enough to report and record the incident and monitor carefully for any further changes. If concerned, ensure thermal and fluid therapy is sufficient and reverse anaesthetic drugs or commence recovery. Atropine/glycopyrrolate (if bradycardia)
Cardiac arrest	Cessation of heart activity	Blood loss, hypercapnia	1. Apply gentle cardiac massage. 2. Administer adrenaline via pre-placed intravenous catheter or intraosseous needle. 3. Crystalloid and/or colloid or blood transfusion fluid therapy
Drop in blood pressure	Regular readings show progressively or acutely reduced values. May be accompanied by reduced cardiac output. Weak pulse	Blood loss, length of anaesthesia, hypothermia	Increase fluid rate and include colloid or blood transfusion where severe blood loss has occurred. Provide additional heat support and carefully monitor temperature. Continue to monitor blood pressure
Excessive salivation, mucoid or porphyrin production	Crackling and fluid sounds from upper airway and possibly in the lungs. Rodents show red/brown porphyrin discharge from eyes, nose and mouth	Stress or irritant response to anaesthetic gases. If occurring past the induction stage may suggest inadequate anaesthetic	Use non-noxious gas (such as sevoflurane) in species predisposed to the reaction, e.g. rodents. Anticholinergic drugs to reduce secretions
Hypothermia/ hyperthermia	Thermometer probe readings show increase or decrease in body temperature outside of the species' range and/or individual baseline parameters. Hypothermia leads to decrease in heart rate. Hyperthermia leads to increase in heart rate. Cold extremities and poor blood circulation (reduced CRT)	Severe blood loss, poor provision or monitoring of heat support	Check correct placement of thermometer probe, and battery life. Crystalloid and/or colloid or blood transfusion fluid therapy. Therapy for hypothermia: external heat support, warm fluids, etc. Therapy for hyperthermia: gently reduce external heat support
Seizures	Convulsions, rigidity of limbs, cardiac fluctuations may follow	Hypoglycaemia and hypocalcaemia	Diazepam, glucose or CaEDTA administration, fluid therapy (concentration will depend on species and severity). Reverse or turn off anaesthetic as soon as possible

7.29 (continued) The most common problems encountered before, during and after anaesthesia of mammal patients. (continues) ▶

Problem	Signs	Main causes	Corrective strategies
Recovery			
Dyspnoea	Respiratory movements become shallower and/or irregular, open-mouth breathing or collapse	Airway obstruction (e.g. bronchial secretions) or lungs compressed (poor handling/positioning techniques), heat stress	Immediate adjustment of handling/positioning. Administer oxygen. Quiet stress-free environment. Administer anticholinergic drugs (atropine/glycopyrrolate) to reduce secretions. Re-intubation and IPPV if required
Regurgitation or vomiting	Stomach contents visible in the mouth, fluid sounds during respiration, apnoea	Inadequate starve times, poor positioning or excessive manipulation of stomach	Hold head lower than the body. Swab material out of mouth and use pipette/syringe to access narrow mouths such as those of rodents, rabbits and insectivores. Take particular care with unintubated patients. See also corrective strategies for apnoea
Seizures	Convulsions, rigidity of limbs, cardiac fluctuations may follow	Hypoglycaemia and hypocalcaemia	Diazepam, glucose or CaEDTA administration. Fluid therapy (concentration will depend on species and severity). Reverse or turn off anaesthetic as soon as possible
Anaemia	Pale mucous membranes, visible oozing or haemorrhage, prolonged recovery	Internal haemorrhage, sutures/ligatures slipping or removed by patient, self-inflicted injury on excitable recovery (particularly wildlife). Low PCV	Immediate haemorrhage site compression. Re-anaesthetize for re-suturing or surgical repair. PCV assessments if concerned but severity not immediately obvious. Fluid loss replacement (crystalloids/colloids/blood transfusion). Administer local anaesthetic, BiteNot or Elizabethan collars
Hypothermia / hyperthermia	Thermometer probe readings show increase or decrease in body temperature outside of the species' range and/or individual baseline parameters. Hypothermia leads to decrease in heart rate. Hyperthermia leads to increase in heart rate. Cold extremities and poor blood circulation (reduced CRT)	Severe blood loss; poor provision or monitoring of heat support	Check correct placement of thermometer probe, and battery life. Crystalloid and/or colloid or blood transfusion fluid therapy. Therapy for hypothermia: external heat support, warm fluids, etc. Therapy for hyperthermia: gently reduce external heat support

7.29 (continued) The most common problems encountered before, during and after anaesthesia of mammal patients.

Problems	Signs	Main causes	Corrective strategies
Pre-anaesthesia (in all cases patients should be stabilized and fully assessed for suitability prior to anaesthetizing)			
Anorexia and hypoglycaemia	Poor body condition, weakness/lethargy, ataxia	Poor nutrition, pain/discomfort, disease, stress	Give supportive nutrition and investigate underlying cause
Dehydration	Wrinkled skin around eyes in some species, sunken eyes, basilic vein increased refill time	Lack of access to fluid, disease, heat stress	Intraosseous, subcutaneous, oral or intravenous fluid administration
Ileus	Distended crop, no recent faeces passed, weakness and depression	Chronic/acute stress or poor husbandry	Remove crop contents (to prevent fermentation). Provide prokinetics and fluid and nutritional therapy
Dyspnoea	Respiratory movements become shallower and/or irregular, open-mouth breathing or collapse	Stress, pain or disease, airway obstruction or keel and air sacs (poor handling techniques)	Immediate adjustment of handling. Administer oxygen. Quiet, stress-free environment
Stress and fear	Trying to hide, aggression, elevated respiratory rate, regurgitation of food, vocalization	Travel effects, handling, pain or physically compromised, unaccustomed to close human contact	Allow to calm down in a warm, darkened and quiet enclosure. Minimize handling. Avoid contact or close proximity to predator species. Investigate causes of pain or discomfort

7.30 The most common problems encountered before, during and after anaesthesia of bird patients. (continues) ▶

Problems	Signs	Main causes	Corrective strategies
During anaesthesia (anaesthetic equipment and heart rate should be checked first)			
Reduced respiration	Respiratory movements become shallower and/or irregular	Airway obstruction or air sacs compressed, reduced cardiac output, anaesthetic gases or drugs	Reduction, cessation or reversal of anaesthetic drugs. Oxygen provision and occasional keel compressions/IPPV and reflex stimulation, e.g. toe or wing pinch. Check positioning of patient; lateral recumbency produces the least resistance. Ensure correct placement of ETT. Place an air sac tube if indicated
Apnoea/ respiratory arrest	Respiratory movements cease, pale mucous membranes or cyanosis, poor or low reading on pulse oximeter	Airway obstruction, air sacs compromised, ETT in too far (entered a single bronchus), hypercapnia, anaesthetic overdose	1. Create a stimulus, e.g. toe pinch or reposition. 2. Turn off anaesthetic gases and/or give reversible drugs. 3. Attempt quick intubation or replace blocked ETT. 4. Apply IPPV via ETT or tight-fitting mask, and gentle keel compressions. Hindlimbs can be gently flexed in a cranial-caudal motion. 5. Apply doxapram. 6. Place an air sac cannula. 7. Check monitoring equipment and verify the situation by evaluating the patient
Dysrhythmia	Irregular heart rate (tachycardia/bradycardia) and rhythm	Disease, inappropriate or overdose of anaesthetic, pain or too close to consciousness	If other reflexes and signs are stable it may be enough to report and record incident and carefully monitor for any further changes. If concerned, ensure fluid therapy is sufficient and reverse anaesthetic drugs or commence recovery
Cardiac arrest	Cessation of heart activity	Blood loss, hypercapnia	1. Apply gentle external cardiac massage. 2. Administer adrenaline via pre-placed intravenous catheter or intraosseous needle. 3. Crystalloid and/or colloid or blood transfusion fluid therapy
Drop in blood pressure	Regular readings show progressively or acutely reduced values. May be accompanied by reduced cardiac output. Weak pulse	Blood loss, length of anaesthesia, hypothermia	Increase fluid rate and include colloid or blood transfusion where severe blood loss has occurred. Provide additional heat support and carefully monitor temperature. Continue to monitor blood pressure
Hypothermia / hyperthermia	Thermometer probe readings show increase or decrease in body temperature outside of the species' range and/or individual baseline parameters	Severe blood loss, poor provision or monitoring of heat support	Check correct placement of thermometer probe and battery life. Change to oesophageal readings. Crystalloid and/or colloid or blood transfusion fluid therapy. Therapy for hypothermia: external heat support, warm fluids, etc. Therapy for hyperthermia: gently reduce external heat support
Seizures	Convulsions, rigidity of limbs, cardiac fluctuations may follow	Hypoglycaemia and hypocalcaemia	Diazepam, glucose or CaEDTA administration. Fluid therapy (concentration will depend on species and severity). Reverse or turn off anaesthetic as soon as possible
Recovery			
Dyspnoea	Respiratory movements become shallower and/or irregular, open-mouth breathing or collapse	Stress, pain or disease, airway obstruction (e.g. bronchial secretions) or pressure on keel and air sacs (poor handling techniques)	Immediate adjustment of handling. Clear airways. Administer oxygen. Quiet, stress-free environment. Re-intubation and IPPV if required
Regurgitation or vomiting	Crop contents visible in the mouth, fluid sounds during respiration, apnoea	Inadequate starve times, poor positioning or excessive manipulation of crop	Hold head lower than the body. Swab material out of mouth and use pipette/syringe for easy access. Take particular care with unintubated patients. See also corrective strategies for apnoea
Seizures	Convulsions, rigidity of limbs, cardiac fluctuations may follow	Hypoglycaemia and hypocalcaemia	Diazepam, glucose or CaEDTA administration. Fluid therapy (concentration will depend on species and severity). Reverse or turn off anaesthetic as soon as possible

7.30 (continued) The most common problems encountered before, during and after anaesthesia of bird patients. (continues)

Problems	Signs	Main causes	Corrective strategies
Recovery (continued)			
Anaemia	Pale mucous membranes, visible oozing or haemorrhage, prolonged recovery	Internal haemorrhage, sutures/ligatures slipping or removed by patient, self-inflicted injury on excitable recovery (particularly wildlife), low PCV (assessment if concerned but severity not immediately obvious)	Immediate haemorrhage site compression. Re-anaesthetize for re-suturing or surgical repair. PCV assessments. Fluid loss replacement (crystalloids/colloids/blood transfusion). Administer local anaesthetic, BiteNot or Elizabethan collar
Hypothermia/hyperthermia	Thermometer probe readings show increase or decrease in body temperature outside of the species' range and/or individual baseline parameters	Severe blood loss, poor provision or monitoring of heat support	Check correct placement of thermometer probe and battery life. Change to oesophageal readings. Crystalloid and/or colloid or blood transfusion fluid therapy. Therapy for hypothermia: external heat support, warm fluids, etc. Therapy for hyperthermia: gently reduce external heat support

7.30 (continued) The most common problems encountered before, during and after anaesthesia of bird patients.

Problems	Signs	Main causes	Corrective strategies
Pre-anaesthesia (in all cases patients should be stabilized and fully assessed for suitability prior to anaesthetizing)			
Anorexia and hypoglycaemia	Poor body condition, weakness/lethargy	Poor nutrition, pain/discomfort, disease, stress. Often husbandry-related	Give supportive nutrition and investigate underlying cause
Dehydration	Sunken eyes, wrinkled skin, dry/tacky mucous membranes	Lack of access to fluid, disease, heat stress	Warm water bath for 10–20 minutes, with rehydration formula in it such as Reptoboost (depth depends on how weak the patient is). Intraosseous, intracoelomic, subcutaneous or oral fluid administration
Ileus	Distended coelomic cavity, increased gas or ingesta felt on palpation, no recent faeces passed	Hypothermia, hypocalcaemia, gastrointestinal tract disease, prolonged anorexia	Stabilize and treat underlying issues. Provide heat and fluid therapy. Diagnostic tests required prior to anaesthesia
Dyspnoea	Respiratory movements become shallower and/or irregular, gaping mouth breathing or collapse	Stress, pain or disease, airway obstruction (poor handling techniques)	Immediate adjustment of handling. Quiet, stress-free environment. >40% oxygen administration is not advised as it may result in respiratory depression
Stress and fear	Trying to hide, aggression or elevated respiratory rate, regurgitation (in snakes), sudden passing faeces and urates	Travel effects, handling, pain or physically compromised, unaccustomed to close human contact	Allow to calm down in a warm, darkened and quiet enclosure. Minimize handling. Avoid contact or close proximity to predator species. Investigate causes of pain or discomfort
During anaesthesia (anaesthetic equipment and heart rate should be checked first)			
Reduced respiration	Respiratory movements become shallower and/or irregular, but this is typical for reptiles under anaesthesia	Airway obstruction or lungs compressed, reduced cardiac output, anaesthetic gases or drugs	To be expected and therefore IPPV is always required. Sternal recumbency is best. Reflexes such as toe pinch, jaw tone or Bauchstreich reflex
Apnoea/respiratory arrest	Respiratory movements cease, pale mucous membranes or cyanosis, poor or low reading on pulse oximeter	Airway obstruction, lungs compromised, ETT in too far (entered a single bronchus), hypercapnia, anaesthetic overdose	1. Create a stimulus, e.g. toe/tail pinch or reposition. 2. Turn off anaesthetic gases and/or give reversible drugs. 3. Attempt quick intubation or replace blocked ETTs. 4. Apply IPPV via ETT or tight-fitting mask, and limb movements can be instigated for chelonians and lizards. 5. Apply doxapram. 6. Check monitoring equipment and verify findings by evaluating the patient

7.31 The most common problems encountered before, during and after anaesthesia of reptile patients. (continues) ▶

Problems	Signs	Main causes	Corrective strategies
During anaesthesia (anaesthetic equipment and heart rate should be checked first)			
Dysrhythmia	Irregular heart rate (tachycardia/bradycardia) and rhythm	Disease, inappropriate or overdose of anaesthetic, pain or too close to consciousness	If other reflexes and signs are stable it may be enough to report and record incident then carefully monitor for any further changes. If concerned ensure fluid therapy is sufficient and reverse anaesthetic drugs or commence recovery
Cardiac arrest	Cessation of heart activity	Blood loss, hypothermia	1. Warmed crystalloid and/or colloid or blood transfusion fluid therapy. Apply thermal therapy and careful thermoregulation, e.g. heated table, water circulating heat mats, hairdryer, etc. (Adrenaline is not useful in reptiles owing to cardiac shunting)
Drop in blood pressure	For larger lizards and chelonians particularly, regular readings show progressively or acutely reduced values. May be accompanied by reduced cardiac output. Weak pulses. Difficult to assess in snakes	Blood loss, length of anaesthesia, hypothermia	Evaluate patient particularly as readings can be variable in reptiles. Increase fluid rate and include colloid or blood transfusion where severe blood loss has occurred; provide additional heat support and carefully monitor temperature
Hypothermia/ hyperthermia	Thermometer probe readings show increase or decrease in body temperature outside of the species' range and/or individual baseline parameters	Severe blood loss, poor provision or monitoring of heat support	Check correct placement of thermometer probe, and battery life. Change to oesophageal measurements. Crystalloid and/or colloid or blood transfusion fluid therapy. Therapy for hypothermia: external heat support, warm fluids, etc. Therapy for hyperthermia: gently reduce external heat support
Seizures	Convulsions, rigidity of limbs, cardiac fluctuations may follow. (Rarely seen in chelonians or snakes)	Hypoglycaemia and hypocalcaemia	Diazepam, glucose or CaEDTA administration, fluid therapy (concentration will depend on species and severity), reverse or turn off anaesthetic as soon as possible
Recovery			
Dyspnoea	Respiratory movements become shallower and/or irregular, gaping mouth breathing or collapse	Stress, pain or disease, Airway obstruction (e.g. bronchial secretions) or lung movement restricted (poor handling/positioning techniques)	Immediate adjustment of handling /positioning. Clear airways. Quiet stress-free environment. >40% oxygen administration not advised as may result in respiratory depression. Re-intubation and IPPV if required
Regurgitation or vomiting	Gastrointestinal contents visible in the mouth, fluid sounds during respiration, apnoea	Inadequate starve times, poor positioning	Hold head lower than the body; swab material out of mouth and use pipette/syringe for access. Care particularly with unintubated patients. See also corrective strategies for apnoea
Seizures	Convulsions, rigidity of limbs, cardiac fluctuations may follow. (Rarely seen in chelonians and snakes)	Hypoglycaemia and hypocalcaemia	Diazepam, glucose or CaEDTA administration, fluid therapy (concentration will depend on species and severity), reverse or turn off anaesthetic as soon as possible
Anaemia	Pale mucous membranes, visible oozing or haemorrhage, prolonged recovery	Internal haemorrhage, sutures/ligatures slipping or removed by patient, self-inflicted injury on excitable recovery (particularly wildlife). Low PCV	Immediate haemorrhage site compression. Re-anaesthetize for re-suturing or surgical repair. PCV assessment if concerned but severity not immediately obvious. Fluid loss replacement (crystalloid/colloids/blood transfusion). Administer local anaesthetic, BiteNot or Elizabethan collars
Hypothermia/ hyperthermia	Thermometer probe readings show increase or decrease in body temperature outside of the species' range and/or individual baseline parameters	Severe blood loss; poor provision or monitoring of heat support	Check correct placement of thermometer probe, and battery life. Change to oesophageal readings. Crystalloid and/or colloid or blood transfusion fluid therapy. Therapy for hypothermia: external heat support, warm fluids, etc. Therapy for hyperthermia: gently reduce external heat support

7.31 (continued) The most common problems encountered before, during and after anaesthesia of reptile patients.

Problems during anaesthesia

With pre-existing and underlying problems controlled or minimized (see earlier), anaesthesia may commence. There are common trends and typical problems that potentially arise during anaesthesia and surgical procedures; these are often respiratory or cardiovascular, or temperature-associated.

Respiratory problems

- Apnoea can occur during lengthy anaesthesia or when patients receive an anaesthetic overdose, but it is also frequently encountered during small mammal chamber inductions using isoflurane. The use of the less noxious sevoflurane for induction may avoid apnoea. In small mammals and birds, cardiac arrest will rapidly follow apnoea and there will need to be an immediate and methodical response. In contrast, reptiles can remain hypoxic and use anaerobic respiration for 4 to >24 hours, hence the need for their intubation and manual ventilation.
- Respiratory obstruction may also occur from excessive oral secretions that have dried into 'plugs', or the presence of food particles in the mouth. The risk from both these sources may be minimized by intubating animals. (See Figure 7.5 for fasting and re-feeding times.)
- Hypersalivation is regularly seen in chinchillas and guinea pigs, often triggered by the use of isoflurane chamber inductions, where mucous membranes are irritated. This creates a threat of aspiration pneumonia. Anticholinergic drugs such as atropine or glycopyrrolate can be given before or during the occurrence of this problem.
- Recumbency of the patient during anaesthesia can compromise respiratory efficiency, particularly in species such as rodents and rabbits with large hindguts. Recumbency of birds can also pose threats to circulating ventilation; therefore, where possible, a bird should be positioned laterally, as dorsal or sternal recumbency restricts major air sacs, even if IPPV is being supplied.
- Early signs of hypercapnia and hypoxia may go undetected; therefore, it is essential that patients are intubated wherever possible and connected to a capnograph monitor. Regular checks of mucous membrane colour and capillary refill time and occasionally 'sighing' the circuit re-breathing bag will help identify and treat any early signs. The use of a capnograph in intubated patients will provide essential information to assist with finely tuned anaesthesia.
- Poor provision of analgesia (see Recognition of signs of pain, earlier).

Birds and reptiles do not have a diaphragm and rely on other musculature movements (including intercostal, pectoral and abdominal muscles) to circulate air around their respiratory tissues; thus classic chest compressions may not be effective. As small mammals possess diaphragms, classic gentle chest compressions can be employed but should be 'circumferential' with pressure applied to both sides of the chest. Rocking the animal (e.g. posterior end gently tilted up then down) may also create a more natural respiratory motion as the diaphragm is flattened by the weight of the hindgut.

Cardiovascular problems

Cardiac arrest may occur for a variety of reasons, most commonly overdose of anaesthetic agent, hypovolaemia and/or blood loss. Constant monitoring of heart rhythm and rate, blood pressure and oxygen saturation will offer warnings, which should be acted upon efficiently.

Temperature fluctuations

- Hypothermia is one of the most common problems encountered during sedation or anaesthesia. Species highly susceptible to hypothermia include mammals weighing <1 kg, birds weighing <300 g and all reptiles.
- Hyperthermia, although not as commonly seen as hypothermia, can be a threat. Scalds, burns or even death can also be caused by overzealous heating.

Machines can sometimes malfunction and display incorrect values, or they may be misinterpreted. Monitoring devices should therefore be checked regularly to ensure they are functioning properly and are provided with adequate power.

Problems during recovery

The recovery stage should be acknowledged for posing significant risks to patients. 'Problem' recoveries may be prolonged or excitable, whereby the patient may suddenly start moving and panicking. Regular assessments should be made until the patient is satisfactorily able to support its body position and is eating, and baseline parameters have returned.

Respiration

Patients that have been successfully intubated should have their airway maintained to provide IPPV until voluntary ventilation and swallowing reflexes have returned. This provides immediate accessibility to support respiration or resuscitation, and is protection against potential obstruction from oral secretions. Some individuals (particularly birds) may require rapid re-intubation after an apparent recovery. In reptiles, extubation can be delayed while heart rate is monitored using a Doppler probe and the patient is periodically ventilated or 'sighed' (one to four breaths every 30 seconds) with room air, using a resuscitator bag or resuscitation unit.

Respiration can also be compromised during recovery due to restriction of lung and air sac movement. Birds should be gently held or propped upright until they are able to perch (see Figure 7.25). Rabbits and rodents should be maintained in sternal recumbency with the chest slightly raised to avoid pressure from the hindgut on the diaphragm.

Aspiration/inhalation of crop or stomach contents can occur if the patient was not starved sufficiently prior to anaesthetizing, or if food was offered before the patient had sufficiently recovered post-anaesthesia. If this occurs the patient's mouth should immediately be cleared of any food debris using a cotton bud or suction device (e.g. a syringe) and, where appropriate, the buccal cavity and airway should be observed to ensure the debris is cleared. In general, food and water bowls should be returned to enclosures when the patient has regained coordinated movement.

Cardiovascular changes

- Ferrets can develop a massive fall in blood pressure following an apparently successful recovery, especially where there has been blood loss. This is thought to be due to histamine release that triggers the vagal reflex (also lowering temperature and cardiovascular output). Circulatory efficiency will be optimized with minimal use of cardiovascular depressive drugs, and by maintaining fluid therapy throughout procedures and slow recoveries.
- Surgical wounds and capillary refill time must be monitored after surgery for early signs of haemorrhage caused by slipped ligatures. Adequate analgesia and fluid therapy must also be provided. Where haemorrhage has occurred PCV should be monitored to assess the fluid requirements.

Thermoregulation

During recovery the patient's temperature should be closely monitored, particularly in mammals and reptiles. In some of the small mammal species it is challenging to acquire repeated rectal temperatures. A thermometer can therefore be placed near to the patient and monitored for changes. In some patients a small soft probe can be placed in the rectum for prolonged recoveries (Figure 7.32). Thermal support should be adjusted to provide comfortable and optimal recovery environments for the patient.

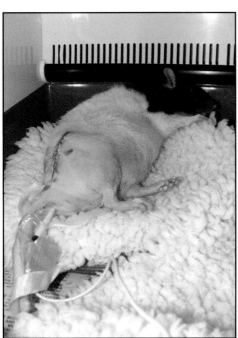

7.32 A rat in recovery in an incubator having its temperature assessed.

Nutritional support

If procedures are prolonged there may be problems regarding the patient's nutritional balance. Guidelines on nutritional support and starving and re-feeding times are given earlier in this chapter (see Figure 7.5).

Pain or discomfort

If inappropriate or insufficient analgesia has been administered then the patient is likely to show signs of pain and discomfort prior to gaining full consciousness. This can be demonstrated in various ways, including writhing, thrashing, biting the focal area of pain, jumping or sudden movements, vocalization, skin colour changes in some reptiles, abnormal position or muscle tension (Figures 7.33 and 7.34), and aggression towards others (Bays *et al.*, 2006).

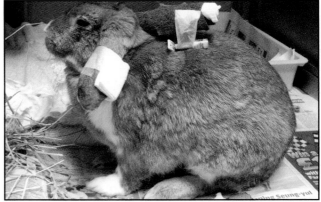

7.33 Abdominal discomfort in a rabbit patient suffering from gut stasis and gastric bloat. Note the upright, hunched or tense posture.

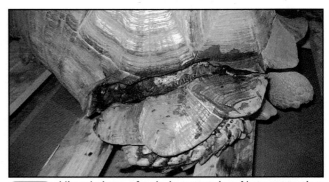

7.34 Visual signs of pain in a tortoise. Note retraction of the head and limbs tucked up against the body. (Courtesy of Matthew Rendle)

Discomfort can initiate highly excitable responses and aggravate pre-existing conditions such congenital epilepsy in gerbils, and this should be anticipated prior to recovery (Hollamby, 2009). If a bandage or other physiological alteration has been implemented then this can often provoke a panicked response, and care should be taken to minimize this by ensuring bandaging is comfortable and the recovery environment is quiet and darkened. Other causes of discomfort are related to surgical site preparation and include the application of chlorhexidine or ultrasound gel, or irritation from clipper blades. Irritable applications should be removed before the patient regains consciousness, and skin irritation treated.

Case study: A lame fox

Case presentation

A wildlife warden presents a wild red fox to the practice after a suspected road traffic accident. Observations from a distance show that the animal is tachypnoeic, with increased respiratory effort. It is 10/10ths lame on the left hindlimb, and blood is present on the fur of this limb. The fox is otherwise bright, alert and responsive. It is decided that diagnostic imaging is necessary to investigate for potential respiratory pathology and fractures; this will require general anaesthesia.

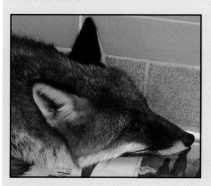

Considerations

- The respiratory signs could be related to thoracic trauma (e.g. resulting in pulmonary contusions or fractured ribs) or a ruptured diaphragm. Care should be taken to reduce stress and to provide airway support in the form of oxygen and intubation as soon as possible.
- Many wild animals show signs of distress in captivity; the tachypnoea could be related to this rather than to overt respiratory disease.
- Attempts to restrain the animal should avoid further trauma to the lame leg, and should also avoid restriction of respiratory movements where possible. Any restraint is liable to cause stress to the fox.
- The degree of haemorrhage should be assessed if feasible, to try to determine whether the patient is likely to be suffering from hypovolaemic shock after acute blood loss.
- Of primary concern is the safety of staff members in the vicinity. The fox is a wild animal and is prone to aggression if cornered or restrained. Staff should receive training in handling before dealing with such animals.
- Foxes frequently carry several zoonotic conditions, including ringworm, sarcoptic mange and leptospirosis, Lyme disease (*Borrelia*), tuberculosis (mammalian or avian), yersiniosis (including *Yersinia enterocolitica*, *Y. pseudotuberculosis* and *Y. pestis*) and various gastrointestinal bacteria (including *Salmonella*, *Escherichia coli* and *Campylobacter*). In countries other than the UK, foxes are also a major reservoir for rabies.

Restraint and handling

- In order to minimize stress to the fox, it should be housed in a quiet darkened area of the clinic and disturbance kept to a minimum. All drugs and equipment should be collated before commencing the procedure.
- Wild foxes behave similarly to feral dogs, and comparable procedures can be used to restrain them initially, e.g. the use of a dog-catcher (taking care not to traumatize the respiratory tract further when holding the neck), a broom to pin the neck to the ground, or a squeeze cage.
- To minimize the physical restraint period (reducing the risk to staff and the stress to the animal), intramuscular injectable anaesthetics are preferred. These require only brief restraint to administer. A disadvantage is that control of the anaesthetic is reduced compared to intravenous or inhalational drugs. Where possible, an accurate weight should be obtained (e.g. by weighing the fox in its arrival container and then deducting the container's weight once the fox has been removed) to enable correct dosing.
- All staff should wear appropriate PPE when handling the fox, to reduce the risk of zoonotic disease transference. As a minimum this should include disposable gloves. Staff should also practise good hygiene, washing hands after handling the fox.

Anaesthetic protocol

- The protocol of choice will probably be an alpha-2 agonist with ketamine, hand-injected intramuscularly. Although this combination is suboptimal for the animal's unknown health status, the regime is a compromise between animal and staff safety. The alpha-2 agonist can be reversed with atipamezole at the end of the procedure. For an animal that is more dyspnoeic or has reduced mental status, the doses used should be lowered, or induction with an inhalational agent contemplated. In moribund animals, examination may be permitted without the use of anaesthetic agents (although it would be advisable to muzzle a fox to protect staff).
- After induction, the animal should initially be muzzled to reduce the risk of trauma to staff. Once the fox is anaesthetized, it should be intubated (but only when it is safe to do so) and gaseous agents used to top-up anaesthesia if required.
- The alpha-2 agonist can be reversed using atipamezole. During recovery the animal should be maintained in a quiet darkened area. Once recovered it should be provided with food and water. Dog food is suitable but if that is not recognized as food, carcasses such as day-old chicks or quail should be offered.

References and further reading

Bailey JE and Pablo LS (1998) Anaesthetic monitoring and monitoring equipment: application in small exotic pet practice. *Seminars in Avian and Exotic Pet Medicine* **7**(1), 53–60

Bays TB, Lightfoot T and Mayer J (2006) *Exotic Pet Behaviour: Birds, Reptiles and Small Animals,* p. 360. Elsevier Saunders, St. Louis

Bennett RA (1998) Reptile anesthesia. *Seminars in Avian and Exotic Pet Medicine* **7**, 30–40

Brunson DB (1997) Pharmacology of inhalation anesthetics. In: *Anesthesia and Analgesia in Laboratory Animals,* ed. DF Kohn, *et al.,* pp. 29–41. ACLAM and Academic Press, New York

Carpenter JW (2005) *Exotic Animal Formulary, 3rd edn.* Elsevier, St. Louis

Chinnadurai SK, Wrenn A and DeVoe RS (2009) Evaluation of noninvasive oscillometric blood pressure monitoring in anaesthetized boid snakes. *Journal of the American Veterinary Medical Association* **234(5)**, 625–630

Chitty J (2010) Birds of prey. In: *BSAVA Manual of Exotic Pets, 5th edn,* ed. A Meredith and C Johnson-Delaney, pp. 200–220. BSAVA Publications, Gloucester

Curro TG (1993) Evaluation of the isoflurane-sparing effects of butorphanol and flunixin in psittaciformes. *Proceedings of the Association of Avian Veterinarians,* pp. 17–19

Curro TG, Brunson D and Paul-Murphy J (1994) Determination of the ED$_{50}$ of isoflurane and evaluation of the analgesic properties of butorphanol in cockatoos (*Cacatua* spp.). *Veterinary Surgery* **23**, 429–433

Degernes L (2008) Anaesthesia of companion birds. *Compendium* (cp.vetlearn.com), pp. 1–11

Eatwell K (2010) Lizards. In: *BSAVA Manual of Exotic Pets, 5th edn,* ed. A Meredith and C Johnson-Delaney, pp. 273–293. BSAVA Publications, Gloucester

Edling TM (2005) Anaesthesia and analgesia. In: *BSAVA Manual of Psittacine Birds, 2nd edn,* ed. N Harcourt-Brown and J Chitty, pp. 87–96. BSAVA Publications, Gloucester

Feldberg W and Symonds HW (1980) Hyperglycaemic effect of xylazine. *Journal of Veterinary Pharmacology and Therapeutics* **3**,197–202

Flecknell PA (1996) *Laboratory Animal Anaesthesia. 2nd edn.* Academic Press, New York

Flecknell PA (2000) Anaesthesia and perioperative care. In: *BSAVA Manual of Rabbit Medicine and Surgery, 2nd edn,* ed. A Meredith and P Flecknell, pp. 154–165. BSAVA Publications, Gloucester

Flecknell PA (2009) Anaesthetic management. In: *Laboratory Animal Anaesthesia, 3rd edn,* p. 81. Elsevier, St. Louis

Fraser MA and Girling S (2009) *Rabbit Medicine and Surgery for Veterinary Nurses.* Wiley-Blackwell, Oxford

Girling S (2003) *Veterinary Nursing of Exotic Species.* Blackwell Publishing, Oxford

González-Gil A, Silván G, García-Partida P *et al.* (2006) Serum glucocorticoid concentrations after halothane and isoflurane anaesthesia in New Zealand white rabbits. *Veterinary Record* **159**, 51–52

Harkness JE and Wagner JE (1989) *The Biology and Medicine of Rabbits and Rodents, 2nd edn.* Lea and Febiger, Philadelphia

Heard DJ (1993) Principles and techniques of anesthesia and analgesia for exotic practice. *Veterinary Clinics of North America*: *Exotic Animal Practice* **23**, 1301–1327

Heard DJ (2001) Reptile anaesthesia. *Veterinary Clinics of North America: Exotic Animal Practice* **4**(1), 83–117

Hedenqvist P and Hellebrekers LJ (2003) Laboratory animal analgesia, anesthesia, and euthanasia. In: *Handbook of Laboratory Animal Science, 2nd edn,* ed. J Hau and GL Van Hoosier, pp. 413–455. CRC Press, Boca Raton

Hernandez-Divers SJ (2008) Triage of sick Boids (Boas and Pythons). Exotics – Reptiles. *NAVC Conference 2008.* pp. 1757–1761

Hollamby (2009) Rodents: neurological and musculoskeletal disorders. In: *BSAVA Manual of Rodents and Ferrets,* ed. E Keeble and A Meredith, pp.161–359. BSAVA Publications, Gloucester

Huckabee JR (2000) Raptor therapeutics. *Veterinary Clinics of North America: Exotic Animal Practice* **3**, 91–116

Jepson L (2009) *Exotic Animal Medicine: A Quick Reference Guide.* Saunders Elsevier, Edinburgh

Johnson-Delaney CA (2009) Ferrets: anaesthesia and analgesia. In: *BSAVA Manual of Rodents and Ferrets,* ed. E Keeble and A Meredith, pp. 245–253. BSAVA Publications, Gloucester

Lawton MPC (1992) Anaesthesia. In: *BSAVA Manual of Reptiles,* ed. PH Beynon *et al.,* pp. 170–183. BSAVA Publications, Cheltenham

Lawton MPC (1996) Anaesthesia. In: *BSAVA Manual of Psittacine Birds,* ed. PH Beynon, *et al.,* pp. 49–59. BSAVA Publications, Cheltenham

Lierz M and Korbel R (2012) Topics in medicine and surgery: Anaesthesia and analgesia in birds. *Journal of Exotic Pet Medicine* **21**, 44–58

Longley LA (2008) *Anaesthesia of Exotic Pets,* p. 314. Elsevier Saunders, Edinburgh

Longley L (2010) *Saunders Solutions in Veterinary Practice: Small Animal Exotic Pet Medicine.* Saunders Elsevier, Edinburgh

Lord B, Boswood A and Petrie A (2010) Electrocardiography of the normal domestic pet rabbit. *Veterinary Record* **167**, 961–965

Ludders JW (2006) Respiratory physiology of birds: Considerations for anesthetic management. *Seminars in Avian and Exotic Pet Medicine: Anesthesia and Analgesia.* **7**(1), 3–9

Lukasik VM (1999) Premedication and sedation. In: *BSAVA Manual of Small Animal Anaesthesia and Analgesia,* ed. C Seymour and R Gleed. BSAVA Publications, Gloucester

Machin KL and Caulkert NA (1996) The cardiopulmonary effects of propofol in mallard ducks. *Proceedings of the American Association of Zoo Veterinarians,* pp. 149–154

Meredith A and Johnson-Delaney C (2010) *BSAVA Manual of Exotic Pets, 5th edn.* BSAVA Publications, Gloucester

Nevarez JG (2005) Monitoring during avian and exotic pet anaesthesia. *Seminars in Avian and Exotic Pet Medicine,* **14**(4), 277–283

Olson ME, Vizzutti D, Morck DW *et al.* (1993) The parasympatholytic effects of atropine sulphate and glycopyrrolate in rats and rabbits. *Canadian Journal of Veterinary Research* **57**, 254–258

Patel SS and Goa KL (1996) Sevoflurane: a review of its pharmacodynamic and pharmacokinetic properties and its clinical use in general anaesthesia. *Drugs* **51**, 658–700

Paul-Murphy J (2006) Pain management. In: *Clinical Avian Medicine, No.1,* ed. GJ Harrison and TL Lightfoot, pp. 233–239. Spix Publishing, Palm Beach, Florida

Redrobe S (2004) Anaesthesia and analgesia. In: *BSAVA Manual of Reptiles, 2nd edition,* ed. SJ Girling and P Raiti, pp. 131–146. BSAVA Publications, Gloucester

Reusch B and Boswood A (2003) Electrocardiography of the normal domestic rabbit. *Journal of Small Animal Practice* **44**, 514

Richardson C and Flecknell P (2009) Rodents: anaesthesia and analgesia. In: *BSAVA Manual of Rodents and Ferrets,* ed. E Keeble and A Meredith, pp. 63–72. BSAVA Publications, Gloucester

Schumacher J and Yelen T (2006) Anesthesia and analgesia. In: *Reptile Medicine and Surgery, 2nd edn,* ed. DR Mader, pp. 442–452. Saunders Elsevier, St. Louis

Short CE (1987) *Principles and Practice of Veterinary Anesthesia.* Williams and Wilkins, Baltimore

Sladky KK and Mans C (2012) Topics in medicine and surgery: clinical anaesthesia in reptiles. *Journal of Exotic Pet Medicine* **21**, 17–31

Smith A and Swindle M (1994) *Research Animal Anesthesia, Analgesia and Surgery,* p. 25. Scientists Center for Animal Welfare, Greenbelt, MD

Stanford M (2004) Practical use of capnography in exotic animal anaesthesia. *Exotic DVM: Proceedings from the International Conference on Exotics,* Volume 6.3

Strombek DR and Guildford WG (1991) Hepatic necrosis and acute hepatic failure. In: *Small Animal Gastroenterology.* pp. 574–592. Wolfe Publishing, London

Self-assessment questions

1. In which of the following animals would it not be appropriate to use a corneal reflex?
   a. Cornsnake
   b. African grey parrot
   c. Fox
   d. Hermann's tortoise
2. If apnoea occurs during hamster anaesthesia, which of the following actions should be taken?
   a. Inform the vet and check other reflexes. If cardiac output is compromised, turn anaesthetic off, begin resuscitation and administer emergency drugs
   b. Don't bother the vet until you are sure all possible life signs are not detectable
   c. Turn off anaesthetic gas or give adrenaline, suggest the vet finishes the procedure, begin chest compressions
   d. Inform the vet and check other reflexes. Give the animal a fighting chance to start breathing itself; wait until the heart rate has slowed further before commencing chest compressions and administering emergency drugs
3. Which of the following animals has complete tracheal rings and would therefore be potentially damaged when using an ETT with an inflatable cuff?
   a. Royal ball python
   b. Hedgehog
   c. Amazon parrot
   d. Rabbit
4. Which of the following species possess atropinesterases?
   a. Cockatiel
   b. Rabbit
   c. Red-eared terrapin
   d. Degu
5. How would you induce anaesthesia in a tortoise?
   a. Ketamine – alfaxalone – intubation – IPPV with isoflurane or sevoflurane
   b. Induction chamber and Ayre's T-Piece delivering sevoflurane or isoflurane – intubation – IPPV
   c. Ketamine – intubation – IPPV with isoflurane or sevoflurane
   d. Mask and Ayre's T-piece delivering sevoflurane or isoflurane
6. How would you perform cardiopulmonary resuscitation in an anaesthetized bird?
7. Which of the following statements about analgesia in birds is incorrect?
   a. Birds do not show any signs of pain
   b. Bupivacaine and lidocaine can be administered simultaneously
   c. Butorphanol is a good analgesic
   d. The non-steroidal anti-inflammatory agent meloxicam has been used in birds
   e. Provision of a calm environment will reduce analgesic requirements
8. What health and safety considerations should be given to anaesthesia of a wild badger?

Diagnostic imaging

Suzetta Cameron and Judith Churm

This chapter is designed to give information on:

- Radiographic positioning and obtaining diagnostic radiographs of exotic patients
- Ultrasonography of exotic species and the limitations and modifications to be noted in different species
- Diagnostic endoscopy, including anaesthetic and positioning requirements and care of the equipment

---

Introduction

Exotic animals are less likely to reveal anything on clinical examination than are dogs and cats. Diagnostic imaging is therefore an important part of obtaining a diagnosis.

In many practices it is the role of the nurse to assist the veterinary surgeon in performing procedures such as radiography, ultrasonography and endoscopy. It is essential that the nurse has the basic knowledge and skills to carry out their role, as suitable restraint and correct positioning are integral to producing a safe and successful outcome.

The amount of information that can be acquired in radiography is directly related to the quality of an image.

Considerations prior to imaging include:

- Species
- Clinical health and age
- Requirement for chemical restraint
- Anatomical area of interest
- Requirement for multiple views
- Health and safety of staff.

Diagnostic radiography

Equipment

Radiography machine

The radiography machine should have a capacity of 300 milliamperes (mA) at 1/60 of a second or less and a kilovolt peak (kVp) range of at least 40–100 kV.

It is useful to have an X-ray machine with a tube that can be rotated so that it is at 90 degrees to the table surface, enabling horizontal beam radiography. This allows lateral and craniocaudal views to be obtained without disturbing the natural position of the organs, and also reduces the need for chemical immobilization. This is especially helpful in chelonians where there is no muscular division between the abdomen and the thorax, meaning that rotating the animal significantly affects the positioning of internal organs.

> ⚠️ **WARNING**
> There are health and safety and radiological safety considerations that need to be addressed before using a horizontal beam.

Film selection and exposure factors

To ensure a high-quality radiographic image it is essential to use the appropriate film type.

Mammography film

Mammography film is recommended for smaller patients, where fine detail is needed. This is used in conjunction with a single-screen rare earth cassette. Unlike standard radiographic film, mammography film has emulsion on only one side of the base. It produces highly detailed images. Care must be taken when filling the cassette to ensure that the emulsion side of the film lies next to the screen.

Mammography film also has a low exposure latitude, which enhances small differences in contrast.

Due to the fine grain in mammography film, which also facilitates the production of highly detailed images, it is termed a slow to ultra-slow film.

Dental film

Non-screen dental film is useful for obtaining intraoral radiographs of the maxillary and mandibular incisor teeth and is also useful for evaluating the cheek teeth in larger rodents. The small size of these films facilitates intraoral radiography in smaller patients. Dental film also has the ability to highlight fine detail. It is best used with a cone attached to the X-ray tube head, to improve collimation and to prevent scatter of the primary beam.

Collimation and exposure factors

Careful collimation over the area of interest is particularly important to reduce scatter, which would negatively affect image quality, and ensures the safety of the personnel involved. A grid may be used in larger species to reduce scatter. As with dogs and cats, a grid should be used when the thickness of the area of interest exceeds 10 cm.

When using slower cassette and film combinations it is necessary to increase the X-ray exposure. Milliampere second (mAs) values may need to be increased by up to four times. However, to reduce movement blur, mA should be increased and time reduced.

Normal radiographic film is typically developed using a rapid access processor and the development time is usually 90 seconds. With mammography film, a rapid access processor can still be used but it should be set to a slow speed so that the development time is increased to 120–130 seconds.

Digital radiography

Digital radiography is becoming increasingly popular within veterinary practice and has a number of advantages in exotic species. Digital radiography uses a specialized digital plate instead of a conventional cassette. The resulting images can be viewed immediately on a computer and can be transferred between computers when referring cases, for example. Images can be digitally manipulated to correct exposure factors and this has the potential to reduce radiation doses. Areas of interest can be magnified, which is particularly useful in very small patients. As with other species, the use of digital radiography eliminates the need for film storage.

Mammals

Restraint

Small mammals such as rabbits, guinea pigs, chinchillas, degus and sugar gliders are increasingly popular pets and so are seen with increasing frequency in general practice. If the health of the patient allows, anaesthesia is usually required in these species to obtain diagnostic radiographs. It facilitates correct positioning, enables standard comparable views to be taken and decreases the number of repeat exposures.

Radiographic views and positioning

Radiography can be used in these patients to evaluate the skull, thorax, abdomen, limbs and spine.

Skull

Evaluation of the skull is a common requirement in these species because of the high incidence of dental abnormalities, inner ear disease and eye problems. Five radiographic views are typically obtained: dorsoventral (or ventrodorsal); lateral (right or left); right lateral oblique; left lateral oblique; and rostrocaudal. With care, these can all be taken on one cassette.

Dorsoventral view

The dorsoventral view is particularly useful for comparing the tympanic bullae and dental arcades. The patient is positioned in sternal recumbency, with the head overlying the cassette (Figure 8.1). Care should be taken to minimize head rotation and it may be necessary to tilt the nose up with a foam wedge. The primary beam should be centred midway between the eyes.

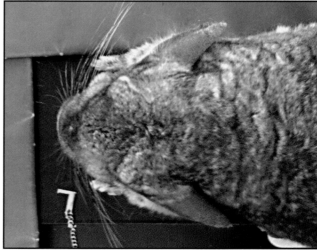

8.1 Positioning of a chinchilla for a dorsoventral view of the skull.

Lateral (right or left) views

The lateral view is useful for evaluating the occlusal plane of the cheek teeth, the occlusion of the maxillary and mandibular incisor teeth, and overgrowth of incisors. The patient is positioned in lateral recumbency, with the head overlying the cassette. The patient's nose is slightly raised so that the median axis is parallel to the cassette. A foam wedge can be placed under the mandible to minimize rotation, although this is not always necessary. The primary beam is centred over the cheek teeth.

Right and left lateral oblique views

It is important to take both right and left lateral oblique views to enable comparison of both sides of the mouth (Figure 8.2). Correct positioning should allow visualization of the mandibular cheek teeth of one side and the maxillary cheek teeth of the opposite side. By taking both right and left lateral oblique views, separation of the root shadows of all of the teeth is obtained.

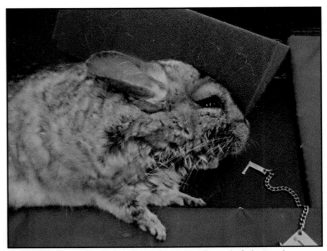

8.3 Positioning of a chinchilla for a left lateral oblique view of the skull. The patient's nose is slightly raised so that the median axis is parallel to the cassette.

evaluated. In addition, overgrown cheek teeth may be observed curving laterally on this view.

The patient is placed in dorsal recumbency. A cradle can be used if necessary. The head is positioned perpendicular to the body and is secured in place by taping the nose to the sides of the cradle. The primary beam is centred over the incisor teeth.

Thorax, abdomen and spine

Although not ideal, it is common to image the whole patient in order to evaluate the thorax, abdomen and spine. Dorsoventral (or ventrodorsal) and lateral views are used for this purpose.

Dorsoventral (or ventrodorsal) view

The patient is positioned on the cassette in sternal recumbency (dorsal recumbency for the ventrodorsal view). The fore- and hindlimbs are gently extended and secured to the cassette using radiolucent tape or light sandbags. The primary beam is centred on the midline at the thoracolumbar vertebral junction (Figure 8.4).

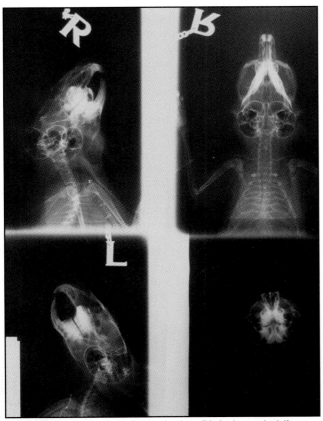

8.2 From upper left clockwise: Right lateral oblique radiograph of a chinchilla which highlights the upper right and lower left molar teeth. A dorsoventral radiograph of a chinchilla. Rostrocaudal view of a chinchilla skull, highlighting the orbits and sinuses. Lateral view of a chinchilla skull showing normal dentition.

The patient is positioned in lateral recumbency, with a foam wedge placed under the maxilla and the nose slightly raised (Figure 8.3). The wedge should rotate the skull by 10–20 degrees. It can be useful to take this view with the mouth open, thus allowing greater separation of the dental arcades. An effective technique is to use a needle cap cut to size and positioned between the upper and lower incisors. Again, the primary beam is centred over the cheek teeth.

Rostrocaudal view

The rostrocaudal view is useful for visualizing the temporomandibular joint and frontal sinuses. This is essential if the skull is to be completely and thoroughly

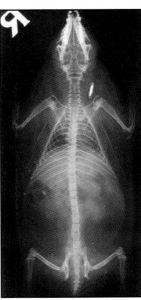

8.4 Dorsoventral radiograph of a tenrec. The identichip can be seen implanted to one side of the neck.

Lateral view

The patient is placed on the cassette in right lateral recumbency. The forelimbs are pulled cranially and taped to the cassette using radiolucent tape or are tied using a soft tie. The hindlimbs are secured caudally, to enable the abdomen to be imaged without superimposition (Figure 8.5).

The primary beam is centred over the caudal border of the scapula.

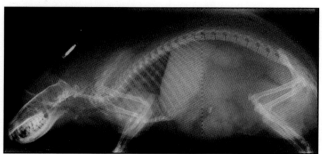

8.5 Lateral radiograph of a tenrec, with good contrast allowing clear distinction between soft tissue and bony structures. Ideally the fore- and hindlegs should be pulled forwards and backwards, respectively, to stop them obscuring the chest and abdomen.

Limbs

The limbs are typically imaged using two views: dorsoventral (dorsopalmar or dorsoplantar, depending on location); and lateral. Positioning is undertaken as for dogs and cats.

Contrast studies

Gastrointestinal tract

Positive contrast studies of the gastrointestinal tract can be undertaken in small mammals using either barium sulphate or iodide compounds. The contrast medium is typically administered via a gastric or oesophageal tube under general anaesthesia. Oral administration can occasionally be undertaken by introducing contrast medium slowly into the mouth prior to anaesthesia, but great care must be taken to prevent aspiration.

- Barium sulphate is the most commonly used contrast agent and is given at about 10–15 ml/kg. If there is suspicion of gastric outflow blockage or severe tympany (dilation of the gut with gas and or fluid), a smaller amount should be instilled to prevent stomach rupture.
- The use of organic iodides is recommended if gut perforation is suspected. Both ionic and non-ionic compounds can be used but, as with other species, ionic compounds will draw water into the gastrointestinal tract. Special care therefore needs to be taken in debilitated or dehydrated patients, or their condition can deteriorate.

It should also be remembered that the contrast medium will become progressively diluted as it travels through the gastrointestinal tract, resulting in reduced opacity.

Nasolacrimal ducts

Positive contrast studies of the nasolacrimal ducts can be undertaken in the larger species by cannulating the ducts and introducing iodine-based contrast media.

Urinary tract

Retrograde studies of the urinary system can be undertaken in small mammals using organic iodides such as Gastrografin (diatrizoate meglumine and diatrizoate sodium). This can be administered into the urinary tract using a small-diameter catheter inserted into the urethra. For positive contrast studies the bladder is distended with positive contrast medium. For double contrast studies a small volume of positive contrast medium is introduced and the bladder subsequently distended with air.

Excretory urography has been undertaken in rabbits and ferrets by administering iodide compounds intravenously via the cephalic vein. Both ionic and non-ionic compounds can be used for this purpose but ionic compounds can be associated with nausea, vomiting and hypotension following rapid intravenous injection.

Spinal cord

Myelography can be performed in guinea pigs, rabbits and ferrets. The technique is similar to that described for dogs, but it is wise to consult an anatomy text as significant anatomical differences may exist. A non-ionic iodide such as Omnipaque (iohexol) should always be used for myelography, as ionic iodides are irritating to the brain and spinal cord. The two sites that can be used for injection are the atlanto-occipital space or between the fifth and sixth lumbar vertebrae.

Common findings in small mammal radiography

- Gastrointestinal disorders.
- Skeletal deformities/fractures.
- Respiratory disease.
- Dental malocclusion.
- Ileus.
- Otitis media.

Birds

In most cases of illness and where skeletal problems are suspected, radiography is generally advised. Radiography is also essential prior to coelomic endoscopy because the presence of organ enlargement or ascites may alter the site of the entry portal or preclude endoscopy altogether.

Since birds have a relatively high respiratory rate, short exposure times should be chosen to minimize movement blur. At least two radiographic (orthogonal) views should be obtained, with the ventrodorsal and lateral being most common.

Restraint

Birds should be anaesthetized for radiography, to avoid stress and injury to the patient and to ensure that standard, well positioned views are produced. Some practitioners have advocated the use of 'X-ray boards', which restrain conscious birds. These can be used but, with recent advances in anaesthesia, they are seldom necessary.

Radiographic positioning

Correct positioning is important because fractures of bones such as the clavicle or coracoid can be easily missed on poorly positioned radiographs (Figure 8.6). In addition, accurate assessment of the coelomic organs and air sacs is only possible in non-rotated radiographs.

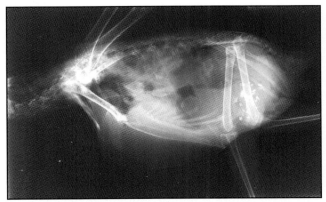

8.6 In this lateral radiograph of a bird the coracoid bones are superimposed and a ventrodorsal view would be needed to identify any pathology.

8.7 (a) A kestrel positioned for a ventrodorsal view. (Courtesy of C. Rice) (b) Ventrodorsal radiograph of a bird with a fractured ulna (arrowed).

Ventrodorsal view

The bird is placed in dorsal recumbency. The legs are extended caudally and secured with tape. The wings are then spread out and taped down symmetrically in order to minimize rotation (Figure 8.7). The primary beam is centred on the keel.

Lateral view

The bird is positioned in lateral recumbency, with its lower leg taped down and pulled caudally. Its upper leg is extended cranially at an angle of 45 degrees and its wings are extended above its back and taped in position (Figure 8.8) or held down with a light sandbag. This position should not be maintained while waiting for film processing, as stretching the wings can cause radial nerve damage. Once the exposure has been made, the wings should be released.

Contrast studies

In birds, the air sacs act as natural negative contrast, highlighting the internal organs.

Gastrointestinal tract

Contrast studies are most commonly used for imaging the gastrointestinal tract in order to identify radiolucent foreign bodies, intraluminal masses, displacement of bowel loops by extraluminal space-occupying lesions, and gut enlargement.

Barium sulphate is the most commonly used contrast medium (Figure 8.9). A 30–50% solution is

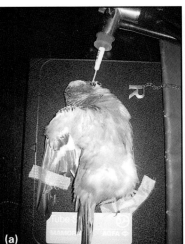

8.8 (a) A budgerigar positioned for a lateral view. (b) Lateral radiograph of the skull of a macaw showing normal anatomy.

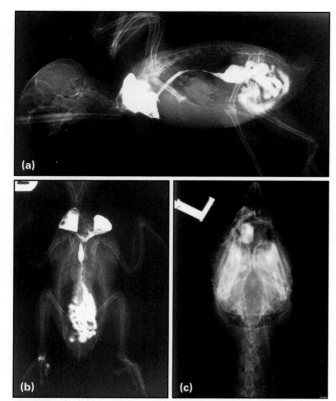

8.9   **(a, b)** Lateral and ventrodorsal radiographs of a bird, showing barium contrast medium in the crop and gastrointestinal tract. **(c)** Dorsoventral radiograph of a bird skull, showing contrast medium in the nasal sinus.

administered via a crop tube at approximately 20 ml/kg bodyweight. The timing of exposures will depend on the size of the bird but, as a general guide, transit times are much quicker in birds than in mammals. In African grey parrots the crop will be empty after approximately 1 hour, the contrast medium will reach the large intestine in 1.5–2 hours (although some contrast will remain in the stomach at this stage) and the stomach will be empty after about 6 hours, when the contrast medium will be approaching the distal gut.

It is also possible to perform gastrointestinal studies using water-soluble organic iodides. These are associated with faster transit times and are the agents of choice when a ruptured bowel is suspected. Gastrografin (diatrizoate meglumine and diatrizoate sodium) is an ionic high-osmolar compound that will draw fluid into the gastrointestinal tract. This causes dilution of the contrast material and can also dehydrate the bird; it is therefore rarely recommended. A non-ionic, low-osmolar compound such as Omnipaque (iohexol) can be used at 10 ml/kg bodyweight.

Cloaca

Barium sulphate can be administered directly into the cloaca in order to demonstrate cloacal and colonic masses. Care must be taken that barium sulphate is not introduced into the oviduct or ureters using this technique.

Urinary tract and heart

Excretory urography and non-selective angiography have been described in birds. They involve the intravenous administration of an organic iodide. Both ionic and non-ionic compounds can be used, but ionic compounds can be associated with nausea, vomiting and hypotension following rapid intravenous administration. A dose of 2 ml/kg, warmed to body temperature, is administered via the brachial vein. Rapid sequence exposures are required because of the short circulation time in these species: the contrast medium reaches the kidneys 30–60 seconds after injection.

Excretory urography can be used for delineating the ureters prior to cloacal surgery and is indicated for identifying renal masses, ureteral obstructions and abnormalities in renal excretion. Angiography can be used for delineating the cardiac chambers when cardiomyopathy is suspected.

Spinal cord

Myelography can be performed in birds but is rarely undertaken in general practice. A technique has been described in which the contrast agent (a non-ionic iodide) is introduced into the thoracolumbar region. Lumbar puncture is not possible in birds because of the fused synsacrum. Injection into the cerebellomedullary cistern is not recommended because it is not always achievable, and trauma to the spinal cord at this level can result in death.

Common findings in bird radiography

- Enlarged organs, e.g. liver, heart, proventriculus.
- Skeletal deformities/fractures (Figure 8.10).
- Foreign bodies.
- Pneumonia/air sacculitis.
- Abscesses.
- Ascites (Figure 8.11).
- Eggs (Figure 8.12).

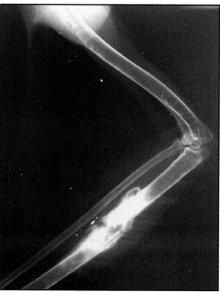

8.10   A fractured ulna in a bird.

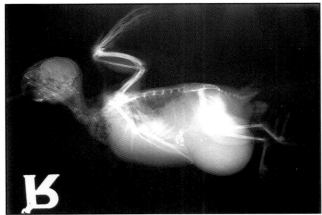

8.11 Radiograph demonstrating ascites in a budgerigar.

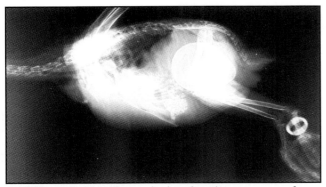

8.12 Lateral radiograph showing the presence of an egg in the reproductive tract of an egg-bound bird.

Reptiles

Restraint

Lizards

It is not always necessary to anaesthetize or chemically restrain lizards for radiography. Larger lizards can be immobilized using the ocular vasovagal response. This involves applying gentle but firm digital pressure to both eyes using clean, dry cotton wool. A bandage can then be wrapped around the head to hold the cotton wool in place (Figure 8.13). This will cause the lizard to remain quiet and still until stimulated by noise or positional changes. It must be appreciated, however, that this technique can cause a drop in blood pressure and so the use of a Doppler ultrasound monitoring probe is recommended. Some lizards will remain immobile if the head is covered with a small cloth.

Very active lizards (particularly smaller lizards) may be restrained by placing them into a suitably sized transparent container. Although this will not immobilize them, it will limit movement enough to obtain diagnostic radiographs. The exposure must be taken when the lizard is still. The use of other mechanical restraint devices such as sandbags and ties is difficult in these patients and is not recommended.

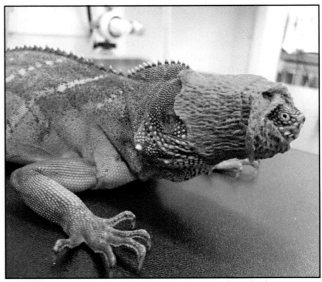

8.13 Demonstration of the vasovagal technique on a water dragon.

Snakes

Chemical restraint of snakes is not always necessary for radiography but is often beneficial to facilitate positioning and eliminate the spinal curvature associated with normal muscular contractions.

Chelonians

Chelonians can usually be imaged successfully without the use of chemical or physical restraint.

Radiographic positioning

Lizards

Two orthogonal views should be obtained in these species, with dorsoventral and lateral being the most common.

Dorsoventral view

The lizard is positioned in sternal recumbency (Figure 8.14). In small patients it is common to image the whole patient, with the beam centred on the spine midway between the fore- and hindlimbs.

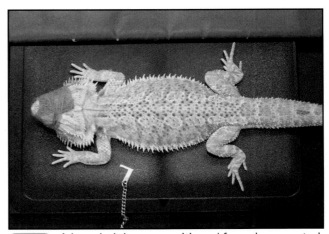

8.14 A bearded dragon positioned for a dorsoventral view.

Lateral view

The lateral view can be obtained in one of two ways. In larger lizards, particularly those with a calm temperament, horizontal beam radiography is ideal and has the advantage that the organs are maintained in their natural positions. It is a useful view for assessing the lungs and even follicles but is only appropriate when the lizard can be adequately immobilized, either chemically or using the vasovagal response.

- A shelf must be securely mounted on the wall adjacent to the X-ray machine.
- The cassette is positioned on the shelf in an upright position against the wall and supported in a suitable stand.
- A lead sheet should be placed between the cassette and the wall to comply with health and safety regulations.
- The lizard is then placed on a raised platform on the shelf, with its median plane parallel to the cassette (Figure 8.15).
- The X-ray tube is rotated 90 degrees to the surface of the table and the primary beam centred on the mid portion of the lizard.

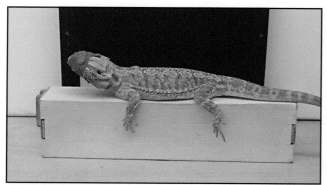

8.15 A bearded dragon positioned for a lateral view using a horizontal X-ray beam.

If horizontal beam radiography is not available or appropriate, standard vertical beam radiography can be undertaken (Figure 8.16). The lizard is positioned in lateral recumbency on top of the cassette and maintained in this position using two foam wedges. Again, the primary beam is centred on the mid portion of the lizard, and the legs should be extended away from the field of interest.

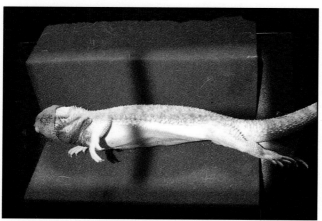

8.16 A bearded dragon positioned for a lateral view using a vertical X-ray beam.

Contrast studies

The most common contrast studies undertaken in lizards are gastrointestinal, and barium sulphate is the most commonly used contrast agent (Figure 8.17). A 30–50% solution is administered via a gastric tube at 20 ml/kg bodyweight. Oral dosing is not recommended because it can be associated with aspiration and loss of barium sulphate through the nose and mouth.

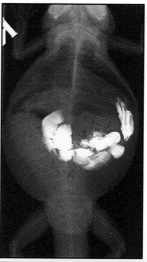

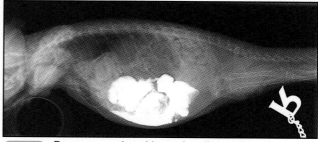

8.17 Dorsoventral and lateral radiographs of a lizard, showing barium in the gastrointestinal tract.

Gut transit time is very slow in lizards, ranging from approximately 24 hours to 2–3 weeks in some herbivorous species. Transit can also be further delayed in sick animals. In addition, barium sulphate can become desiccated in the gastrointestinal tract, particularly in patients suffering from ileus or dehydration, and so special care needs to be taken in such patients.

Water-soluble organic iodides (ionic and non-ionic) can be used in place of barium and are the agents of choice if gut perforation is suspected. Iodides are associated with faster transit times than barium sulphate. When using ionic compounds, care needs to be taken in debilitated and dehydrated animals for the reasons already outlined. Ionic compounds are administered by stomach tube at a dose of 10 ml/kg bodyweight. It should also be remembered that ionic iodides such as Gastrografin (iohexol) will be progressively diluted as they pass through the gastrointestinal tract, resulting in reduced opacity.

Direct cloacal administration of contrast medium can be used for identification of distal intestinal obstructions and caudal abdominal masses. Care needs to be taken not to rupture a diseased intestine, and the volume of agent needed should therefore be estimated prior to administration; back pressure on the syringe should not be relied upon.

Double contrast studies can be performed on the upper gastrointestinal tract and provide better mucosal detail than do single contrast studies. A contrast agent is first administered via a gastric tube. The volume of agent administered should be between one-third and one-half of the gastric volume. The stomach is then gently distended with air, allowing improved contrast.

Myelography cannot be performed in lizards because reptiles do not have a true subarachnoid space.

Common findings in lizard radiography

- Metabolic bone disease.
- Skeletal deformities/fractures.
- Reproductive abnormalities.
- Soft tissue calcification.
- Gastrointestinal impaction.

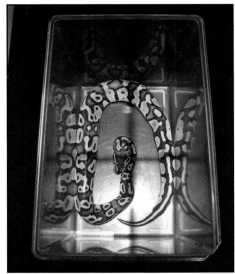

8.18 A conscious royal python positioned in a clear container for the dorsoventral view.

Snakes

Due to the elongated anatomy of these animals, it is useful to be able to estimate where the major organs are situated. This is best achieved by mentally dividing the snake into three sections: the cranial third contains the oesophagus, trachea and heart; the middle third contains the lungs, liver, stomach and cranial air sac; and the caudal third contains the intestines, kidneys, gonads, fat body and cloaca (see Chapter 4).

At least two orthogonal views should be obtained; dorsoventral and lateral views are the most common.

Dorsoventral view

Non-coiled dorsoventral views can be obtained in conscious patients using radiolucent acrylic tubing. A tube can also be made from developed X-ray film, plugged at one end to prevent escape. The snake should be gently guided into the tube, which is then taped directly on to the cassette to prevent movement. The primary beam is centred on the mid-section of the snake. The kV will need to be increased slightly to compensate for the tubing.

Radiographs of conscious snakes in coiled positions may give a general impression but do not allow accurate visualization of internal organs or the spine due to positional artefacts. Such views can be obtained by placing the snake into a suitably sized transparent container, which is then placed directly on to the cassette (Figure 8.18). It is important to position the snake so that its body is curled around in a neat, non-rotated manner. Rotation will compromise the symmetry of the spine and ribs (Figure 8.19). The primary beam is centred over the middle of the box.

Chemical restraint is necessary for obtaining dorsoventral views of specific anatomical areas. Many snakes are too long for even the largest cassettes; therefore sectional views must be taken. The snake is stretched across the cassette in sternal recumbency and multiple exposures are taken, working from proximal to distal until all portions of the snake have

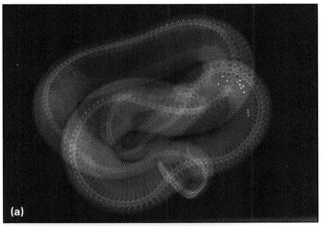

(a)

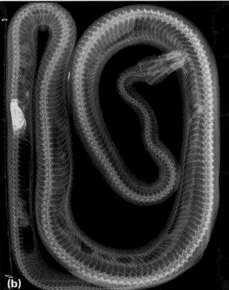

(b)

8.19 Dorsoventral radiographs of coiled snakes. **(a)** The snake is badly positioned, with its body overlying itself and obscuring the image. **(b)** Good positioning with as little superimposition as possible allows the anatomy to be seen more clearly. (Courtesy of C. Rice)

been imaged. Lead sheets should cover unexposed areas of the cassette. Labelled markers taped to the patient can assist in obtaining accurate sequential views and can assist in the correlation of radiographic findings with their anatomical location (Figure 8.20). The primary beam is centred over the mid-section of each portion.

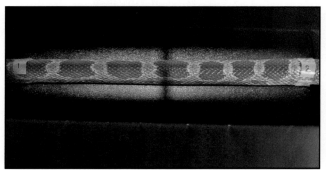

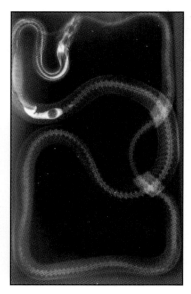

8.22 Dorsoventral view of a conscious snake with barium in the gastrointestinal tract.

8.20 An anaesthetized cornsnake positioned for a dorsoventral view. Radiopaque marker tape can be used to identify various positions along the snake.

Lateral view

Chemical restraint is necessary for obtaining lateral views of snakes. The principles are as described above for the DV view, except that the snake is positioned in lateral recumbency (Figure 8.21).

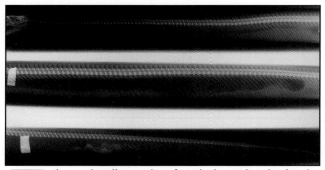

8.21 Lateral radiographs of a whole snake obtained by imaging sections in turn.

Contrast studies

The principles of contrast studies in snakes are largely the same as those for lizards. Gastrointestinal studies (Figure 8.22) can be undertaken using barium- or iodine-based contrast agents delivered by stomach tube.

Common findings in snake radiography

- Egg binding.
- Skeletal deformities/fractures.
- Osteomyelitis.
- Lower respiratory tract disease.
- Tumours.
- Gastrointestinal disorders.

Chelonians

The type of X-ray cassette selected and the exposure required will depend on the size of the chelonian and the density of its shell. Compared with other exotic species, higher kV values are needed to obtain good quality images because of the density of the carapace.

At least two radiographic views should be obtained: the dorsoventral and lateral or rostrocaudal views are most common. The rostrocaudal view allows comparison of the lung fields.

Dorsoventral view

The tortoise or turtle is placed in sternal recumbency on top of the cassette (Figure 8.23). A large piece of tape secured over the shell can be used for physical restraint but is rarely necessary. It may be necessary to immobilize a more active patient by placing it on a foam block – no larger than the plastron – with its limbs unsupported. The disadvantage to using this technique is that it causes magnification of the image and decreases sharpness. It is normal to image the whole patient with the primary beam centred over the centre of the carapace.

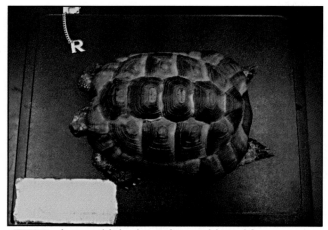

8.23 A spur-thighed tortoise positioned for a dorsoventral view.

Lateral view

As for lizards, the lateral view can be obtained in one of two ways.

Horizontal beam radiography is ideal, as the organs are maintained in their natural positions, allowing for accurate examination of the skeletal system, lungs and digestive tract. As retained eggs are a common problem in chelonians, good abdominal contrast is essential. The patient is positioned on a raised platform on a shelf adjacent to the X-ray machine, with its median plane parallel to the cassette. It is useful if the platform is smaller than the plastron and the legs are unsupported to aid immobilization (Figure 8.24). The X-ray tube is rotated 90 degrees to the surface of the table, with the primary beam centred over the mid portion of the carapace.

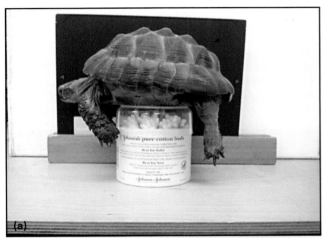

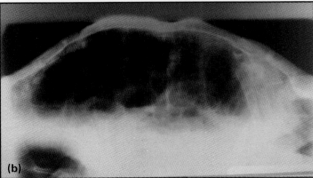

8.24 (a) A spur-thighed tortoise positioned for a lateral view using a horizontal X-ray beam. (b) Lateral radiograph of a tortoise, showing normal lung fields but with some old pyramid changes to the spine and shell.

If horizontal beam radiography is not available or appropriate, the lateral view can be obtained using standard vertical beam techniques. In this case, the patient should be secured to a block using tape and the block/patient positioned so that the animal is in lateral recumbency. In the authors' experience it is necessary to use a block of reasonable weight to maintain the animal's position, particularly with the larger chelonians. Again, the primary beam is centred over the mid portion of the carapace.

Rostrocaudal view

As with the lateral view, the rostrocaudal view can be obtained in one of two ways. For the reasons mentioned earlier, horizontal beam radiography is ideal. The patient is positioned on a raised platform on a shelf adjacent to the X-ray machine. It is again useful if the platform is smaller than the plastron and the legs are unsupported. For this view, the median plane of the patient should be perpendicular to the cassette, with the head nearest to the X-ray machine (Figure 8.25). This will allow the primary beam to pass in a rostral to caudal direction. The primary beam should be centred midline over the ventral border of the carapace.

If horizontal beam radiography is not available or appropriate, the rostrocaudal view can be obtained using standard vertical beam techniques. Again, it is necessary to secure the patient to a block with tape. The block/patient is then positioned vertically with the head pointing skywards. The primary beam is centred as for the horizontal beam view.

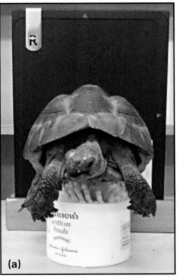

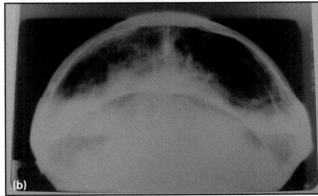

8.25 (a) A spur-thighed tortoise positioned for a rostrocaudal view using a horizontal X-ray beam. (b) Rostrocaudal radiograph of a tortoise with mild inflammatory changes to the right lung.

Contrast studies

Contrast studies in chelonians (Figure 8.26) follow the same principles as for lizards. A particular problem in chelonians is the prolonged gut transit time (up to 2 weeks in larger tortoises). This can be reduced by administering prokinetic agents such as metoclopramide but is best addressed by ensuring adequate hydration. As previously described, transit time can also be reduced by using iodide compounds instead of barium sulphate.

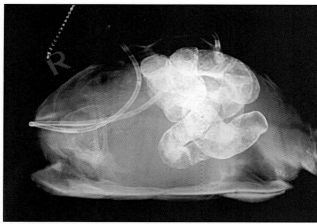

8.26 Lateral radiograph of a tortoise, showing barium in the gastrointestinal tract.

Common findings in chelonian radiography

- Egg binding (Figure 8.27).
- Skeletal disorders including metabolic bone disease.
- Soft tissue calcification.
- Lower respiratory tract disease.
- Uroliths.
- Gastrointestinal disorders.

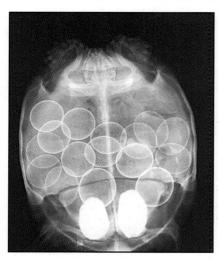

8.27 Dorsoventral radiograph showing the presence of retained eggs in a tortoise. The two white areas near the tail are old methyl methacrylate supports attached to the plastron. (Courtesy of C. Rice)

Diagnostic ultrasonography

Ultrasound waves are high-frequency sound waves produced when a manufactured crystal is deformed by an electrical impulse, causing a piezoelectric effect. The waves are transmitted and then reflected by interfaces of tissues of varying densities. The returning waves are displayed on a monitor in shades of grey, according to the strength of the wave. The degree of weakening of the wave as it passes through tissues is called attenuation.

- Lower-frequency ultrasound will penetrate further (less attenuation) but the resolution of the returning image will be poorer.

- Higher-frequency ultrasound waves will attenuate more quickly and so will penetrate less deeply, but the image resolution will be better.

Many exotic patients are of relatively small size and so higher-frequency transducers (7–10 MHz) should be used. A small sector scanner transducer is necessary to allow close contact of the probe with the small exotic patient or in restricted areas such as the prefemoral fossa of tortoises.

Indications for use of ultrasonography

- Non-invasive diagnostic imaging.
- Examination of soft tissue and fluid-filled structures (Figure 8.28).
- Pregnancy diagnosis.
- Sexing monomorphic species.
- Intraocular and retrobulbar examination.

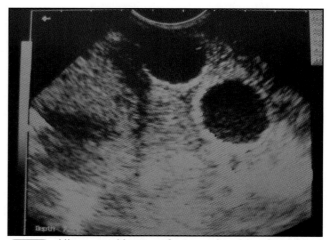

8.28 Ultrasound image of a terrapin with a fluid-filled gastrointestinal tract.

Mammals

Mammals must be prepared by clipping their hair and cleaning the skin. Applying coupling gel at least 5 minutes before examination enhances the contact with the probe. Generally, exotic mammals are examined in a similar fashion to dogs and cats. They are positioned in lateral recumbency and, for cardiac and abdominal examination, an area is prepared that will allow the veterinary surgeon to scan all appropriate organs. Depending on the species, sedation or general anaesthesia is likely to be required.

Examples of indications for ultrasonography include the detection of: tumours (e.g. in ferrets with adrenal disease); retrobulbar abscesses in rabbits; and cystic ovaries in guinea pigs.

Birds

Different tissues have individual resistances to the sound waves, called acoustic impedance. Where two tissues of differing acoustic impedance are adjacent to each other (e.g. bone and soft tissue or gas and soft tissue) most of the beam is reflected and the deeper tissues are shaded and so cannot be visualized clearly. Thus, the air sacs of birds act as a shield to ultrasound, making it less useful diagnostically. It can, however, be used in conditions such as ascites and for cardiac and ocular examination. Coupling gel can be used and, although in some cases feathers need to be removed, it is generally possible to scan successfully by parting the feathers or using naturally occurring featherless sites (Figure 8.29).

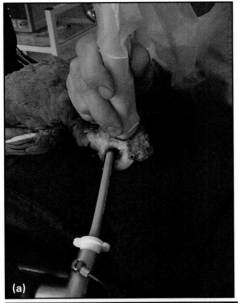

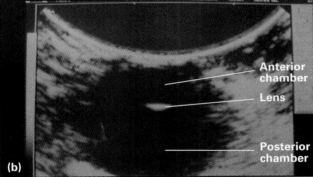

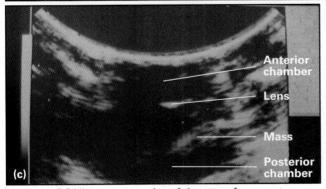

8.29 **(a)** Ultrasonography of the eye of a parrot. **(b)** Ultrasound image of a normal bird's eye. **(c)** Ultrasound image of a bird's eye with a soft tissue mass in the posterior chamber.

Reptiles

Ultrasonography is very useful in reptiles, especially when radiography fails to distinguish between soft tissue structures. The best example of this is for the detection of follicles in tortoises and lizards with preovulatory follicular stasis. Good contact with the reptile's skin is desirable; ultrasound gel should be applied at least 5 minutes before ultrasonography begins. Contact will be enhanced if the reptile's skin is cleaned thoroughly first. Imaging can usually take place without the need for a general anaesthetic.

Lizards can be imaged along the length of their body. It is preferable to avoid acoustic shadowing by the ribs if possible.

Snakes can be scanned for evaluation of organs but avoidance of acoustic shadowing by the ribs is difficult. Very approximately: the cranial third of snakes contains the head, trachea, oesophagus and heart; the middle third contains the liver, lungs, stomach, small intestine and splenopancreas and the caudal third contains the urogenital tract, intestine, kidneys and cloaca. The image deteriorates if a snake is about to shed, as there is an air space between the skin layers.

Chelonians can be held in sternal recumbency and imaged via the prefemoral fossa. The hindlimb is pulled caudally (Figure 8.30a). From this position the liver, kidneys, bladder and reproductive tract may be imaged. The three-chambered heart can be visualized by placing the probe between the shoulder and the neck and directing it caudally (the cervicobrachial approach; Figure 8.30b). The thyroid glands, great vessels and liver can also be imaged using this method.

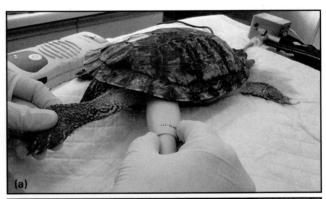

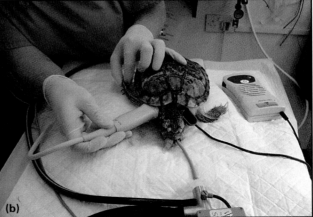

8.30 Positioning the ultrasound probe in chelonians. **(a)** The terrapin is held in sternal recumbency and imaged via the prefemoral fossa, with the hindlimb pulled caudally. **(b)** The probe is placed between the shoulder and the neck of the terrapin and directed caudally (the cervicobrachial approach).

Some probe heads are too large to fit into the prefemoral fossa. Where this is the case, there are three options:

■ A 'stand-off' is used – this is usually a celluloid block or fluid-filled latex glove, which provides an acoustically transmitting space between the probe and the body
■ The fossa is filled with coupling gel – this bridges the gap between the probe and the body and allows at least a partial picture to be obtained
■ The probe (in a waterproof sleeve if necessary) and the back end of the tortoise are immersed in water. Putting portions of the animal into water and using this as an acoustic coupling medium is done very commonly, e.g. for small aquatic turtles.

Diagnostic endoscopy

The use of endoscopes is a very important part of diagnostic imaging of exotic species. The small size of many exotic animals and their ability to hide and mask disease mean that visualization and endoscopic biopsy of internal organs is often the most informative diagnostic procedure undertaken. It is of particular importance in birds.

Basic equipment required for endoscopy

■ Rigid endoscope (30 degree 2.7 mm; Figure 8.31) plus protection sheath.
■ Operating sheath with ports for air or water and operating instruments.
■ Light source and cable (ideally plus video camera and monitor).
■ Endoscopic biopsy instruments.
■ Surgical instruments.
■ Sterile drapes.
■ CO_2 insufflator for reptile and mammal endoscopy.

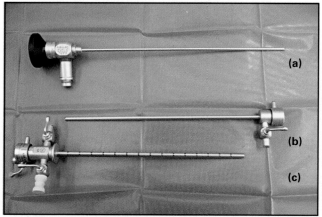

8.31 A rigid endoscope **(a)** with two sheaths **(b, c)**. The sheaths protect the delicate endoscope from damage and they also have portals, which allow water, air or operating instruments to be inserted alongside the endoscope. The lower sheath (c) has ingress ports for gas insufflation.

Cleaning and sterilization of endoscopy equipment

Endoscopes are delicate instruments; although many are now autoclavable, this can over time shorten their usable life. Endoscopy equipment should be cleaned immediately after use to prevent the drying of tissue fluids, which can be difficult to remove.

How to clean endoscopy equipment

1. Soak equipment in a neutral pH enzymic cleaner and clean the sheaths carefully, using suitable brushes.
2. Either gas-sterilize equipment using ethylene oxide (EtO) or cold-sterilize equipment by soaking it in an appropriate solution (glutaraldehyde is a carcinogen and has been largely replaced by safer chemicals including quaternary ammonium products and halogenated tertiary amines). Soaking endoscopes or cameras for longer than 45 minutes is not recommended.
3. Rinse equipment with sterile water and dry using sterile swabs.

These are general recommendations and the manufacturer's guidelines should always be followed.

Surgical instruments

An endoscopy kit should be prepared, and should include the following:

■ One small pair of straight Metzenbaum scissors
■ One pair of rat-toothed and one pair of atraumatic forceps
■ One blade (size 15)
■ One pair of small artery forceps
■ One gauze swab.

This kit is suitable for gaining surgical entry to the body cavity of interest.

Disposable and clear plastic sterile drapes (Figure 8.32) are very useful as they are lightweight and enable good observation of the patient and therefore easier anaesthetic monitoring.

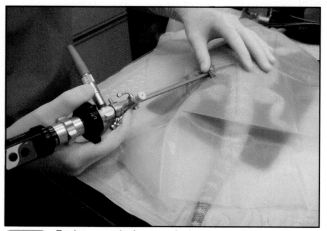

8.32 Endoscopy being carried out on a bearded dragon.

Carbon dioxide insufflation

Unlike birds, the only potential air spaces in reptiles and mammals are the coelom and abdomen, respectively. A gas needs to be inserted to allow the viscera to be seen. Oxygen carries the risk of air embolism and is also combustible. Air can be used for imaging the gastrointestinal tract but carbon dioxide is generally the best choice as it is cheap and safe; any left in the animal is absorbed into the blood and expelled through the lungs. An insufflator is a machine that delivers CO_2 from a cylinder to the patient and regulates the flow and pressure of the gas in the body cavity. The gas is usually delivered through a Veress needle, which has a sharp outer cannula but a blunt inner needle through which the gas passes. It is designed to prevent accidental damage to internal organs.

Mammals

Endoscopy is particularly useful for examination of the oral cavity of rabbits (Figure 8.33), guinea pigs and chinchillas. Care must be taken to use a gag during the procedure. Abdominal examination must be done with air or CO_2 insufflation. Endoscopy is an increasingly useful diagnostic tool due to its minimally invasive nature.

The hair must be shaved and the skin aseptically prepared. The approach depends on the procedure but is generally undertaken with the patient in dorsal recumbency, making an incision to one side of the midline.

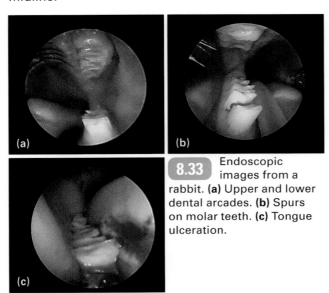

8.33 Endoscopic images from a rabbit. **(a)** Upper and lower dental arcades. **(b)** Spurs on molar teeth. **(c)** Tongue ulceration.

Birds

Endoscopy is useful for examination of the cloaca and it can also be used, with care, to examine the trachea and syrinx.

Birds should be anaesthetized and intubated prior to endoscopy. They should be placed in right lateral recumbency, with their wings held above their backs using a light sandbag or tape. The uppermost left leg is usually held caudally, either manually or secured by tape (some veterinary surgeons prefer to position the leg cranially). The site of insertion is an area between the end of the rib cage, the caudally held femur and the spinal column. The feathers should be gently plucked from the site and aseptic preparation of the skin performed. Care should be taken not to over-wet the site as this will exacerbate heat losses under anaesthetic.

The endoscope can be inserted either between the last two ribs or behind the last rib, depending on the size of the bird and the preference of the veterinary surgeon. The endoscope should then enter the caudal thoracic or abdominal air sac. Birds must be ventilated during anaesthesia as the air sacs have been breached. Once the procedure is finished there is usually no need to suture the hole and the bird should be allowed to wake up in the normal manner.

Examples of endoscopic images from birds are given in Figure 8.34.

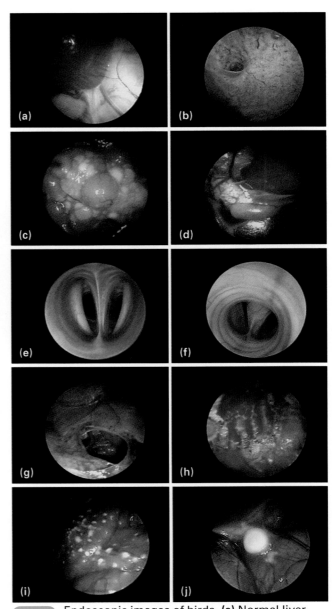

8.34 Endoscopic images of birds. **(a)** Normal liver. **(b)** Normal lung. **(c)** Active ovary. **(d)** Testicle, adrenal gland and kidney. **(e)** Normal syrinx. **(f)** Occluded syrinx. **(g)** Air sacculitis. **(h)** Lung haemorrhage. **(i)** Aspergillosis in an air sac. **(j)** *Aspergillus* granuloma.

Reptiles

Endoscopy is used to visualize and biopsy internal organs, as well as to evaluate the interior of the gastrointestinal tract and respiratory tracts.

Reptiles should be anaesthetized and intubated prior to endoscopy. Reptiles require air or CO_2 insufflation to allow good visualization of the coelom. Care must be taken with IPPV or ventilation when insufflation is being used, as reptiles have no diaphragm.

The coelomic cavities of snakes are less commonly examined by endoscope, unless a specific organ needs examining or sampling as this requires multiple incision sites. Endoscopy can also be used to examine the gastrointestinal tract; a flexible endoscope can be used in this case.

For a coelioscopic approach, lizards should be placed in either sternal (e.g. geckos, bearded dragons, green iguanas) or lateral recumbency (e.g. chameleons). Lizards should have their upper hindlimb taped caudally to the tail. A paralumbar area should be aseptically prepared. In lizards this will be bordered by the caudal ribs, dorsally by the spine and caudally by the hindlimb.

Chelonians should be supported in lateral recumbency. In chelonians, the incision site is the prefemoral fossa, which is the area just cranial to the hindleg. In chelonians, the upper hindlimb should be taped or held caudally.

Examples of endoscopic images from reptiles are shown in Figure 8.35.

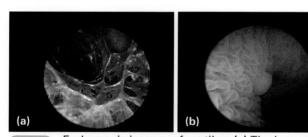

8.35 Endoscopic images of reptiles. **(a)** The lung of a monitor lizard. **(b)** The cloaca of a snake.

Diagnostic imaging of wildlife

Diagnostic imaging is used with wildlife casualties for rapid triage (Figure 8.36). It is important that animals that may be in great distress are assessed as to the feasibility of their release and survival. Injuries that may heal well in one type of animal may result in a slow death in the wild for another. Most imaging is performed under a general anaesthetic but some animals (e.g. swans) may remain still long enough for survey pictures to be taken.

Examples of factors that can be assessed by imaging include the following.

- **Fractures:** Coracoid fractures may heal well in pigeons, but any resulting stiffness in the shoulder of sparrowhawks will mean they cannot hunt successfully.
- **Metabolic bone disease:** This is commonly seen in wood pigeons and can cause pathological fractures of bones.

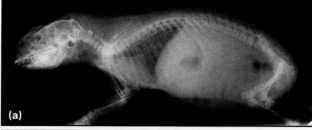
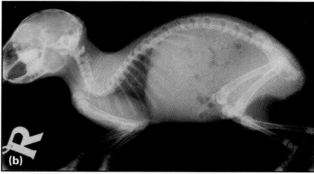

8.36 **(a)** Lateral radiograph of a hedgehog. **(b)** Lateral radiograph of a young wild rabbit. (Courtesy of the RSPCA)

- **Gastrointestinal tract disorders:** *Trichomonas* can be found in the mouth and oesophagus of birds and, if not treated, will spread to other birds and cause weight loss and starvation.
- **Foreign bodies:**
  - Pieces of radiopaque metal in the gizzard of waterfowl may indicate lead poisoning, which can cause weakness and death.
  - Fishing hooks can get caught in the oesophagus and gastrointestinal tract of waterfowl and may cause suffering and starvation (Figure 8.37a).
  - Air gun pellets (Figure 8.37b) may be important or can be an incidental finding.

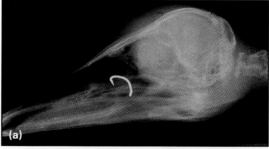
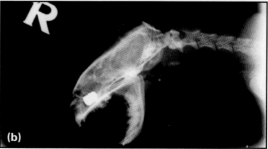

8.37 Diagnostic imaging of wild animals is useful for the investigation of foreign bodies. **(a)** A swan with a hook embedded in its mouth. **(b)** A polecat with an air gun pellet in its skull. (Courtesy of the RSPCA)

■ **Road traffic accidents:** Foxes, badgers and hedgehogs all try to cross roads at night. It is easy to miss fractures, e.g. jaw and pelvis fractures in hedgehogs. Badgers that have been involved in a road traffic accident often curl up and must be assessed by radiography under anaesthesia for spinal injury and head trauma.

■ **Insidious disease:** If seabirds become stressed while hospitalized they are very prone to developing fungal disease such as aspergillosis. This may not be apparent until the animal fails to thrive or dies. Diagnosis by endoscopy is usually instant and definitive.

References and further reading

Capello V and Gracis M (2005) Radiology of the skull and teeth. In: *Rabbit and Rodent Dentistry Handbook*, ed. AM Lennox, pp. 67–70. Zoological Education Network, Florida

Chamness C (2008) Instrumentation. In: *BSAVA Manual of Canine and Feline Endoscopy and Endosurgery*, ed. P Lhermette and D Sobel, pp. 11–30. BSAVA Publications, Gloucester

Ewers R (2007) Getting the best results from radiography. *In Practice* **29**, 464–469

Girling SJ (2002) Mammalian imaging and anatomy In: *BSAVA Manual of Exotic Pets, 4th edn*, ed. A Meredith and S Redrobe, pp. 2–10. BSAVA Publications, Gloucester

Girling SJ (2006) Diagnostic imaging. In: *BSAVA Manual of Rabbit Medicine and Surgery, 2nd edn*, ed. A Meredith and P Flecknell, pp. 52–58. BSAVA Publications, Gloucester

Harcourt-Brown NH (2005) Diagnostic imaging. In: *BSAVA Manual of Psittacine Birds, 2nd edn*, ed. NH Harcourt-Brown and J Chitty, pp. 97–101. BSAVA Publications, Gloucester

Helmer P (2006) Advances in diagnostic imaging. In: *Clinical Avian Medicine, Volume 2*, ed. GJ Harrison and TL Lightfoot TL, pp. 653–658. Spix Publishing, Florida

Hernandez-Divers S (2004) Diagnostic and surgical endoscopy. In: *BSAVA Manual of Reptiles, 2nd edn*, ed. S Girling and P Raiti, pp. 103–114. BSAVA Publications, Gloucester

Hernandez-Divers S and M Lafortune (2004) Diagnostic imaging techniques – endoscopy. In: *Medicine and Surgery of Tortoises and Turtles*, ed. S McArthur *et al.*, pp. 212—227. Blackwell Publishing, Oxford

Raiti P (2004) Non-invasive imaging. In: *BSAVA Manual of Reptiles, 2nd edn*, ed. SJ Girling and P Raiti, pp. 87–102. BSAVA Publications, Gloucester

Silverman S and Tell LA (2005) *Radiology of Rodents, Rabbits and Ferrets: An Atlas of Normal Anatomy and Positioning*, pp. 4–8. Elsevier Mosby, St. Louis

Wilkinson R (2004) Diagnostic imaging techniques – ultrasonography. In: *Medicine and Surgery of Tortoises and Turtles*, ed. S McArthur *et al.*, pp. 187–195. Blackwell Publishing, Oxford

Zody K (2000) Exotic animal radiography. In: *Practical Diagnostic Imaging for the Veterinary Technician, 2nd edn*, ed. CH Han and CD Hurd, pp. 158–186. Mosby, St. Louis

Useful websites

Clinical examination of reptiles: http://priory.com/vet/vetrept2.htm

Digital radiography: http://rpop.iaea.org/RPOP/RPoP/Content/InformationFor/HealthProfessionals/1_Radiology/DigitalRadiography.htm

---

Self-assessment questions

1. Why is mammography film useful in exotic animal radiography?
2. Why are two orthogonal views recommended in radiography?
3. Give some examples of indications for contrast studies in birds.
4. Why is care needed with some contrast agents in gastrointestinal studies of sick animals?
5. List three non-chemical methods of restraint in reptiles.
6. Why might rabbits with dental disease need skull X-rays?
7. Why is carbon dioxide gas used as a way of inflating the body cavities of animals during endoscopy?
8. Why is ultrasonography of more limited use in birds?
9. Why is it important to clip the fur and clean the skin of mammals before ultrasonography?
10. Why are survey X-rays recommended in all wildlife casualties?

Surgical nursing

Donna Brown and Romain Pizzi

This chapter is designed to give information on:

- The role of the surgical nurse before, during and after surgery
- The different hygiene and sterility procedures required when treating exotic pets
- The use and maintenance of microsurgical and endoscopic equipment
- Suture and needle selection
- The methods of dressing wounds and the types of products chosen and why

The role of the nurse

Nurses should be responsible for the following:

- Cleaning the operating theatre and preparation room
- Checking the anaesthetic machine and equipment is functional
- Preparing all instruments and equipment, including the sterilization and disinfection of equipment and adjusting operating table height
- Preoperative care
- Positioning the patient for surgery
- Avoiding hypothermia and hyperthermia
- Postoperative care.

Separation of roles

Ideally, surgical theatre roles should be separate, as in human surgical theatres, with an anaesthetist, a surgeon, a surgical assistant nurse (scrubbed nurse) and a non-sterile circulating theatre nurse.

- The **scrubbed nurse** is a nurse who has scrubbed in to the operation and assists with swabbing, lavage, suction, retraction of tissues, suturing, instrument selection and maintaining an organized instrument trolley.

- The **circulating theatre nurse** is responsible for organizing the surgical theatre, preparing the patient for surgery, attending to the non-sterile equipment and providing the equipment in a sterile manner to the operating surgeon.

This separation of roles may not be necessary for minor procedures and, in many practices, is not possible for the majority of procedures.

While some practices employ separate dedicated anaesthetists for monitoring and maintaining patients, in other practices veterinary nurses are expected to perform the duties of anaesthetist and circulating theatre nurse simultaneously; although nurses are not permitted to induce anaesthesia, they can monitor and maintain anaesthesia and supervise recovery. This requires forward planning, organization and the ability to predict potential problems. If a veterinary nurse is maintaining anaesthesia they must not allow the veterinary surgeon to send them out of theatre to fetch equipment and they must not assist with the operation.

A list for theatre should be prepared the day before with the order of operations to be performed. Dirty procedures (e.g. dentals and procedures involving infected wounds) and any potentially infectious cases should be performed last or preferably in a separate theatre. This avoids any possibility of contamination of clean surgical procedures. Different species do not need to be treated in a specific order.

Safe surgery checklist

The World Health Organization has initiated a safe surgery checklist, which has been found to reduce postoperative morbidity and mortality notably in human patients. Despite appearing very simple, and a little tedious, it has been shown to reduce errors and misunderstandings considerably. A modified version is given in Figure 9.1. More information can be found at: www.who.int/patientsafety/safesurgery.

Before anaesthesia	Before surgical incision	Before leaving theatre
(at least nurse)	*(all theatre staff)*	*(at least surgeon and nurse)*

Before anaesthesia *(at least nurse)*

Confirm:
❏ Patient identity
❏ Procedure
❏ Consent form signed

Check:
❏ Medications given
❏ Anaesthetic machine
❏ Axillary surgical equipment
❏ Instruments sterilized

Date:

Signed:

Before surgical incision *(all theatre staff)*

❏ **Team have introduced themselves**

Confirm:
❏ Patient identity
❏ Procedure
❏ Suitability of clip
❏ Bladder empty (abdominal operations)
❏ Specific preoperative preparations
❏ Antibiosis if required
❏ Other perioperative medication

Anticipated critical steps

Surgeon:
❏ What are the critical steps?
❏ Anticipated time to completion

Anaesthetist/nurse:
❏ Anaesthetic specific concerns

Nurse/surgical assistant:
❏ Sterility of instruments
❏ Any equipment concerns
❏ Essential radiographs displayed

Before leaving theatre *(at least surgeon and nurse)*

Nurse verbally confirms:
❏ Swab count
❏ Sharps accounted for
❏ Specimen labelling *(read aloud)*
❏ Any equipment issues to be addressed

What are the key concerns for recovery and postoperative management?

Specific medication and care

Notes:
(turn over if needed)

9.1 Veterinary surgery safety checklist, modified from the World Health Organization (WHO) surgical safety checklist. (© Romain Pizzi, Zoological Medicine Ltd)

Cleaning the operating theatre and preparation room

All members of staff entering the surgical suite should ideally wear scrub suits, facemasks, surgical hats and suitable footwear that is not used anywhere else. The surgical suite should be fully wiped down with the appropriate cleaning solutions at the start and end of each day. A regular cleaning schedule should include the cleaning of operating lights, windows, floors, walls, tables and also any equipment that may be needed in the theatre suite during the surgeries performed, such as suction machines, electrocautery units and laparoscopic equipment. The operating table should be cleaned thoroughly after every patient and new padding or table drapes used for each animal. The floor should be mopped between patients, especially if any contamination has occurred and particularly if this is due to haemorrhage from the previous procedure.

Within the preparation area, tables should be wiped down, any clinical waste disposed of and clippers cleaned between patients, and the area prepared for the next patient.

More information on cleaning schedules for surgical areas can be found in the *BSAVA Manual of Small Animal Practice Management and Development*.

With any potentially infectious agents or zoonotic diseases, extra care should be taken within the surgical suite to eliminate cross-infection to other patients or to theatre staff. The use of a fogging system may be helpful for this, with chemicals such as F10, but care needs to be taken regarding the clearing time of the chemical and whether ventilation of the area is adequate. See also Chapter 5.

Checking the anaesthetic equipment

Vaporizers should be topped up with volatile anaesthetic agents ideally at the end of the day when the surgical suite is quieter, so as to reduce the risk of accidental exposure to gaseous vapours. There may, however, be occasions, where a vaporizer will need to be filled during the day, particularly if the operations are long and only one vaporizer is available; this must take place in a well ventilated area with the correct key fillers for the agents and vaporizers. If changing a vaporizer over, the new one must be locked into place.

The amount of oxygen in the machine must be checked; an operation must not take place with only a limited amount of oxygen as there may be an emergency, requiring intermittent positive pressure ventilation (IPPV), or a procedure may take longer than originally anticipated.

The following checks must also be made:

- Spare cylinders must always be available or, if using piped gases, there must be a back-up bank
- Cylinders must be connected properly and, when turned on, there must be no gas leak, especially around the Botok seals
- The flow meter must be working correctly, with the bobbin moving freely within the gauge itself
- The circuits, induction chambers and endotracheal tubes should be checked for breakages, disconnections or blockages by connecting the circuit to the machine and looking for any leaks
- With small patients or those with a high metabolic rate, some means of maintaining body temperature must be employed and this should be checked and made ready for use
- Monitoring equipment should be set up and checked
- Emergency drug doses should be calculated and drawn up for each individual patient, working on an accurate weight measurement.

For more information see References and further reading.

Preparation of instruments and equipment

It is important to have a well organized theatre and adequate organized storage so that different surgeons and nurses can locate items easily and rapidly.

All equipment for sterile procedures should be prepared in advance, including intravenous catheters, tapes, fluids, ECG pads, a stethoscope (or oesophageal stethoscope), clippers and scrub solution for patient preparation, bandage or tape for securing the endotracheal tube, and a laryngoscope suitable for exotic patients. This preparation saves a lot of time and ensures that full attention is paid to the patient during surgery.

If the procedure is not one that occurs regularly in practice, the surgeon should be consulted regarding the instruments they may need and checks should be made that these are in stock. How to sterilize the equipment should also be checked, so that it is not accidently melted or broken when sterilized using an incorrect method. Particular care should be taken with endoscopy equipment, cameras and light cables, as well as electrocautery handpieces. Various methods of sterilization are available (see later). Once sterile, all instruments should be laid on a sterile trolley drape in a methodical manner, ideally starting with the instruments the surgeon will need first.

Operating table height

The surgical nurse should adjust the operating table height to suit the surgeon. It is important to ensure that the table is of an adequate height, not only to prevent the surgeon from stooping, which can, over time, lead to back and neck injuries, but also to allow the surgeon to rest his/her forearms on the table during fine surgical procedures. This allows the major muscle groups to be rested and offers better fine muscle control and precision.

Preoperative care

It is very important for the nurse to gain as much information as possible from the owners prior to admission to the hospital ward. A knowledge of the diet, normal behaviour and routines of the patient, as well as general welfare considerations, is key to aiding a full recovery.

Patients that are compromised by dehydration, blood loss, cachexia, anorexia or infection pose a greater anaesthetic risk than those that are clinically normal; a complete pre-anaesthetic assessment and stabilization before surgery (if possible) is therefore especially important. Correct bodyweight measurements should be obtained to allow accurate drug dosing. Blood analysis should be performed (minimum PCV, total protein, blood urea nitrogen or uric acid, and glucose) to assess the health status of the patient, along with radiography and ultrasonography if indicated.

Some exotic species do not need to be starved prior to general anaesthesia (see Chapter 7). This is particularly true for rabbits, as they cannot vomit due to their powerful cardiac sphincter. Other species, including small rodents and birds, have such high metabolic rates that it can be detrimental to their health if they are starved for long periods; food can therefore be taken away 1–2 hours before induction. This also helps reduce the presence of food particles within the oral cavity, which could inhibit intubation. The patient should always be pre-oxygenated if there is suspected or possible airway compromise.

Assessing the patient, stabilization and limiting surgical risk

Adequate surgical assessment before surgery is vital, bearing in mind that many exotic pets are prey species and hence have a propensity to mask signs of illness. Just as in other species, with the exception of severe haemorrhage or penetrating abdominal or coelomic wounds, it is generally advisable to stabilize patients adequately before undertaking anaesthesia and surgery. Provision of warmth, correction of fluid deficits (even if this is by simply providing oral fluids) and correction of a catabolic/cachexic state help to reduce perioperative mortalities.

Preparing the patient for surgery

Once the patient has been anaesthetized, a protective ocular lubricant should be applied to both eyes. This will prevent corneal desiccation from the bright theatre lighting and will also prevent abrasions due to drapes, as patients will have no blink reflex under anaesthesia.

Current studies in humans and dogs have demonstrated that using chlorhexidine-based surgical skin preparations rather than iodine-based skin preparations leads to lower postoperative wound infection rates. There is no notable evidence of this for exotic patients, and the chosen preparation usually depends on the individual surgeon's preferences. Except for amphibians and fish, the same solutions used in cats and dogs at the same dilution rates are appropriate. For amphibians and fish, the skin has a delicate mucous coating and scrub solutions may be irritant or toxic, so skin preparation is usually confined to cleaning with sterile saline.

Clipping and feather removal should be carried out in the 'prep' room. Placing an incontinence pad under the patient (rather than laying it directly on a smooth table surface) can help to reduce the dispersal of removed fur or feathers. The size of the clip area should always be checked with the veterinary surgeon prior to starting the scrub procedure, as it is a lot harder to clip wet fur. No more feathers than necessary should be plucked. Any loose feathers or fur should be vacuumed or swept up to avoid contamination of the scrub site. The incontinence pad is then discarded before the scrub process.

Mammals

Well lubricated clipper blades are less likely to clog, will clip more effectively, and are less likely to traumatize delicate regions of skin. The nurse performing the clip should always check the clipper blades for any broken or missing teeth, which can cause quite severe lacerations (see Figure 9.4).

Birds

For the majority of surgical procedures, feathers are plucked and not cut or clipped. Plucking results in rapid regrowth of the removed feathers in the weeks following surgery, whereas if feathers are cut they will not be lost until the next naturally occurring moult, which may be many months later.

An exception is made for the large flight feathers of the wing. The primary and secondary feather follicles are firmly attached to the periosteum of the bones of the wing. Removal is difficult, painful, and can also result in damage to feather follicles and regrowth of abnormal feathers. Cutting may therefore be a more suitable alternative where necessary.

Remaining feathers may be positioned out of the surgical field using tape such as Micropore (3M) (Figure 9.2).

Reptiles

While reptiles do not have fur to be clipped or feathers to be plucked, crevices between and beneath the scales can trap debris and bacteria; a much more thorough scrub is therefore necessary. Toothbrushes are ideal for this purpose. Good mechanical cleaning of reptile skin is essential to prevent debris entering surgical wounds, leading to later sterile granulomatous reactions. Retained skin scales (dysecdysis) should preferably be removed before surgery by frequent warm water soakings rather than by overly aggressive scrubbing.

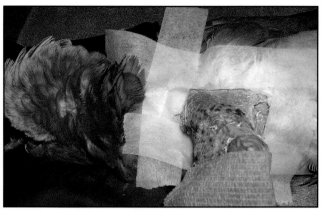

9.2 Note the use of Micropore tape (3M), atraumatically holding feathers back, preventing them from protruding into the sterile field before draping in this galah parrot. (© Romain Pizzi, Zoological Medicine Ltd)

Amphibians

It must be borne in mind that most disinfectants used for standard surgical preparation are highly toxic to amphibians. In the majority of cases, copious flushing with sterile isotonic fluids and gentle cleaning, as well as prophylactic antibiosis, should instead be performed.

Positioning the patient for surgery

Care must be taken when positioning the patient for surgery. Many procedures require that the patient is positioned on its back (i.e. in dorsal recumbency). This can have implications with regard to respiration, especially if the limbs are abducted from the chest as this will limit chest wall movement, particularly in birds. If the patient is lying flat there is the potential for abdominal organs to cause compression of the lungs; this can be avoided by slightly raising the head and thorax if possible (depending on the type of surgery that is being performed).

Paper tape should be used rather than braided ties, as it is less constrictive and therefore minimizes any damage to the surrounding area.

During the surgery an awareness of how much weight or force is being applied to the drapes is required. Resting heavy instruments on top of drapes close to the patient can increase the pressure placed on the patient, which could compromise respiration. This is particularly true for birds as they need to have unrestricted movement of the keel to be able to breathe. Nurses should also be aware that when surgeons lean on drapes they may be applying pressure to the patient.

Avoiding hypothermia and hyperthermia

Most exotic patients are small, with a higher body surface area to mass ratio than dogs and cats, and hence are prone to losing heat rapidly. It is important to balance the need for a sufficiently large clip with the need to reduce excessive heat loss, not just during surgery but also upon recovery. Use of warm disinfectant solutions for the surgical preparation is also helpful, with sparing use of alcohol.

> ⚠ **WARNING**
> **Many exotic pet procedures involve electrosurgery or radiosurgery. It is essential to check first with the surgeon before any alcohol-based skin preparation is applied, to avoid disastrous flammable results.**

Numerous inexpensive methods are practical for maintaining the body temperatures of small exotic patients during even long surgical procedures (Figure 9.3). These include:

- Heat pads
- Hot water bottles
- Latex examination gloves filled with hot water
- Commercially available microwavable pads
- Bags containing beans, split peas or sand and heated in the microwave
- Re-usable hand-warmers (available from outdoor shops).

Heat loss can also be limited using bubble wrap, kitchen foil, cloths or foil survival blankets. Clear plastic drapes do not prevent heat loss very well.

> ⚠ **WARNING**
> - **Chinchillas evolved in the cold, dry climate of the Andes and do not tolerate overheating. With their extremely dense fur and lack of skin sweat glands, they have difficulty losing excess heat.**
> - **While hypothermia is the major risk, small birds are easily overheated, which may manifest as prolonged periods of panting upon recovery from anaesthesia.**

For additional information on fluid therapy, assisted feeding and supportive care; please see Chapter 6.

Postoperative care

Immediate postoperative care

Once the surgery has been completed, the surgical nurse should clean the surgical site with an antiseptic solution (e.g. 0.1% chlorhexidine) to remove any blood and debris, and to avoid any contamination of the wound. If needed, a small dressing can be placed on to the wound (e.g. Melolin (Smith and Nephew), Hypafix (3M) or Allevyn Thin (Smith and Nephew)). If there is excess wetting of the fur or feathers, the patient should be dried as much as possible so that it does not become hypothermic on recovery.

Analgesia should have been administered before and during surgery to help eliminate any postoperative pain (see Chapter 7). Following the procedure, opioid medication can be used for the first 24–28 hours, followed by non-steroidal anti-inflammatory drugs (NSAIDs) for a further 5–7 days, following the instructions of the veterinary surgeon.

An assessment should be made by the veterinary surgeon as to whether fluid therapy should continue postoperatively or be stopped on recovery. Ideally, the intravenous or intraosseous catheter that was placed before the induction of anaesthesia should be left in place until the patient has fully recovered.

The nurse should ensure that the patient is returned to a warm, quiet environment where it should remain until fully recovered. The ambient temperature should be between 21 and 23°C for mammals and birds (heat stroke can occur at temperatures >27°C) and for reptiles should be within the POTR (preferred optimum temperature range) for the species. Incubators and vivaria are invaluable immediately after surgery, especially those that allow

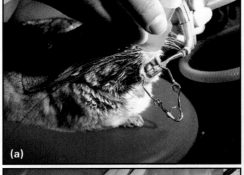
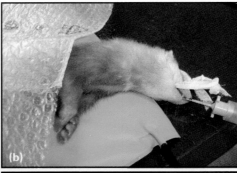
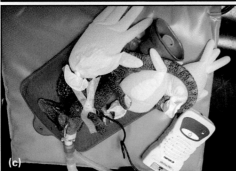
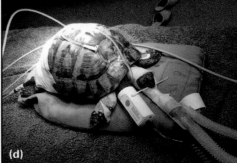

9.3 **(a)** A chinchilla on a microwavable heat mat. Unlike most small mammal pets, chinchillas are prone to overheating under anaesthesia. **(b)** This ferret has been covered in bubble wrap to prevent heat loss before the start of surgery. **(c)** A hot water bottle and latex gloves filled with hot water are used to prevent hypothermia during surgery on this veiled chameleon. **(d)** This tortoise has been placed on a beanbag, pre-heated in a microwave oven, to help prevent perioperative hypothermia. Note that heat sources should be insulated to avoid thermal burns unless they are confirmed to be at a suitable temperature prior to use. (© Romain Pizzi, Zoological Medicine Ltd)

for the addition of oxygen if needed. Old hospital incubators can be used, although they are often too large for many of the smaller species seen in practice and can be difficult to keep clean. Units designed for the veterinary market are easier to maintain and clean and are of a more suitable size (e.g. AICU Animal Intensive Care Unit by Animal Care Products; Brinsea TLC 4M Intensive Care Unit). Fleece bedding (e.g. VetBed), towels or incontinence pads can be used in the recovery cage to add comfort and warmth, and to soak up any exudates or urine from the patient.

The patient's heart and pulse rate, respiratory rate and temperature should be closely monitored and recorded until it has fully recovered from anaesthesia. It may also be beneficial to have the lights dimmed to minimize the stress levels of the patient and therefore promote an uneventful recovery.

Once fully recovered from anaesthesia it is important for the patient to start eating as quickly as possible, as this stimulates gastrointestinal motility and avoids hepatic lipidosis, as well as aiding the healing process and increasing the likelihood of the patient making a full recovery. If the patient is not showing signs of eating it may be necessary to syringe-feed or consider placing a feeding tube (see Chapter 7).

For patients that are unable to stand, extra padding and rolled up towels can be used to prop them up so that they are not lying flat. It is important to ensure adequate access to food and water for these patients.

General postoperative nursing

The patient should be examined daily by the nurse, checking the heart rate, pulse rate, respiratory rate and temperature, as well as the general demeanour. The more critical the case or the smaller the patient, the more frequently checks should take place.

> **Things to consider when examining the patient:**
>
> - Is the patient moving around or is it sitting in the back of the kennel?
> - Is there vocalization when moving?
> - Is the patient eating?
> - Is the patient passing faeces and urine normally?

All information should be recorded on the hospitalization sheets. Any changes should be brought to the veterinary surgeon's attention:

- An increase in heart, pulse or respiratory rate can be indicative of pain
- An increase in temperature can be indicative of infection or pain.

Being able to assess whether a patient is in pain or discomfort is an invaluable skill and one that a nurse uses daily; however, this is more difficult in exotic species, and prey species in particular, as they will often hide clinical signs. If the patient can be observed unobtrusively this will enable a better understanding of their condition.

> **Indications of pain in exotic species:**
>
> - Aggression
> - Vocalization
> - Overgrooming or lack of grooming
> - Inactivity
> - Hiding
> - Hunched posture or pushing abdomen on to the floor
> - Self-trauma
> - Grinding of the teeth (bruxism)
> - Anorexia
> - Extension of the head
> - Abnormal movement.

Wounds should also be examined daily and checked for:

- Reddening of the skin – indicates possible infection
- Heat locally around the wound – indicates possible infection
- Pain – indicates possible infection
- Swelling – a small amount of swelling is expected initially after surgery but should subside
- Alteration of function – particularly if the sutures are too tight to allow movement or if there is too much tissue tension around the wound
- Discharge – the type (e.g. serosanguineous, blood, pus) should be monitored, as well as the amounts produced if possible
- Separation of the wound edges – indicates poor blood circulation and possibility of wound dehiscence.

If a discharge is seen then the wound should be cleaned as frequently as necessary to minimize contamination. Diluted povidone–iodine or diluted chlorhexidine should be used for this, ensuring that the wound itself is clean as well as the surrounding area and the fur or feathers; this will help to prevent any skin scalding and matting, which would augment the irritation and discomfort experienced by the patient and increase the likelihood of self-trauma. Barrier creams can be applied sparingly to protect the skin from damage caused by discharges; however, care must be taken not to coat fur or feathers with cream. If the wound is open then it can be flushed using sterile saline on a daily basis, ensuring that the area around it is kept as dry as possible to decrease the risk of hypothermia.

Equipment and surgical instruments for exotic patients

Clipper blades

It is preferable to use a size 50 clipper blade when clipping the fur of small mammals. The teeth are closer together than those of the regular size 40, which is the blade most often used in practice, and so are less likely to traumatize the skin. This is a particular risk when clipping the thin skin of a rabbit's perineum and groin region (Figure 9.4).

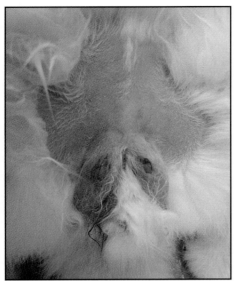

9.4 The skin over this rabbit's scrotum has been traumatized by poorly maintained clippers with broken teeth. Similar injuries can, however, be caused even by well maintained clippers if care is not taken. (© Romain Pizzi, Zoological Medicine Ltd)

Drapes

Plastic drapes have the advantage of being light and not hindering the patient's breathing, while allowing the monitoring of breathing or any movement during anaesthesia (Figures 9.5). They also limit heat loss and, being impervious, do not allow strike-through. Recent human and veterinary studies have demonstrated that adhesive povidone-impregnated cut-through drapes actually increase the risk of post-operative wound infections in mammals (Osuna *et al.*, 1992; Webster and Alghamdi, 2007; Owen *et al.*, 2009); this appears to be because they keep the wound edges moist and warm, which allows bacterial proliferation. Plastic drapes can, however, still be used if a

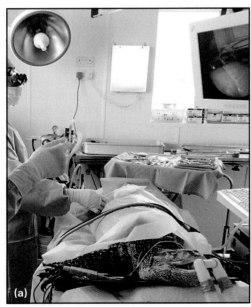

9.5 (a) Clear plastic drapes can cover the patient and table for this endoscopic procedure, but still allow visual monitoring of this ornate monitor lizard. (© Romain Pizzi, Zoological Medicine Ltd) (continues) ▶

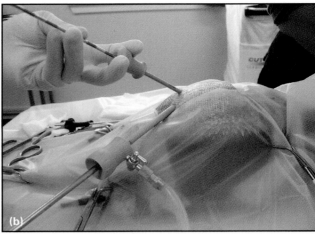

9.5 (continued) (b) For smaller patients, such as this bearded dragon, clear plastic drapes are particularly useful for monitoring anaesthesia under the large draping needed for endoscopic procedures. (© Romain Pizzi, Zoological Medicine Ltd)

window is cut in the drape prior to the surgery in order to keep the drape away from the incision site (Figure 9.6) (as opposed to making the incision directly through the drape). They have the advantage of keeping fur and feathers away from the surgical site.

Adhesive drapes can be useful in reptiles to prevent drape movement during surgery. Traumatic towel clamps should be used with care in reptiles as, unless their skin is mechanically cleaned (scrubbed) very well before surgery, they risk introducing skin particles (even if sterile) beneath the skin, which can lead to sterile granuloma formation.

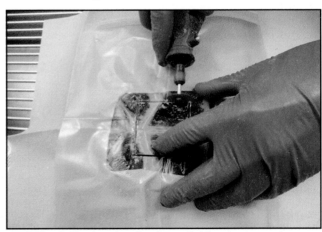

9.6 Adhesive draping is useful for the transplastron coeliotomy in this tortoise. It prevents strike-through despite flushing of the diamond cutting disc with sterile water during the procedure. (© Romain Pizzi, Zoological Medicine Ltd)

Magnification loupes

Magnification loupes not only allow magnification of small structures encountered in exotic patients (Figure 9.7), but can also help compensate for the normal ageing changes in the surgeon's eye. As humans age, the lens of the eye undergoes nuclear sclerosis, becoming less flexible and so less able to accommodate and focus in the near field.

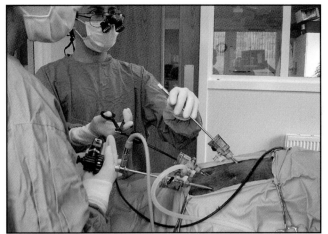

9.7 Magnification loupes are useful for visualizing small incisions and structures, such as during the initial placement of the laparoscopic surgery ports in this seal pup. They also allow the surgeon to see over the top, similar to bifocal spectacles. (© Romain Pizzi, Zoological Medicine Ltd)

Head-mounted light sources

A head-mounted light source may be helpful to the surgeon for visualizing small structures without suffering eye or neck strain.

Retractors

Retractors help to limit the size of wound required for adequate visualization of surgery. While the use of retractors replaces the need for a pair of sterile hands for retraction, their main advantage in small patients is that a flat retractor does not impede visualization or instrument access. The most useful retractor in exotic animal surgery is the Lone Star ring retractor (ARK Surgical Ltd) (Figure 9.8), which is made of autoclavable plastic, with elastic stays that are available with atraumatic ends of different sizes. Alm and eyelid retractors can also be useful, but have more limited applications.

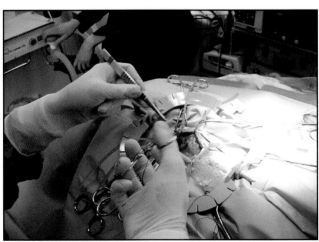

9.8 Ventriculotomy to remove a lead weight in a swan. The low-profile autoclavable Lone Star ring retractor avoids interference from hands holding larger retractors. (© Romain Pizzi, Zoological Medicine Ltd)

Endoscopes and endoscopic instruments

Minimally invasive surgical biopsy and organ examination is not only preferable in many exotic patients, due to their small body size, but is essential for many procedures involving entry into the coelomic cavity of birds. A variety of rigid endoscopes and instruments is available. All should be handled with care, as they are fragile and costly to repair and replace.

Radiosurgery unit

Radiosurgery is the use of high-frequency radiowaves produced by a commercial unit to cut tissue and coagulate blood flow, thereby causing reduced tissue trauma and less potential for haemorrhage. Compared to larger patients such as dogs and cats, small exotic patients are much less tolerant of haemorrhage before it becomes life-threatening. Radiosurgery allows controlled haemostasis (Figure 9.9), with a lower risk of burns than when using standard monopolar electrocautery. This is a particular concern in small patients with dense fur (e.g. rabbits; Figure 9.10), for which there may be poor contact with the ground plate unless the patient is shaved.

There is growing current scientific evidence to support the use of radiosurgery in exotic patients over other modalities such as carbon dioxide laser surgery (Hernandez-Divers, 2008).

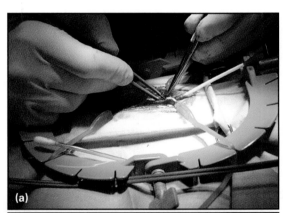

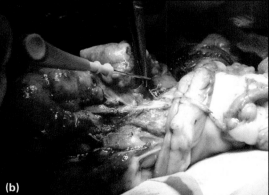

9.9 (a) Use of bipolar radiosurgery and sterile cotton tips to ensure accurate haemostasis in a rabbit undergoing spinal surgery. (b) Monopolar radiosurgery for accurate haemostasis during removal of an abdominal abscess from a rabbit. (© Romain Pizzi, Zoological Medicine Ltd)

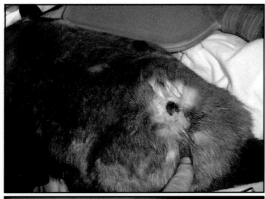

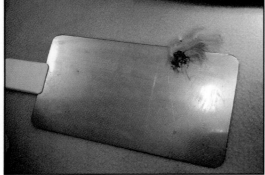

9.10 Monopolar electrosurgery groundplate burn in a rabbit, due to poor contact from the dense fur. (© Romain Pizzi, Zoological Medicine Ltd)

Small swabs

Fine surgery calls for accurate haemostasis. Fine surgical cellulose spears, as used in ophthalmic surgery, are ideal. Cotton buds are slightly smaller and less expensive and the majority of brands with plastic sticks are autoclavable. However, they are less ideal than cellulose spears as, if care is not taken, there is a risk of cotton threads remaining in a surgical site and eliciting a granulomatous reaction, similar to that seen in a dog if a swab is left in the abdomen after surgery.

Microsurgical instruments

These include the fine-tipped instruments often designed for human ophthalmic or vascular surgery. There are no recognized standard sets of instruments for exotic animal surgery, but individual surgeons have their own preferences as to specific instruments. The miniature tip and often rounded handle of microsurgical instruments allows the surgeon to roll them between the fingers gently rather than forcing the instruments and changing the grip.

Box-joint instruments are stronger and longer-lasting than instruments with normal joints, although they have a disadvantage in that box-joints cannot be tightened using a fine screwdriver if they become loose.

Castroviejo needle-holders (Figure 9.11) are a popular choice with exotic animal clinicians. It is important to check the manufacturer's specifications for the maximum diameter needle that can be used, as grasping larger diameter needles, such as the 3 metric (2/0 USP) needles used in dogs and cats, may

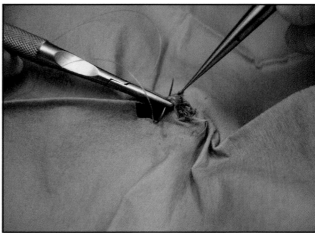

9.11 The use of microsurgical instruments in a gerbil (atraumatic loop-tipped forceps and Castroviejo needle-holders). (© Romain Pizzi, Zoological Medicine Ltd)

bend the jaws out of alignment. Some needle-holders can only be used with 0.7 metric (6/0 USP) needles or smaller. While tungsten-insert jaws are more resilient to wear, these are also easily damaged by grasping larger diameter needles, which will result in permanent grooves in the jaw surfaces.

Iris scissors are also useful for fine and sharp dissection in small patients. There are some materials that should **not** be cut with fine scissors, including:

- Suture material, as this rapidly results in blunting as well as loosening the joints
- The thick skin of reptiles such as the green iguana
- Bones (even those as small as the toes of a leopard gecko).

As for all fine instruments, iris scissors should always be laid flat, even when soaking or cleaning; they should never rest on their tips, as this may bend them. Storage in protective cases and the use of plastic protective instrument tip covers will prolong the lifespan of these fine instruments. They are easily damaged if used inappropriately, handled roughly or cleaned incorrectly.

Equipment sterilization and disinfection

The term sterilization means the removal or destruction of all living microorganisms, including bacterial spores; whereas disinfection is the removal or destruction of pathogenic microorganisms but not necessarily bacterial spores. Some disinfectants do have the advantage of being able to destroy bacterial spores but close attention needs to be paid to dilution rates and contact time.

Hot air ovens

Hot air ovens are useful for the sterilization of glassware and cutting/ophthalmic instruments, and have the advantage of causing less damage and blunting to fine instruments than other sterilization methods. There are, however, disadvantages, which include the following:

- There is a long cooling time and cycle
- There is a risk that materials may become scorched
- This method cannot be used for the sterilization of heat-sensitive items.

Care must be taken not to overload the oven, as this limits the circulation of hot air, and sterility may not be achieved. The machine works by raising the drum temperature to 160°C for 1 hour.

Autoclaves

Autoclaves are used for the sterilization of most instruments and material/paper drapes, but are not suitable for delicate items such as endoscopes, adhesive and non-adhesive plastic drapes, some electrocautery handpieces and light cables. Autoclaves use both heat and pressure to complete the sterilization process; most machines have a variety of cycles and drying functions, depending on whether the instruments are packaged or laid on trays.

Although many endoscopes are described as autoclavable, standard veterinary autoclaves undergo rapid changes in pressure and temperature (so called 'flash' autoclaves), which lead to a markedly shortened lifespan of the endoscopes in comparison to when they are sterilized using other methods.

If instruments are sterilized in packets then they can be put on to a trolley in theatre and opened accordingly, along with anything else that may be needed, including extra swabs, drapes and different sizes of equipment, i.e. screws, plates, pins and drill bits (especially for orthopaedic work). If the available autoclave is not large enough for fully wrapped packs, individual items can instead be placed in the autoclave.

If instruments are autoclaved on trays with no wrapping, they should be left in the autoclave until the patient is in theatre. If in drums, these should stay sealed until the surgeon is ready for them, at which point the drum should be opened briefly and items removed aseptically; Cheattle forceps are ideal for this procedure, or the veterinary surgeons themselves should be allowed to remove instruments, ensuring no accidental break in sterility occurs.

Chemicals

Chemical sterilization is useful for delicate instruments such as endoscopes and for electronic or plastic parts that can be damaged by heat and moisture. When using liquids, care must be taken to ensure that the unit is submersible and that endoscopes are 'soakable'. Care must also be taken to ensure that no air locks are present, as these would result in incomplete sterilization of the lumen.

Quaternary ammonium products and halogenated tertiary amines are most commonly used in practice (glutaraldehyde is a carcinogen and has been largely replaced by safer alternatives). For full sterilization the articles should ideally remain in contact with these chemicals for 10 hours in order for all spores to be killed, whereas as little as 10 minutes' contact is required for disinfection. Delicate equipment such as endoscopes or cameras should be soaked for no more than 45 minutes, or less if the manufacturer's instructions advise this.

Gases can also be used, such as ethylene oxide (EtO) or paraformaldehyde. Health and safety protocols must be strictly adhered to when working with gases; they are extremely flammable and toxic and so should only be used in a controlled environment. If using ethylene oxide the articles must be allowed to aerate for 24 hours before they can be used; this makes the process for quick-turnaround sterilization impossible and limits the use of EtO for sterilizing endoscopy equipment, which is frequently used in exotic veterinary practice.

Cleaning and maintenance of instruments

Wherever possible, blood, debris and bodily fluids should not be allowed to dry on instruments; they should ideally be cleaned immediately after use, but if that is not possible they can be sprayed using an enzymatic foam spray to stop the foreign material from drying on.

- For **automated cleaning**, only CE marked or validated washer/disinfector machines should be used, with low-foaming, non-ionizing cleaning agents and detergents of maximum pH12 and neutral pH for rinsing. Manufacturer's instructions must always be followed. Instruments should be handled carefully and placed into the instrument cleaner with all hinges and joints open, to ensure adequate and thorough cleaning. Heavier instruments should be placed on the bottom of the tray, avoiding overloading, with all concave surfaces placed pointing downwards to prevent pooling of any water. All lumens and cannulas should be flushed before the cleaning cycle begins. Soft, high-purity water must be used for the final flushing and rinsing stage.
- For **manual cleaning**, a double sink system should be used so that instruments can be washed and rinsed in separate areas. The water should not exceed 35°C. The instruments must first be soaked in an approved cleaning solution and then gently cleaned, paying particular attention to the serrations, joints, hinges, teeth and ratchets (in both open and closed positions). Wire brushes should never be used for cleaning due to their abrasive nature, as they can cause pitting of the surface of instruments. Sufficient abrasion can be achieved using a soft-bristled children's toothbrush and applying gentle pressure. In the second sink, the instruments should be rinsed with soft, high purity water and then carefully dried by hand.

The instruments should be checked to ensure they are thoroughly clean and that there has been no accidental damage or wear from surgical usage. All instruments showing signs of damage or wear and tear should be removed and replaced.

The following things should be checked when cleaning instruments:

- All cutting edges should be straight and without nicks, presenting a continuous edge
- All articulated items should move freely without excessive play
- Ratchets should fasten securely and close easily
- Long slender instruments should not be distorted in any way
- Apposing ends should meet squarely.

Regular lubrication of the joints with surgical silicone lubricant spray or instrument 'milk' is recommended. This coats surfaces and displaces water, and should take place before instruments are autoclaved.

Procedures

The Veterinary Surgeons Act 1966 (Schedule 3 Amendment) Order 2002 allows for listed veterinary nurses to perform minor surgery that does not involve entry into a body cavity. While some surgical procedures are specifically excluded in Part II of the schedule, such as castrations of dogs, cats, horses and farm animals, as well as removal of deer antlers in velvet, the Act does not define 'any medical treatment or any minor surgery that does not involve entry into a body cavity'. Ultimately, the interpretation of this wording would be for the courts to decide. The animal must be under the care of a veterinary surgeon and the treatment must be carried out at the veterinary surgeon's direction. The veterinary surgeon must also be satisfied that the veterinary nurse is qualified to carry out the surgical procedure involved. Again, 'qualified' is open to interpretation.

Skin incisions

The skins of mammals, birds and reptiles have different handling properties due to their different collagen contents and thicknesses. There is also variation between species (e.g. the skin of a leopard gecko is much thinner than that of a common iguana) and between body regions (e.g. ferrets have very thick skin over their necks but thin perineal skin).

When incising avian skin, it is best to avoid cutting directly through feather follicles where possible. Many species have featherless tracts (apterylae) that can be selected and prepared for surgical approaches.

Reptile skin is generally thicker than that of mammals and birds of the same size and is much stronger, with a better suture-holding capacity, due to its high collagen content. In comparison, the underlying coelomic muscles are much thinner than those of mammals and, while more force is needed to cut reptile skin, underlying tissues may be injured more easily.

PRACTICAL TIP
When incising reptile skin, it is best to cut between rather than through scales, even if this results in a jagged appearance to the incision.

Smaller scalpel blades (either on a No.3 scalpel handle or a beaver blade handle) are most suitable for the majority of exotic patients. The small curved No.15 blade is well suited to surgery on birds and small mammals, while the pointed triangular No.11 blade is useful for accurately cutting dense reptile skin between scales. Fine ophthalmic-type handles and blades are preferred by some surgeons for small exotic patients.

Sutures

In exotic animals, as for all veterinary patients, sutures are placed:

- To facilitate healing, by the approximation of tissues
- For haemostasis, e.g. the ligation of vessels.

Sutures may also be used temporarily as stays to hold tissues atraumatically.

There are other ways to achieve these aims without the use of suturing. Radiosurgery, electrocautery, laser surgery and chemical styptics, such as potassium permanganate or silver nitrate, can all accomplish haemostasis to varying degrees without the need for sutures. Tissue approximation for healing may also be accomplished with bandages or tissue adhesives, and the need for tissue approximation may be reduced by using less invasive surgical techniques such as endoscopic or laparoscopic surgery.

Sutures are, in essence, foreign bodies in a wound. They can delay healing, induce an inappropriate inflammatory response and lead to wound infection. Human studies have demonstrated that wounds held together with tape heal faster than wounds that have been sutured. For these reasons, the fewest number of sutures of the smallest diameter and made from the least reactive material to support wounds or ligate vessels adequately should be aimed for in all species.

Needle selection

Mammals

Reverse-cutting needles are most suitable for suturing skin wounds in small mammals, as their skin contains a mix of elastic fibres and collagen. Rabbit skin is very variable in thickness: it is very thin and friable over the ventral abdomen, inguinal region, perineum and scrotum, but extremely thick over the dorsal shoulders and neck, especially in uncastrated males. Larger rigid reverse-cutting needles are needed for suturing thicker skin.

Birds

For the thin skin of birds, taper-point needles are generally more suitable than cutting needles, which may tear through to the wound edges and result in a lacerated wound. Other soft tissues may also tear with cutting needles. Swaged-on needles produce less trauma than re-usable needles and are also sharper. Reverse-cutting needles can be used in raptors for the tendons and for the thicker skin over the legs and feet.

Reptiles

Reptile skin has a high collagen content and is responsible for the holding power of repaired coelomic wounds. It is also relatively rigid and inelastic. Reusable needles are not recommended, as the hole formed by the needle will be much larger than the suture (in contrast to the hole formed by a swaged-on needle) and can act as a portal for entry of infection. In most lizards and tortoises, reverse-cutting needles are the easiest and least traumatic to pass through the strong rigid skin. In small delicate species such as leopard geckos, round-bodied needles are best used so as to prevent inadvertent tearing of wound edges.

Rigid *versus* malleable needles

Two of the main manufacturers of individually packed sutures with swaged-on needles are Ethicon and Tyco. Ethicon needles are strong and rigid, whereas Tyco needles are more malleable but have a sharp point. Selection is based on the surgeon's preference, but each has advantages in certain scenarios. Rigid needles are much more useful for suturing the thick skin found over the base of the neck in intact buck rabbits and for closing coeliotomy skin wounds in large iguanas, while malleable needles can be useful when suturing inside the body cavity of small patients with limited access, such as guinea pigs, because the needle can be bent as needed to place a suture in a difficult position.

Suture material selection

> **The perfect suture material would have the following characteristics:**
>
> - Adequate tensile strength
> - Good knot security
> - Easy to handle
> - Non-reactive
> - Non-capillary
> - Non-allergic ▶

- Non-toxic
- Not promote bacterial growth or adherence
- Absorbable at a dependable rate once healing has occurred.
- Inexpensive
- Simple to sterilize.

While no suture material meets all of these requirements, materials can be chosen depending on which of these factors is most important in the exotic species undergoing surgery (Figure 9.12).

Catgut

Catgut is the least suitable suture material commonly available and should **never** be used in exotic animals.

Catgut is manufactured from ovine intestinal submucosa or bovine intestinal serosa, which is treated or tanned similarly to leather with chrome salts, in an attempt to give a more controlled absorption. Unlike the other absorbable suture materials, which rely on hydrolysis to be absorbed, catgut relies on a two-stage process involving the macrophages. Acid hydrolysis and collagenolysis break molecular bonds and the proteins are removed by phagocytosis. As a foreign protein, it illicits a strong inflammatory response; because this may vary widely depending on wound conditions, even in healthy animals, trauma, infection, loss of tensile strength and absorption are very variable. Catgut is no longer used in human surgery, partly due to fears of transmissible spongiform encephalopathies. It is the suture material associated with the highest risk of postoperative complications such as dehiscence and infection in veterinary surgery across all species.

While rabbits do have neutrophils, their cells do not appear to be as able to cope with catgut as those of dogs and cats. On several occasions the author (RP) has found catgut and associated granulomas in rabbits where it has been used after ovariohysterectomy. Absorption tends to be very variable and unreliable, with sutures often present several months and even years after surgery. On one occasion, catgut and associated abdominal granulomas were present more than 2 years after surgery in a rabbit (RP). Catgut appears to result in a much higher risk of postoperative abdominal adhesions in rabbits. Not only are rabbits particularly predisposed to adhesion development (they are used as a laboratory model for human research on adhesions), the

Species	Suture material	Suture pattern	Needle
Small mammals	Monofilament rapid absorbable (poliglecaprone)	Intradermal or subcutaneous simple continuous sutures	Reverse-cutting needle (taper point needles for areas with thin skin)
Birds	Monofilament rapid absorbable (poliglecaprone). If using cutaneous sutures, also monofilament non-absorbable suture (nylon, polypropylene)	Intradermal or subcutaneous simple continuous sutures (simple interrupted cutaneous sutures in thin skin)	Taper-point round needle
Reptiles	Monofilament non-absorbable (nylon, polypropylene)	Everting interrupted sutures – horizontal mattress	Reverse-cutting needle

9.12 Suture and needle selection for skin closure in exotic animals.

use of catgut in this species is also more likely to result in chronic clinical problems such as recurrent colic, in contrast to dogs and cats. When used subcutaneously or intradermally, the resultant inflammatory response can cause severe irritation and result in wound interference and even mutilation in rabbits and rodents (Figure 9.13).

In birds and reptiles, catgut is often not absorbed. The lack of proteases and other enzymes in bird and reptile heterophils compared with mammalian neutrophils appears to result in insufficient breakdown for macrophages to phagocytose and remove the suture. Catgut will therefore act as a permanent foreign body, and commonly causes sterile granulomas due to the associated macrophage reaction. In one study in pigeons, catgut was still present 120 days after placement (Bennett *et al.*, 1992).

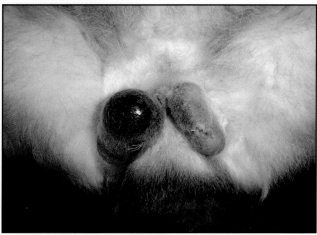

9.13 This rabbit had self-traumatized its scrotum after castration, due to the irritation caused by catgut ligatures. (© Romain Pizzi, Zoological Medicine Ltd)

Multifilament sutures

Absorbable multifilament sutures include polyglactin 910 (e.g. Vicryl), polyglycolic acid (e.g. Dexon) and lactomer (e.g. Polysorb). These are made by twisting or braiding many small strands of material into a larger diameter suture. These materials are softer, more pliable, have less memory, and knot more easily than the more rigid monofilament materials, and are hence popular in veterinary practice.

The irregular surface of these sutures causes increased friction or drag when drawn through the tissues, and they can harbour bacteria in recesses too small for leucocytes to gain access, thereby increasing the risk of postoperative infection. They appear to lose their tensile strength rapidly in an alkaline environment, such as rabbit, guinea pig and chinchilla urine, and so should be used with caution in small mammal cystotomy repair. Due to their wicking ability between tissue planes, braided suture materials should not be used in the gastrointestinal tract or in infected structures.

An often-quoted human study demonstrated that a single silk suture decreased the number of staphylococci required to cause a subcutaneous infection by 10,000 times. This is partly due to silk's braided multifilament nature and partly due to it being a foreign protein, inducing an inflammatory response not unlike that caused by catgut. Silk is only indicated in veterinary surgery for the closure of patent ductus arteriosus, where the resultant inflammatory-induced fibrosis is beneficial for ensuring permanent closure of the duct.

A 'coated' braided suture material is still a multifilament material, with wicking ability between tissue planes. The 'soapy coating' (e.g. calcium stearate) reduces tissue drag but does not change the structure of the suture material.

Braided absorbable materials are not ideal for skin suture, as they illicit a more marked inflammatory response than monofilaments. Braided materials can, however, be useful if suturing near the eye, to prevent inadvertent trauma to the cornea. They are also useful when applying a Chinese finger-trap suture to the skin of a tortoise to keep a pharyngostomy tube in place. Braided absorbable materials such as Vicryl, Polysorb and Dexon can also be used in the oral cavity of rabbits, as the rigid ends of a monofilament suture would cause discomfort.

Suture alternatives

Skin staples

These are stainless steel clips that are applied in the manner of simple interrupted sutures. They cause minimal tissue reaction, although in wounds where there is tension they may cause a 'cheese-wire' effect through the skin. Many animals will try to remove staples and they can become a risk if eaten or left in the environment.

Tissue adhesives

Cyanoacrylate glue is often used to close small skin deficits or wounds in exotic patients. Medical grade glue should always be used, rather than 'super glue' preparations. The advantage of tissue glue is that it is quick and easy to apply and is usually well tolerated. However, the heat caused during the 'curing' process can cause thermal damage to delicate tissues, potentially leading to wound dehiscence or self-mutilation due to irritation.

Species-specific considerations

Birds

Monofilament rapidly absorbable poliglecaprone 25 (e.g. Monocryl) and polyglytone 6211 (e.g. Caprosyn) are the most suitable suture materials for general soft tissue and skin surgery of birds. They are more pliable and have less memory, with better knotting ability than other monofilament absorbable suture materials. Wound healing is much more rapid in birds than in mammals. Combined with their small size, this makes slowly absorbable and rigid suture materials such as polydioxanone (e.g. PDS), polyglyconate (e.g. Maxon) and dioxanone (e.g. Biosyn) not only unnecessary but more likely to result in wound complications such as irritation and seroma formation from rigid suture ends. Although rapidly absorbed, multifilament polyglactin 910 and lactomer result in the most pronounced inflammatory response to synthetic absorbable materials in birds. Non-absorbable nylon is stiff and can be associated with irritation; along with stainless steel sutures, nylon may be associated with haematomas and seromas and even sterile granuloma formation.

Birds may preen skin sutures and, although they do not often remove them, this risk increases with pain, as well as with irritation such as that caused by the stiff ends of simple interrupted nylon skin sutures. Parrots are much more likely to remove sutures than are other birds.

Tissue adhesives can be useful for small skin wounds in birds, but care must be taken that they do not enter the wound as this will then prevent healing from occurring. The author (RP) is not a fan of using staples in birds and has found that many parrots seem to rather enjoy removing them.

Reptiles

Reptile skin is relatively strong, with a high content of parallel collagen fibres, and so is usually the primary layer for closing coelomic cavity wounds and surgical incisions. The coelomic membrane and body wall are usually very thin and soft, having little if any suture-holding strength. Reptiles rarely interfere with their wounds, which is helpful as healing is very slow; sutures usually have to remain in place for 4–8 weeks. In lizards and snakes, the skin has a tendency to invert; everting suture patterns such as horizontal (Figure 9.14) or vertical mattress are therefore needed.

Staples are also useful in larger reptiles as they evert the wound edges. Skin wounds closed in this manner often have an exposed raw edge, which may be sealed using tissue adhesive to prevent tissue irritation and entrance of infection.

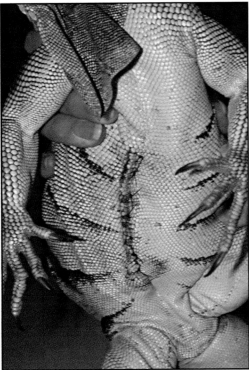

9.14 Horizontal mattress sutures used for wound closure in a green iguana. (© Romain Pizzi, Zoological Medicine Ltd)

Polypropylene and nylon are the most suitable skin suture materials. Catgut should never be used as it appears to cause severe granulomatous reactions and acts as a permanent foreign body. Even modern absorbable suture materials broken down by hydrolysis are absorbed very slowly and variably, and so are best avoided.

The more rapidly absorbed materials such as polyglecaprone 25 (e.g. Monocryl) and polyglytone 6211 (e.g. Caprosyn) may be selected for internal sutures and ligatures. Many surgeons, however, prefer to use inert non-absorbable systems such as Ligaclips or Hemoclips internally.

Tissue adhesive is never sufficient to close any significant wounds in reptiles on its own, even in small geckos, due to the prolonged healing period required. Snakes and lizards will often shed the everted suture line very neatly at the next ecdysis.

Amphibians and fish

Most amphibians have very thin skin. The exception is the ventral skin of giant frogs and toads, which is much thicker and more collagen-rich. Undermining skin and advancing wound edges is also not possible in most locations. For this reason, wound closure can be difficult and suture closure may not be viable, relying instead on second intention healing. Protection with Orabase paste is useful (see later). When sutures are used, as for ventral coeliotomy closure, round-bodied tapered needles are best. Healing may be slow due to the poikilothermic physiology of fish and amphibians (similar to that of reptiles), and non-absorbable polypropylene skin sutures are often the best choice, followed by monofilament slow absorbable materials (e.g. PDS, Biosyn).

Arthropods

It is not possible to use sutures in arthropods (e.g. tarantulas, scorpions, insects, crabs). These animals have a sclerotized rigid cuticle, with brittle plates and flexible joint membranes. Neither joint membranes nor cuticle plates have the ability to hold sutures. A study on wounds in tarantulas found that sutures simply tore through the cuticle and caused larger wounds, resulting in deaths.

In tarantulas and scorpions, wounds are best repaired using tissue adhesives applied in several separate layers. If tissue adhesives are not available, any commercial *liquid* cyanoacrylate glue is suitable. 'Super glue' *gels* are not suitable. In severe trauma cases, limbs can be amputated and the stumps sealed with tissue adhesive. Tarantulas also have the ability to autotomize their limbs (i.e. they can cast off a leg at a breakaway point when it is either pulled or damaged). Grasping the leg firmly with forceps and applying a short sharp dorsal jerk will normally result in the spider autotomizing the leg. Although there is a muscle inserting on the joint membrane that acts to seal the wound, limiting haemolymph loss, it is always safest to apply a tissue adhesive seal. The leg will then regenerate at the next ecdysis and will be of normal size and appearance within three moults.

Needle-holders

Fine **Castroviejo** holders, typically used in ophthalmic surgery, are popular in exotic animal surgery (see Figure 9.11). They are fine squeeze-action needle-holders with a catch. **Ryder** and **Derf** needle-holders are other small fine-tipped instruments that have the advantage of having locking handles.

Gillies needle-holders are designed to be comfortable to hold and are available for either the left or right hands; they incorporate suture-cutting scissors, which is useful for veterinary surgeons who commonly operate without an assistant. They have a slotted tip to allow one to suture away from the surface such as in a deep cavity. The major disadvantage in exotic animal surgery is that they rely on the hand grip to close them and hold the needle, which also fixes the wrist, making fine suturing difficult, especially through tough tissues such as iguana skin. They can also cause hand and arm fatigue more readily than other instruments, and the needle can slip and wobble, making suturing fine structures difficult. In the author's opinion (RP) they are not very suitable for most exotic animal surgery.

McPhail or **Mathieu** needle-holders, similar to large animal instruments, are also occasionally used in small animals, and have a squeeze-release catch. The disadvantage of these and Castroviejo needle-holders, which also have a squeeze action catch release, is that the instrument cannot be grasped firmly with all the fingers of the hand when suturing thick tissues, such as when placing intradermal sutures in rabbit neck skin, otherwise they release the needle.

Olsen-Hegar needle-holders are similar to Mayo-Hegar needle-holders, which lock, but they also incorporate scissors (like Gillies) and so are popular with veterinary surgeons. They can, however, lead to inexperienced surgeons inadvertently cutting the sutures, a similar problem to that encountered when using Gillies. Because the joint is farther from the gripping surfaces as cutting blades are incorporated, they have a smaller mechanical advantage than Mayo-Hegar holders, and grasp needles less firmly. The joints are also prone to loosening over time.

Kilner needle-holders are a small locking instrument similar to Mayo-Hegar holders, but have cranked or offset arms. This helps with natural rotation of the wrist for finer or more delicate suturing, with a smaller arc of needle movement. Their small size also enables them to be supported by the index finger for more accurate and secure needle placement through tough tissues.

Sutured wound strength

It is the tissue that has been sutured, rather than the sutures themselves, that gives repaired wounds their strength. The number of collagen fibres and their orientation in the tissues determines strength.

The main cause of wound dehiscence after procedures carried out by inexperienced surgeons is improperly tied knots. Other common causes include: only taking small bites of the wound edge with sutures, causing the sutures to tear through; and failure to restrict active animals after surgery. This appears to be a particular problem in rabbits after coeliotomy, with 2 weeks' hutch rest recommended after abdominal surgery. Rabbits appear to be poor at protecting their wounds and, as a prey animal, their flight response can be particularly strong and a flying leap may result in linea alba dehiscence.

Suture diameter is much less important for dehiscence in exotic animals than in dogs and cats, due to their small body size.

> **PRACTICAL TIP**
> The aim should always be to use the fewest number of sutures of the smallest diameter made from the least reactive material, placed for the least amount of time required to ensure physiological healing.

Knots with a double first throw, as in a typical surgeon's knot, are only useful in preventing wound edges from springing apart before placing the second throw, when wound edges are under slight tension. The double throw or surgeon's knot is actually slightly less secure, and it is easier for inexperienced surgeons inadvertently to tie a slip knot second throw, or leave a gap.

Single first throws are generally suitable for exotic animals and are safer to place. Tension should always be equal on both suture limbs, to prevent the knot throws tumbling, forming slip knots.

Tissue tearing and knot failure are the main causes of linea alba dehiscence in rabbits. If knotted correctly, continuous sutures are faster and less traumatic to place, reduce anaesthesia time, and are less irritant to rabbits and less likely to result in subcutaneous seromas or knot reactions. It is, of course, essential that knots are square and securely tied. For monofilament absorbable sutures, the first knot should have five single throws and the end knot should have seven single throws.

Information on suture patterns can be found in the *BSAVA Manual of Canine and Feline Surgical Principles: A Foundation Manual* and the *BSAVA Textbook of Veterinary Nursing, 5th edn*.

Drains

Due to the viscous or almost solid nature of pus in many exotic species, drains are not often used in infected wounds. For surgeries where a lot of dead space has been created (e.g. skin advancement flaps) drains may occasionally be placed, and their care follows that for more familiar species (see the *BSAVA Textbook of Veterinary Nursing, 5th edn* for more information). Drains should be monitored regularly and should be removed as soon as serous drainage ceases.

Suture removal

Sutures will need to be removed at different times depending on the nature of the wound, the species involved and the suture material used.

In general terms: where absorbable sutures are used to close skin wounds, removal is not critical unless the patient is chewing the area or infection is a concern. All non-absorbable sutures or staples must be removed. In mammals sutures should be removed at 10–14 days postoperatively. The same principle applies to birds; however, as many bird skin defects are closed with absorbable sutures, this is not necessarily required. Reptile skin takes significantly longer to heal and, if non-absorbable sutures are placed, they should not be removed until 4–8 weeks postoperatively. Wounds closed using absorbable suture material or skin adhesive should be monitored until healing is complete.

Wound management

Wound dressings

Wound dressings and bandaging can reduce pain by restricting movement, eliminating friction and abrasion, and avoiding desiccation of the wound surface. Many exotic animals, including rabbits, rodents and birds, will find dressings stressful. It is therefore essential that dressings are kept as small as possible. In some cases, the use of suture loops to hold dressings in place limits their size while still allowing them to be changed regularly. Adhesive adherent dressings such as Allevyn Thin (Smith and Nephew) can often be applied on their own to wounds in birds. This dressing will adhere to the wound bed and cause rehydration of necrotic tissue, as well as debriding the wound. Some dressings may have a direct analgesic effect on wounds.

Hydrogels

Hydrogels consist of a network of polymer chains that are water-insoluble and in which water is the dispersion medium. They are superabsorbent and can contain >99% water. They are commonly indicated to prevent wound bed desiccation as well as to hydrate necrotic tissue, facilitating wound debridement.

Human studies have shown that refrigerated hydrogels have a noticeable local analgesic effect in wounds. While the direct analgesic effect is difficult to demonstrate conclusively in animals, the effect appears – at least anecdotally – to be similar in a whole host of exotic species. It appears to be especially effective in rabbits and pet rodents, and can be useful in perineal fly-strike wounds.

Hydrogels swell three-dimensionally as they absorb fluid and so do not apply pressure to the wound. Their high absorbency reduces tissue oedema, and the debriding action is atraumatic via rehydration of necrotic tissue. To maintain a moist wound environment they need to be applied under a semi-permeable dressing. If used under a permeable dressing, such as a perforated polyurethane membrane (e.g. Melolin, Smith and Nephew), the hydrogel will dry out, forming crusts in the wound.

In order to reduce the risk of wound cross-infection, tubes should be handled cleanly (the tip of the tube should not contact tissue) and they must not be shared between patients as anaerobic bacteria can grow in the gel. Commercially available products are aimed at the human market and so are generally small single-use containers. If they are to be used more than once, tubes should be labelled; opened tubes should be discarded after a few days, even if refrigerated. There is no harm in refrigerating all of the hydrogels stocked in a practice, to reduce the risk of bacterial growth.

Silver creams and dressings

Silver has been recognized for its antimicrobial properties for over 2000 years; there are records of the ancient Macedonians using it to cover wounds. Silver has numerous antibacterial mechanisms of effect: interaction with nucleic acids inhibits cell division, while interactions with proteins and enzymes and binding to the cell wall affect cellular respiration, cell membrane function and transport of substances across the cell membrane. Silver is particularly useful in reptiles with infections with multi-drug-resistant agents such as *Pseudomonas* (Figure 9.15), or where renal disease may preclude aminoglycoside use.

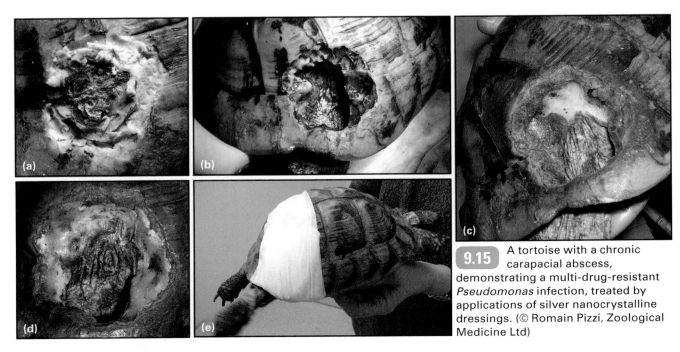

9.15 A tortoise with a chronic carapacial abscess, demonstrating a multi-drug-resistant *Pseudomonas* infection, treated by applications of silver nanocrystalline dressings. (© Romain Pizzi, Zoological Medicine Ltd)

Flamazine (Smith and Nephew) is 1.0% w/w silver sulfadiazine in water emulsion. Because it is a semi-solid oil emulsion it functions as a foreign non-absorbable substance in the wound and may interfere with healing. Thick applications of 3–5 mm are needed for adequate silver levels in most cases, which are not practical. Up to 10% of the sulfadiazine may be absorbed systemically, at least in mammals, and so it should be used cautiously in patients with renal impairment. In large wounds serum sulfadiazine levels may alter the effects of systemically administered drugs.

Numerous commercial nanocrystalline silver dressings are available in a variety of forms. These have the advantage of sustained release. Seven-day active dressings are available, which are suitable for wounds with minimal necrotic debris, reducing costs to the owner, especially for large reptile wounds, which may take months to heal. They can be applied to carapace and plastron bone infections in chelonians, as cavity dressings, and can also be used to debride wounds if applied wet and removed dry. Dressings must be applied moistened with sterile water for silver to be active. Saline should not be used, as this will interfere with silver ion release and prevent its antibacterial effect.

Silver dressings will alter the appearance of wounds, staining them dark brown-black, and this can also cause discoloration of fur in mammals. Humans report a tingling sensation when silver dressings are first applied and, at least anecdotally, there appears to be a similar effect in rabbits and reptiles. In a small number of patients these dressings appear to cause wound irritation, and patients will interfere with them. Silver dressings appear to delay the separation of burn eschars (scabs) in reptiles, and the scabs may need to be removed manually. Other problems are purely practical, such as difficulties attaching dressings in some locations. These dressings are expensive and this is a disadvantage when teamed with the long healing periods of reptile wounds (sometimes months); however, silver dressings remain cost-effective for small wounds.

Dressing shell wounds

Tortoises occasionally incur full-thickness shell wounds due to trauma from dog bites or lawn mowers. As these are always dirty wounds they should never be closed with epoxy resin and similar materials initially, as this will simply result in abscessation. If stabilization is needed for loose fragments, this can be accomplished with plates and screws, wire and screws, or even cable ties and epoxy resin. The majority of wounds, however, are left open and managed with dressings to keep them clean; necrotic material is debrided and the wound is only sealed once it has granulated. Care is required if flushing debris from these wounds, as lung penetration may have occurred or debris could be flushed into the coelomic cavity, resulting in coelomitis.

Topical treatments and applications

Orabase

Orabase (ConvaTec) is a preparation used for the treatment of mouth ulcers in humans. It is a protective paste composed of gelatin, pectin and sodium carboxymethylcellulose in a plasticized hydrocarbon gel, which binds to ulcerated surfaces and mucous membranes, forming a protective layer. It can be mixed with antibiotics and is useful in the treatment of oral ulcerations in chelonians, and for the packing of surgical or traumatic skin wounds in fish and amphibians. It can be mixed with enrofloxacin when applied to fish, to provide initial antibiotic cover to wounds in situations where the patient may be difficult to medicate in a hospital tank.

Topical antibiotics

Topical antibiotics are usually ineffective in most mammals due to dilution by exudates, which also flush them from the wound surface; some studies have demonstrated that fusidic acid-impregnated dressings are associated with higher rates of multiple-drug-resistant infections.

Although the use of topical antibiotics can also lead to resistant wound infections in reptiles and birds, these species typically produce less wound exudate and so topical antibiotics are more useful. The difference is because their heterophils, which perform a similar but not identical role in wound healing and infection to that of mammalian neutrophils, do not contain the same proteases and peroxidases.

Cleansing solutions

Cleansing solutions are probably one of the most misused veterinary products in practice. Dermisol cream (Pfizer) is widely used as a topical treatment for almost any dermatological lesion in all species. It is highly acidic, consisting of malic acid, benzoic acid and salicyclic acid, and can be irritating even to normal rabbit skin, particularly in the perineal region. It is toxic to granulation tissue, should never be used for urine scalds or perineal faecal soiling, and is very painful if misused in fly-strike wounds. Dermisol preparations are intended as debriding agents to cleave the junction between necrotic and vital tissue and so can be used in wounds with a lot of necrotic debris. They are of very limited application in rabbit and rodent wound management. They can be used in the initial management of bird and reptile wounds where there is a large quantity of solid necrotic tissue or scab covering the wound, although this may be better accomplished with surgical debriding and rehydrating dressings.

Barrier films and liquid skin preparations

Barrier films and liquid skin preparations can be useful in exotic animal wounds. Opsite (Smith and Nephew) is a non-stinging barrier film that may be sprayed on to skin to create a waterproof barrier. It can be useful for the short-term prevention or management of perineal urine scalding in rabbits but does need frequent application, ideally once every 24 hours. It simply fragments atraumatically away from skin over a period of time. Liquid skin dressings such as Germolene (Bayer) and New-Skin (Bayer) are also useful for protecting open wounds and for keeping them clean, particularly in small reptiles, where there is no other way of covering wounds to prevent desiccation or contamination.

Poultices

Poultices, such as animal Lintex (Robinson), are occasionally used in rabbit wounds, mainly by large animal veterinary surgeons. These preparations consist mainly of boric acid, which has been banished from human wound care protocols. Boric acid causes vasodilation, oedema and a degree of maceration of tissues, which results in exudate production, believed to 'draw out' infection. None of these irritant actions is desirable in wound healing, and wound healing is delayed by prolonged inflammation. Poultices should not be used in any exotic animal wound.

The use of antiseptics in wounds

Antiseptics are chemical substances that kill or inhibit microorganisms on tissue surfaces. While they have a well recognized role to play in the initial treatment of a fresh wound, they are frequently misused in chronic wounds. Antiseptic flushing of a wound can initially help prevent infection by reducing both the adherence of organisms and the bacterial load in a wound. Dilute solutions of chlorhexidine or povidone–iodine are sometimes advocated for the daily cleaning of wounds. Many studies have shown that these are cytotoxic to fibroblasts and epithelial cells at lower concentrations than those at which they are bactericidal. They are thus more likely to retard wound healing than prevent or treat wound infection. Some studies have found this effect to increase the risk of wound infection because of the detrimental effects on healing.

Hydrogen peroxide has been recommended in older texts as a disinfectant, and also for stomatitis or 'mouth rot' in snakes, but again has very poor antibacterial activity and is highly toxic to fibroblasts, retarding healing, as well as being painful in wounds. In humans there have even been reports of fatal air embolisms associated with its use.

While, in general, antiseptics have little place in the management of infected wounds, as these are best treated with systemic antibiotics and aggressive debridement, 'shell rot' of tortoises is one exception to this rule. This condition may manifest as small chalky white chips or flecks in keratin plates of the plastron and carapace that progress and undermine the keratin and can affect the underlying bones. Opportunistic Gram-negative bacteria such as *Pseudomonas* are common causes. As well as correcting any underlying husbandry problems, debriding and daily scrubbing with povidone—iodine is effective in clearing the infection in mild cases without the need for systemic antibiotics, as the infection is (at least initially) superficially attacking the keratin.

Amphibians and fish are extremely sensitive to disinfectants due to their delicate, permeable skin. Povidone–iodine and chlorhexidine scrubs, as well as quaternary ammonium- and chlorine-based antiseptics, are toxic to amphibians and fish. Clinical signs of toxicity include erythema, petechiation, lethargy, regurgitation, muscle twitching, seizures and death. Wounds should never be treated with these agents and they should not be used as skin preparations before surgery; systemic or topical antibiotics should be used instead.

Analgesia in wound management

Wound interference is a particular problem is some exotic species. Rabbits, rats and parrots all interfere with dressings, removing sutures and even mutilating wounds if pain is not adequately managed. In some animals, pain will also result in a decreased food intake, with resultant delays in wound healing. Analgesia is most effective if given before a painful event such as surgical wound debridement, and multimodal combinations of opioids and non-steroidal anti-inflammatory drugs (NSAIDs) will be more effective than either agent alone. See Chapter 7 for more information.

Local anaesthetics

Local anaesthetic agents are sometimes advocated in an attempt to limit wound interference and mutilation, such as postsurgically in rats. Commonly used agents such as lidocaine (e.g. EMLA cream) have been shown to have an antibacterial effect that can interfere with microbiological culture results of samples taken from wounds. In research in rabbits, EMLA cream was found to reduce significantly the ability to culture bacteria from infected wounds in the laboratory.

Ironically, while local anaesthetic agents have an antibacterial effect on samples for culture, studies in rodents and rabbits have shown that, due to the other adverse effects of these agents on macrophages and fibroblasts in the wound, open wounds repeatedly treated with local anaesthetic have a notably *increased* risk of development of wound infections, as well as delayed healing. If used, local anaesthetics are best applied sparingly before surgery, and only in species likely to interfere with their wounds. Their use should be avoided in chronic or open wounds.

More information on the use of local anaesthesia can be found in Chapter 7.

Bandages

General information on bandaging can be found in the *BSAVA Textbook of Veterinary Nursing, 5th edition*. Some types of bandage are specific to exotic animals.

Many of the exotic patients seen in practice do not tolerate bandages, so reducing patient interference is a key part of the postoperative care given by nurses. This can be achieved by giving the patient (particularly parrots) something else to chew on or extra stimulation by putting radios on in the ward, or a different way of feeding them which keeps them occupied for longer. If bandages are needed they have to be light in weight and not too restrictive for the patient. Simple three-layered bandages can be used but often slip due to short smooth fur and the normal movement of the patient. Casting material can be used for fracture repair but again this has to be light in nature and, due to the anatomical structure of the limbs, can be difficult to apply and secure in place.

Figure-of-eight bandages

Birds

Figure-of-eight bandages are used in birds to stabilize some wing fractures for a few days; this is just enough time for a fibrous callus to form. They should not be left on for long periods due to the risk of joint ankylosis. They are particularly helpful for small birds, where orthopaedic surgery is not a viable option, or in cases where either the radius or the ulna has a simple closed fracture and the other intact bone is already acting as a splint. The bandage material should be placed in contact with the caudal aspect of the humerus and shoulder, and gently wrapped around the wing in a figure-of-eight manner (Figure 9.16). The bandage must not be allowed to slip down to the elbow and rest on the secondary feathers, as that might cause damage to the feathers themselves. The bandage should be strapped gently around the chest if there is a fracture above the elbow.

Lizards

A similar type of bandage is used in lizards for leg fractures. As leg fractures are often secondary to metabolic bone disease due to secondary nutritional hyperparathyroidism, surgical fixation with pins is not an option as the bones are too weak to tolerate implants. In hindleg fractures, the leg is simply bandaged to the tail relatively firmly; this acts as a form of splint and allows enough stability for the slow-forming bridging callus. Correction of any UVB lighting deficit and adequate calcium supplementation must also be provided in order for healing to take place.

Tape splint

Birds

A simple tape splint using Micropore (3M), Transpore (3M) or similar atraumatic material is sufficient to provide external coaptation for fractured legs in small passerine birds and in budgerigars. As the joints above and below need inclusion, this is only suitable for fractures occurring below the knee, i.e. fractures of the tibiotarsus or more distal.

Reptiles

The same method can be applied in small lizards with fractured toes, to make a 'snowshoe'.

Hindleg fractures in small terrestrial chelonians can similarly be allowed to heal by padding the leg with cotton wool before bandaging or taping it firmly into the inguinal fossa. It is, however, important to remove the bandage regularly and check the leg for any signs of pressure sores or movement inside the inguinal fossa, which would prevent healing.

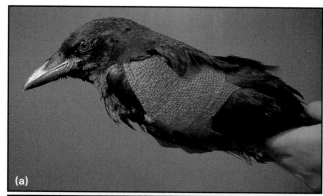

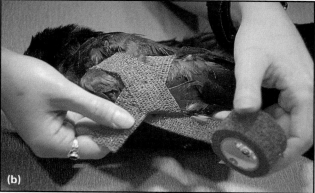

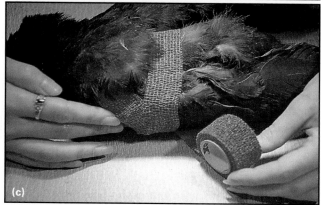

9.16 Bandaging a fracture. **(a)** Carrion crow with figure-of-eight bandage supporting a closed fracture of the ulna (the bandage holds only the carpal and elbow jointed flexed; it does not include the body). **(b)** Conforming bandage used to form a figure-of-eight support for a fractured humerus. The bandage is holding the carpal and elbow joints flexed. **(c)** The humerus is then immobilized by passing the bandage completely around the body, passing beneath the opposite wing. (Reproduced from the *BSAVA Manual of Wildlife Casualties*)

Ball bandages

Bumblefoot in birds is not simply a pododermatitis but is closer in aetiology to a decubital ulcer. It is a particularly common problem in falconry birds that are kept tethered to a perch for long periods. Continued pressure on the foot reduces the vascular perfusion of the tissues, with resultant devitalization of the plantar surface of the foot. While allowing the bird free flight in an aviary, or cleaning perches regularly and covering them with artificial turf, is sufficient to cure very mild cases, more severe cases will require surgical debridement and ball bandaging (Figure 9.17).

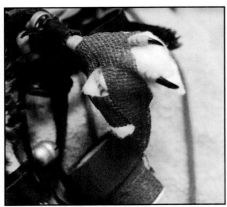

9.17 Ball bandage. A simple bandage with a large wad of cotton wool (some prefer to use half a squash ball) held in place with elasticated cohesive dressing. The bandage must be kept dry and the talons must protrude such that the toes are able to flex and extend slightly, thus preventing adhesions between healing bone and tendon. The bandage should be removed after 3–5 days. (© John Chitty) (Reproduced from the *BSAVA Manual of Raptors, Pigeons and Passerine Birds*)

As its name suggests, a ball bandage is simply a dressing and a large ball of cotton wool followed by the standard gauze and covering layers. This removes direct pressure from the perch on the plantar surface of the foot and spreads weight more evenly. Disadvantages are that only one foot can be bandaged in this way at a time and that some birds do not tolerate the bulking bandage and may peck at or rip it.

Fracture fixation

Fracture repair can be achieved with internal or external fixation. The small size of some patients will limit the techniques and equipment that can be used. Small fixation plates designed for human fingers may be suitable for small rabbits, but this is limited by bone size. Many exotic patients are too small for these, so Kirschner wires can be used as medullary pins and, in larger patients, medullary pins (as for small cats and dogs) and cerclage wires.

Many practices now have the equipment to place external fixators (Figure 9.18); these have the advantage of allowing more use of the limb postoperatively and do not require bandaging. The pins

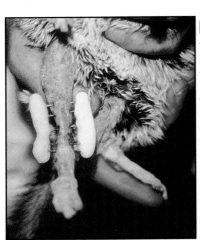

9.18 Type II Kirschner-Ehmer external fixator used to repair a transverse fracture of the tibia in a chinchilla. Small non-threaded K wires were connected using hand-rolled polymethylmethacrylate bars. (Reproduced from the *BSAVA Manual of Exotic Pets, 4th edn*).

and external fixators should be checked on a regular basis to ensure no movement has occurred while the patient is recovering, that there is no infection along the pins' tracts, and that the fracture itself is stable.

Postoperative complications specific to exotic pets

Prevention of postoperative abdominal adhesion formation

Some rabbit texts mention the use of verapamil, a calcium channel blocker, in the prevention of postoperative adhesion formation in pet rabbits. However, the authors of this chapter are not convinced of the benefit of its use, given the limited number of occasions it has actually been documented in this species. An extensive review of peer-reviewed human literature on the prevention of postsurgical abdominal adhesion yields several thousand papers. It is a topic of major importance due to the impact of adhesions on fertility in women. However, among these only two papers on the use of verapamil exist, and these found it to be of little practical benefit; no further research has been performed. In human medicine the emphasis has now changed to limiting the factors and conditions that predispose to adhesion formation in the first place.

When performing a laparotomy on a rabbit, there is often a surprising amount of peritoneal fluid, in contrast to dogs and cats. It is also well known that desiccation and abrasion are important factors in adhesion formation in rabbits. Desiccation and abrasion are mainly caused by the use of dry gauze surgical swabs and rough tissue handling.

Using moistened swabs is relatively simple but is probably the most significant factor in routine laparotomy to reduce adhesion formation. In larger operations lavage and suction are also beneficial in removing pro-inflammatory substances that can initiate adhesion formation. Limited and gentle tissue handling, such as using rat-toothed instead of dressing forceps, avoiding desiccation of viscera by extended exposure, and accurate haemostasis are all also extremely important.

NSAIDs have also been demonstrated as having a notable effect in reducing adhesion formation after abdominal surgery, which is another benefit to giving NSAID analgesia perioperatively.

> **KEY POINT**
> Moistened swabs and perioperative anti-inflammatory drugs are the most important methods of preventing postoperative abdominal adhesion formation in rabbits.

References and further reading

Bennett RA, Yeager M, Trapp A *et al.* (1992) Tissue reaction to five suture materials in pigeons (*Columbia livia*). *Proceedings of the Association of Avian Veterinarians*, pp. 212–218

Hernandez-Divers S (2008) Radiosurgery and laser in zoological practice: separating fact from fiction. *Journal of Exotic Pet Medicine* **17**, 165–174

Longley LA (2008) *Anaesthesia of Exotic Pets*. Saunders, Philadelphia

Osuna DJ, DeYoung DJ and Walker RL (1992) Comparison of an antimicrobial adhesive drape and povidone–iodine preoperative skin preparation in dogs. *Veterinary Surgery* **21**, 458–462

Owen LJ, Gines JA, Knowles TG and Holt PE (2009) Efficacy of adhesive incise drapes in preventing bacterial contamination of clean canine surgical wounds. *Veterinary Surgery* **38**, 732–737

Webster J and Alghamdi AA (2007) Use of plastic adhesive drapes during surgery for preventing surgical site infection. Cochrane Database Systematic Review **17**, 4 [CD006353]

Self-assessment questions

1. What suture material, needle and suture pattern is most suitable for closure of a skin laceration in a green iguana?
2. How can you prevent hypothermia developing in a peregrine falcon that is having a leg fracture repaired?
3. What is the single most important thing you can do to limit postoperative abdominal adhesions developing in a rabbit undergoing an ovariohysterectomy?
4. For how long prior to anaesthesia and surgery should you withhold food from a guinea pig?
5. What is the most practical method of disinfection or sterilization of a rigid endoscope between procedures when performing coelioscopy on different birds on the same day?
6. In which situations would the use of multifilament braided polyglactin be useful for skin wound closure? What are the disadvantages of this suture material's use?
7. When would you consider using a figure-of-eight bandage in a bird?
8. How would you prepare the skin of an Argentinian horned frog for surgery?

10

Laboratory techniques

John Chitty and Nick Carmichael

This chapter is designed to give information on:

- Blood sampling, including skin preparation, needle selection and sample volume, suitable sites for venepuncture, and prioritization and interpretation of blood tests
- Skin sampling techniques, including species-specific information that takes into account feathers, scales, etc.
- Urine collection, tests and interpretation
- Faecal appearance, methods of collection and parasitology
- Bacteriology
- Handling pathological samples, including sample transportation and health and safety considerations

Blood

Blood sample requirements vary between species and it is important that appropriate samples are obtained and handled correctly in order for results to be reliable. The appropriate blood collection tubes for specific blood tests are shown in Figure 10.1.

Sample tube	Tests and suitability
EDTA	Haematology (mammals; not suitable for use in most birds and all reptiles)
Lithium heparin	Biochemistry (mammals). Haematology and biochemistry (birds and reptiles)
Spun heparin gel	Electrolytes and biochemistry (all species)
Clotted	Serology and biochemistry (all species)
Citrate	Clotting studies (all species)
Fluoride–oxalate	Glucose (all species)

10.1 Appropriate blood tubes for blood samples.

Mammals

Skin preparation

Skin preparation is necessary prior to venepuncture. The technique used for clipping and swabbing the skin of ferrets and guinea pigs with a surgical spirit cotton wool ball or gauze swab is similar to that used for dogs and cats. However, care should be taken not to use excessive amounts of spirit as this may induce cooling in small or sick individuals or may be groomed off and result in intoxication.

Needle selection and sample volume

The size of needle and syringe used for collecting blood will vary depending on the size of the animal as well as the site of venepuncture. For example:

- A 2.5 ml syringe and a 23 gauge 5/8 inch needle for collection from the ear or lateral saphenous vein of a 3 kg rabbit

- A 1 ml syringe and a 25 gauge 5/8 inch needle for collection from the ear vein of a smaller rabbit
- A 2.5 or 5 ml syringe and a 23 gauge 1 inch needle for vena cava venepuncture in ferrets and rodents.

Rabbits

Clipper blades should be very sharp. Coarser dog or cat hair will blunt clipper blades, making them unusable in rabbits. Rabbit skin is easier to tear than dog or cat skin; extra care should therefore be taken. A specific set of quiet clippers (as used for cats) should be kept for rabbits.

Spirit may be used on the skin when taking blood from the lateral saphenous or jugular vein; however, when using the marginal ear vein, spirit should be avoided as it may cause cooling and vasoconstriction. Warm dilute chlorhexidine or F10SC (1:250 dilution) may be more appropriate.

Chinchillas

Chinchillas have very thin skin, which is easy to break when clipping. It may, therefore, be more appropriate to pluck fur from the venepuncture site.

Suitable sites for venepuncture

Jugular vein/cranial vena cava

These are the most common sites for blood collection. In tractable animals, the jugular vein (either left or right) (Figure 10.2) may be used; the collection method is similar to that utilized in cats and dogs. However, this site can be very difficult to use in female rabbits with a large dewlap, in ferrets with very thick neck skin, or in guinea pigs with short, stocky necks.

Animals may also find restraint very stressful and for this reason the author (JRC) recommends that venepuncture is carried out under isoflurane anaesthesia. The laboratory should be informed of the use of this anaesthesia for ferrets, as it may result in an alteration of some parameters. Small gauge needles

(23 gauge or smaller) should be used, as thicker needles tend to blunt as they pass through the skin and then simply 'bounce' off the vein (especially in ferrets and some rabbits).

Where jugular venepuncture is difficult, the cranial vena cava should be used instead. This is particularly appropriate in ferrets, where the heart is positioned much more caudally in the thorax compared to dogs, cats, rabbits and rodents.

It can also be used in rabbits and other small mammals, though more care is needed to avoid entering the atria. Venepuncture of the cranial vena cava is generally performed on anaesthetized animals (Figure 10.3), although it may also be carried out in conscious debilitated animals.

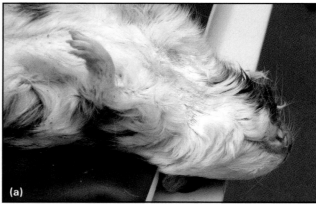

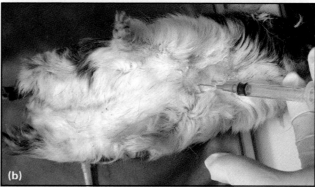

10.3 **(a)** Taking blood from the cranial vena cava of a guinea pig. The sedated animal is in dorsal recumbency with its head over the edge of a table. **(b)** The needle enters the left thoracic inlet, angled toward the right hindleg. (© John Chitty)

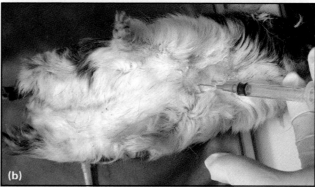

10.2 The right jugular vein of an anaesthetized ferret. (© John Chitty)

Venepuncture of the jugular vein/vena cava in a small mammal

1. The animal is laid on its back with its head pulled ventrally (or resting over the edge of a table.
2. The needle (typically 23 gauge 1.25 inch) is inserted at 45 degrees into the left thoracic inlet (which has already been clipped and prepared aseptically), aiming towards the right hindleg.
3. As the needle is inserted, gentle negative pressure is applied to the syringe until blood is aspirated.
4. As the needle is withdrawn, digital pressure is applied to the thoracic inlet.

Cephalic vein

This site is suitable for drawing small volumes of blood or for insertion of catheters. The position of the vein and the collection technique is similar to that for dogs and cats, although the shortness of the leg does make the technique more difficult in small mammals.

Lateral saphenous vein

The lateral saphenous vein is a very useful vein for drawing small to medium volumes of blood, especially in rabbits (e.g. 1–2 ml from a medium-sized rabbit) (Figure 10.4); unless large volumes of blood are required, this is this author's (JRC) site of choice for conscious rabbits.

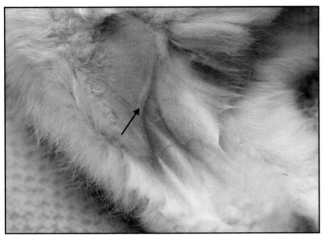

10.4 The lateral saphenous vein of a rabbit (arrowed). (© John Chitty)

The rabbit is held so that its hindleg rests over the edge of a table. The fur is clipped over the lateral region between the stifle and the hock. The assistant restraining the rabbit can then raise the vein by gripping around the stifle.

Marginal ear vein

This site (Figure 10.5) can be suitable for the collection of blood samples from rabbits, although the vein may collapse if large volumes are needed (it would be difficult to obtain more than 1.5 ml from the average sized rabbit using this method). It can be very hard to sample from this site on cold days or in very scared rabbits, due to peripheral vasoconstriction. Application of local anaesthetic cream 15 minutes prior to sampling may facilitate venepuncture by inducing vasodilation and also by reducing the chances of the rabbit jumping as a reaction to the needle insertion.

To take a sample, the fur is carefully clipped along the caudal ear margin and the vein is raised by gripping the ear at its base, specifically on the caudal margin. It is recommended that the vein is raised for at least 1 minute prior to sampling.

The marginal ear vein is widely recommended as a blood collection site in rabbits. In contrast, although some authors claim that the central ear artery is the site of choice for taking larger blood samples, there are claims that an induced arteritis may result in sloughing of the distal ear (Ward, 2006).

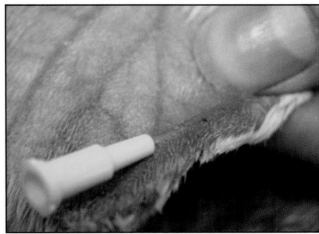

10.5 The marginal ear vein of a rabbit with an intravenous catheter in place (© John Chitty)

Toenail

This site has been used to obtain blood from ferrets for Aleutian disease (AD) serology. However, it is painful for the ferret and multiple sampling can result in nail deformities. For these reasons, coupled with the lack of evidence in favour of AD testing, the National Ferret Welfare Society has condemned the practice of obtaining samples in this manner. In addition, blood collected from this site would not be appropriate for biochemical or haematological analysis because of contamination and tissue fluid dilution.

Birds

Skin preparation

Wetting the skin with a spirit-soaked swab improves visualization of the site; wetting the feathers will also keep them out of the way. However, care must be taken not to over-wet the bird as this may lead to hypothermia. Special care must be taken when preparing the skin of passerine birds as they may preen their feathers immediately after application of preparations.

Restraint

In most cases, two operators are required for bleeding conscious birds, with the exception of very small passerine and psittacine birds (e.g. budgerigars and cockatiels), for which a simple one-handed holding technique greatly facilitates jugular venepuncture.

Needle selection and sample volume

The size of needle and syringe used for collecting blood will vary depending on the size of the bird. For example:

- A 2.5 ml syringe and a 23 gauge 5/8 inch needle for collection from the jugular vein of a 1 kg Harris' hawk or 400 g African grey parrot
- A 1 ml syringe and a 25 gauge 5/8 inch needle for collection from the ulnar vein of a pigeon
- A 0.5 ml normal insulin syringe and a 29 gauge 1/2 inch needle for collection from the jugular vein of a canary.

In general, the largest needle size that can be used safely should be selected where possible, to avoid damage to blood cells as birds' RBCs are nucleated. As for mammals, the volume of blood that may be safely removed is up to approximately 1% bodyweight (e.g. up to 10 ml from a 1 kg Harris' hawk and up to 0.2 ml from a 20 g finch). It is important to note that this figure is for healthy birds; the volume taken should be reduced slightly for sick and/or dehydrated birds.

Collection sites

Blood collection sites for birds, with their advantages and disadvantages, are discussed in Figure 10.6 and illustrated in Figures 10.7 to 10.9.

Restraint	Advantages	Disadvantages	Recommended species	Tips
Right jugular vein (Figure 10.7)				
The bird should be restrained or anaesthetized and the neck extended. Parting of the feathers reveals the vein running under a large apterium (featherless tract). Placement of a digit at the base of the neck raises the vein	Easy. Large volumes can be taken. Haemostasis relatively simple. Restraint may be stressful for sensitive or dyspnoeic birds	Very difficult for left-handed operators, although the left jugular may be utilized in larger species. Handling may be difficult in larger raptors or macaws. Struggling birds may cause laceration of the vein and fatal subcutaneous haemorrhage; general anaesthesia may therefore be appropriate, especially if inexperienced	Not appropriate for pigeons or waterfowl. May be very hard to visualize in poultry. Route of choice in all other commonly seen species	Anaesthesia may be recommended for this technique. Gentle digital pressure applied afterwards to avoid haematoma formation
Superficial ulnar/basilic vein (Figure 10.8)				
The bird is restrained or anaesthetized and placed on its back. One wing is extended and the vein visualized. The operator raises the vein with his/her free hand	Easier for left-handed operators. Restraint relatively simpler than for the right jugular vein, especially in larger species	Fragile vein and may be hard to draw large volumes, especially in smaller birds. Haemostasis can be hard to achieve and the bird should be placed back in the cage to allow it to calm down and its blood pressure to drop. This is preferable to prolonged handling. Unlike jugular venepuncture, haemorrhage is unlikely to be fatal and is readily visible; however, small losses may cause a lot of mess and distress to owners. Occasionally a haematoma may form along with a slight wing drop that may last 1–2 days	Suitable for all except very small passerine and psittacine birds. Method of choice in pigeons and poultry	To facilitate haemostasis a drop of tissue glue may be helpful
Superficial plantar metatarsal/caudal tibial vein (Figure 10.9)				
The bird is restrained and the leg extended. The operator can raise the vein with their free hand. Restraint is normally minimal	Superficial, simple to visualize and raise. In passerine birds can be pricked to allow collection of blood drops	Haemostasis difficult	The short tarsometatarsal of psittacine birds makes this vein difficult to access and use. In raptors it may be difficult to work close to the feet. Method of choice in waterfowl	Tissue glue may facilitate haemostasis or a light temporary dressing may be applied
Toe clip				
		Inappropriate in raptors where damage to talons is undesirable and lack of access to other veins is unlikely. In other species, not recommended due to contamination of collected blood with urates and tissue fluid. While this method has been recommended in the past (and sometimes now), it is not the method of choice		

10.6 Sites for venepuncture in birds.

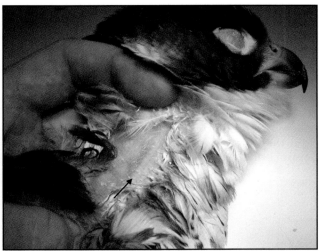

10.7 The right jugular vein of a peregrine falcon (anaesthetized). (Reproduced from the *BSAVA Manual of Raptors, Pigeons and Passerine Birds*; © John Chitty)

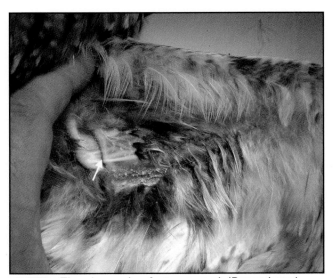

10.8 The ulnar vein of a tawny owl. (Reproduced from the *BSAVA Manual of Raptors, Pigeons and Passerine Birds*; © John Chitty)

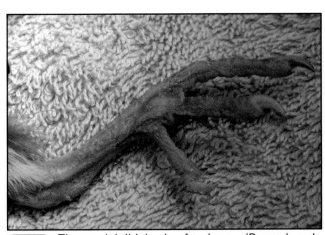

10.9 The caudal tibial vein of a pigeon. (Reproduced from the *BSAVA Manual of Raptors, Pigeons and Passerine Birds*; © John Chitty)

Reptiles

Needle selection and blood volume

As for birds, the largest bore needle appropriate to the size of the lizard or snake size should be used:

- 23 gauge for animals weighing 100–300 g
- 21 gauge for larger lizards and for snakes weighing 300–2000 g
- 19–18 gauge for larger snakes.

The needle should be long enough to penetrate the vertebral bodies or to access the heart, depending on the selected route.
Examples of needle selection:

- Tail vein of a large iguana: 21 gauge 1.5 inch
- Heart or tail vein of an adult bearded dragon: 23 gauge 1 inch
- Heart or tail vein of an adult veiled chameleon: 25 gauge 5/8 inch
- Heart of a large boid snake: 21 gauge 1.5 inch
- Jugular vein of most chelonian species: 23–21 gauge 5/8 inch
- Subcarapacial vein of a chelonian: 23 gauge 5/8 inch in species <80 g; up to 18 gauge and 1–1.5 inch in large terrestrial species >3 kg; and 2 inches or longer in very large leopard tortoises.

As for small mammals and birds, up to 1% of the individual's bodyweight can be taken as a blood sample.

Suitable sites for venepuncture

Lizards

Ventral tail vein

The ventral tail vein is usually most appropriate for blood collection from reptiles (Figure 10.10). The vein lies just ventral to the vertebral body and the needle is inserted mid vertebra. The needle is inserted until bone is contacted. The needle is then gently withdrawn, with negative pressure applied to the syringe until blood flows. It is important to clean the skin adequately before inserting the needle. If the lizard is cold, the tail should first be warmed by placing it in a bowl of warm water to achieve better blood flow.

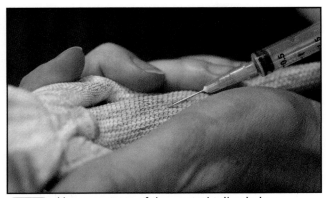

10.10 Venepuncture of the ventral tail vein in a bearded dragon. (© John Chitty)

The same vein may be accessed from the lateral approach by inserting the needle a fraction ventral to the 'lateral' line (where the lateral processes of the vertebrae can be palpated between the epaxial and hypaxial muscle blocks) and 'feeling' the needle between the processes. At this point, slight negative pressure is applied until the vein is entered and blood appears. Owners must be warned of the risk of autotomy (as discussed in Chapter 4) before attempting tail venepuncture in geckos.

Heart

If unable to obtain blood by any other method (or in geckos that may autotomize), the heart may be used. The technique is similar to that described later for snakes. In most lizards seen in practice the heart is located within the pectoral girdle; it is therefore accessed from the ventral midline just caudal to the sternum, with the needle angled cranially. In monitor lizards, the heart is often more caudally placed.

Snakes

Ventral tail vein

The ventral tail vein is often used in larger snakes. The technique is similar to that for lizards (using a ventral approach), although there is a greater risk of lymphodilution. It is also important not to insert the needle too close to the vent, to avoid contamination from hemipenile secretions.

Heart

Alternatively the heart may be used. If the heart cannot be palpated or visualized, an 8 MHz Doppler ultrasound probe can be used to locate it (Figure 10.11). The heart is then fixed between finger and thumb, and the needle is inserted from the caudal direction to ensure entry into the ventricle rather than

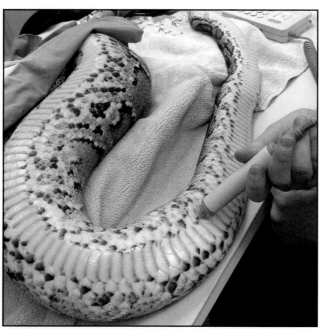

10.11 Locating the heart in a large anaesthetized boa constrictor using an 8 MHz Doppler ultrasound probe. (© John Chitty)

the atria (as there is a risk of atrial laceration). If the ventricle is entered there appears to be little risk of significant iatrogenic damage.

Chelonians

Jugular vein

The jugular vein is the 'gold standard' site for blood collection in chelonians. It is usually larger on the right than on the left, and there are two branches: ventral and dorsal (Figure 10.12).

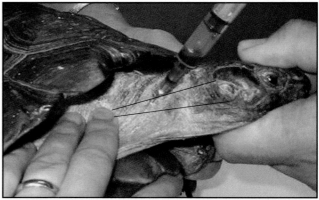

10.12 Venepuncture of the dorsal branch of the right jugular vein of a tortoise. The lines show the two branches of the jugular vein. (© John Chitty)

The vein is very superficial and can be difficult to visualize. There is also a risk of accidentally penetrating the carotid artery, which lies just under the jugular vein; this would result in a large post-venepuncture haematoma. Pressure must therefore be applied to the neck immediately after sampling.

Restraint can be difficult (especially in aquatic species and larger terrestrial chelonians, for which sedation is usually required) and at least two operators are required. In all species 23–21 gauge 5/8 inch needles are appropriate. Longer needles are used in larger specimens.

Subcarapacial vein

As an alternative, the subcarapacial vein may be used (Figure 10.13). Blood from here enters the jugular vein. While there is a higher risk of lymphodilution, restraint is much easier (making it this author's (JRC) technique of choice, certainly for aquatic chelonians).

1. The head is pushed in (using a large cotton-tipped swab for aquatic species).
2. A bent needle is inserted into the ventral midline, where the skin joins the shell.
3. The needle is inserted until the ventral vertebrae are 'hit' and is then gently manoeuvred (while applying gentle negative pressure) until blood is seen.
4. If lymph is withdrawn, the needle should be removed and the procedure started again.

Using this route, it is possible to take blood from even very small (<80 g) tortoises. For this route 23–18 gauge 1–1.5 inch needles are appropriate.

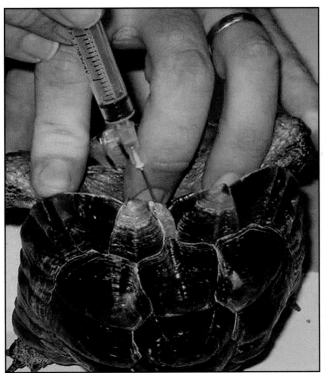

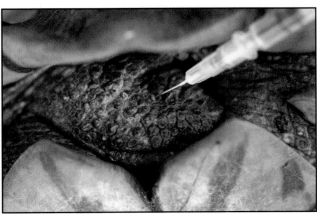

10.13 Venepuncture using the subcarapacial vein. The needle is angled so that it enters the body where the skin joins the shell, dorsal to the head. It then passes dorsally to access the vein just ventral to the vertebrae. (© John Chitty)

Dorsal tail vein

The dorsal tail vein (Figure 10.14) should be reserved until last (other than in giant species, where it may be the only vein accessible without sedation), as there is a very high risk of the sample becoming contaminated with lymph when using this route. The skin should be thoroughly scrubbed with chlorhexidine or povidone–iodine as there is a high risk of contamination, particularly as this site is close to the cloaca. There is little tissue between bone and skin. The needle is inserted into the dorsal midline and gently manoeuvred towards the dorsal spinous processes until blood appears. If using this vein, the laboratory should always be informed due to the likely effects of lymph contamination.

10.14 Venepuncture of the dorsal tail vein of a tortoise. (© John Chitty)

Brachial vein

The brachial vein does not appear clinically useful in the chelonian species routinely seen in UK practice.

Prioritizing blood tests

In many cases it is impossible to take a large enough blood sample to cover all the potential tests required, especially in very small (e.g. 20 g budgerigars) or very sick patients. In these cases it is therefore essential to prioritize the most important tests. While priorities are often set by the differential diagnoses (e.g. checking uric acid in a polyuric bird), the results of other tests may also be important in guiding priorities; for example, if radiography of a vomiting budgerigar reveals metal in the gizzard, heavy metal tests (lead/zinc) may be more important than haematology.

In the generally unwell animal, where there are no specific guiding tests, the clinician should concentrate on more general tests; haematology and protein (albumin/globulin) tests may give more information than, for example, enzyme assays.

Where only tiny samples (a few drops) can be obtained, it is still possible to obtain much vital information, including:

- PCV and buffy coat (Figure 10.15)
- Total solids (total protein as determined by refractometer)
- Blood smears – give an approximate idea of white cell numbers and differential morphology.

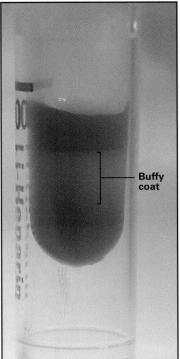

10.15 The large buffy coat in this sample suggests that the patient (a bearded dragon) has leukaemia. Lymphoproliferative disease is common in this species. (© John Chitty)

Buffy coat

⚠️ **WARNING**
Determination of total protein by refractometer can be used in mammals but is considered less accurate in birds and reptiles. Results must therefore be interpreted with care.

Interpretation of blood tests

Interpretation of blood tests is particularly difficult in exotic species.

- Less is known about the types of disease seen and the pathophysiology of disease in these species than in dogs and cats; less is also therefore known about the types and significance of changes likely to be seen in blood samples.
- Less is known about how appropriate many of the tests are for exotic species; the choice of test and its use may be based on historical usage or on conclusions drawn from other species.
- 'Normal' (reference) values may be based on very small sample numbers and so may be skewed by 'outrider' results. While large databases are being built, some (e.g. ISIS) include both sick and healthy animals, which may skew 'normals' where there are small sample numbers.
- As for all species, reference values vary between laboratories and between different analysers and/or techniques. It is therefore always appropriate to seek specialized guidance on the choice of test and on the interpretation of that result (or pattern of results) from that particular laboratory, based on the reference values appropriate to their techniques. Ensuring a good history is provided on the submission form greatly assists in the interpretation of results.

Overall, however, the case clinician is often in the best position to interpret blood results, as the clinical assessment of the patient must be taken into account.

Skin

Small mammals

The skin sampling techniques used in small mammals are identical to those used in dogs and cats, as given in the *BSAVA Textbook of Veterinary Nursing* and the *BSAVA Manual of Canine and Feline Dermatology*. Figure 10.16 gives indications for the various skin sampling techniques.

Technique	Indications
Aspiration	Pustules/cysts – cytology
Coat brushing	Suspected louse, flea or fur/cheyletiellid mite infestation
Hair pluck	Suspected ringworm (dermatophytosis) or louse infestation. Hair may be submitted for ringworm culture or for microscopy
Impression smears	Cytology of exudative (Figure 10.17) or scaling lesions
Acetate tape	Suspected louse (Figure 10.18), flea, fur mite (Figure 10.19) or cheyletiellid mite infestation. May also be used for cytology of exudative or scaling lesions
Skin scraping	Suspected burrowing mite infestation (mange (Figure 10.20) or demodicosis)

10.16 Skin sampling techniques and their applications in small mammals.

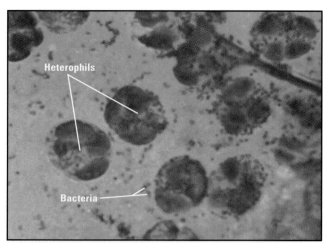

10.17 An impression smear from an exudative skin lesion in a rabbit. The presence of bacteria and heterophils confirms pyoderma. (Diff-Quik stain; original magnification x 1000) (© John Chitty)

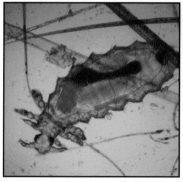

10.18 A rat louse (*Polyplax spinulosa*) (female). (© John Chitty)

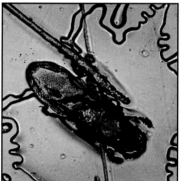

10.19 A *Chirodiscoides* fur mite from a guinea pig. (© John Chitty)

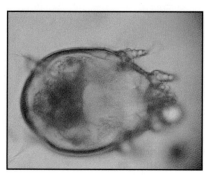

10.20 A sarcoptid mite from a rat. (© John Chitty)

Birds

Skin scrapes

Skin scrapes are taken in birds with crusts or hyperkeratotic lesions suggestive of parasitism. The procedure is the same as that used for dogs or cats, although care must be taken not to cut the very thin skin of the bird inadvertently. The skin sample (scraping) is taken into 10% potassium hydroxide or liquid paraffin. Unlike in mammals, the cells are often present as 'rafts' or 'sheets'.

Feather digests

Feather digests are used where there is evidence of feather damage but no parasites are found on gross examination. They are also useful where changes (e.g. in colour or opacity) in the calamus (feather shaft) indicate possible quill mite infestation. An erupting or damaged feather is digested in warmed 10% potassium hydroxide before centrifugation and microscopic examination.

Pulp cytology techniques

Indicated where birds are chewing large wing/tail feathers (remiges/rectrices) and blood feathers are present:

1. Pull blood feathers from the area that is being chewed. Ideally choose a damaged and an undamaged feather.
2. Clean the calamus using surgical spirit.
3. Incise along the calamus.
4. Gently squeeze the calamus. Small 'pearls' of clear fluid will be seen along the cut. These can be sampled using standard impression smear techniques. Discard blood-tinged fluid.
5. Stain the samples with a standard trichrome stain (e.g. Diff-Quik, Dade).
6. If required, a small sterile swab may be inserted into the pulp and sent for culture and/or the whole feather can be preserved in formol saline and submitted for histopathology. The incision in the calamus allows for good penetration by the fixative.

Indicated when birds are plucking body feathers and blood feathers are present:

1. Using forceps, grasp and remove a blood feather.
2. Gently squeeze the distal end, forcing fluid from the proximal end.
3. Discard the first (blood-tinged) drop. Subsequent clear fluid can then be collected on a microscope slide and stained using a trichrome stain. A bacteriological swab may also be inserted into the collected fluid (prior to staining) to obtain a sample for culture.

Alternatively, the following technique may be used for either presentation:

1. Clean the distal end of a feather (where barbs are emerging from the sheath), with the feather remaining *in situ* on the body.
2. Insert a needle (23 gauge 5/8 inch – syringe attached) into the feather pulp via this site (Figure 10.21). Gently aspirate a single drop of pulp content and place it on a microscope slide. Stain with Diff-Quik (or any other trichrome).
3. This method has the advantage of not requiring another feather to be removed and avoids extraneous contamination with blood.

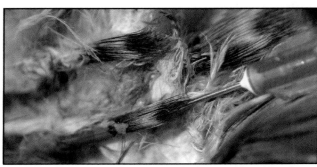

10.21 Collection of feather pulp from a blood feather. (© John Chitty)

Acetate tape samples

Tape samples are indicated where there is excessive scale, where the skin appears 'dry' or where there are exudative, crusting or hyperkeratotic lesions.

Technique for obtaining an acetate tape sample

1. Add one drop of Giemsa stain to a microscope slide.
2. Lay a piece of adhesive acetate tape on the area of the lesion (Figure 10.22).
3. Stick the tape on to the slide, on top of the stain.

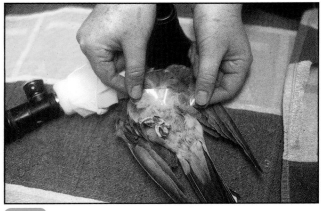

10.22 Acetate strip applied to the skin of a cockatiel.

Reptiles

Because reptiles have a more impervious, scaled skin, tests used in small mammals and birds are therefore of less use; biopsy with histopathology is often more appropriate. Skin sampling techniques and their applications in reptiles are given in Figure 10.23.

Test	Method	Indications
Acetate tape	As for dog/cat	Exudative/crusting/scaling lesions. Suspected ectoparasitic infestations
Aspiration	As for dog/cat	Pustular/cystic lesions
Impression smear	As for dog/cat	Exudative/crusting/scaling lesions (Figure 10.24)
Scale sampling	Loose scales from lesion margins may be removed using forceps and submitted in their entirety for culture/cytology	Any lesion with loose scales
Shed skin examination	Loose shedding skin may be gently removed for cytology	Dysecdysis. Suspected ectoparasitism

10.23 Skin sampling techniques and their applications in reptiles.

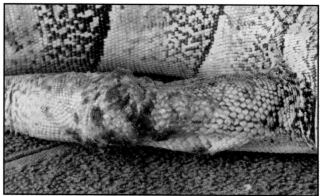

10.24 A scaling lesion on the forelimb of a green iguana. Removal of the superficial scab, followed by an impression smear of the underlying lesion, confirmed a fungal infection. (© John Chitty)

Urine

Small mammals

Collection

Urine can be taken from small mammals in the same way as from dogs and cats. Cystocentesis is commonly performed (usually on anaesthetized animals, although ferrets generally do not require anaesthesia for this). The bladder may be located and stabilized by palpation, although some authors recommend ultrasound guidance due to an increased risk of gut penetration in these species compared to cats and dogs.

'Free catch' or catheterized samples may also be obtained and may be satisfactory for dipstick and specific gravity testing; care should be taken when interpreting bacteriology results in these circumstances. Urine samples should be collected into plain and small boric acid sample pots for submission to the laboratory.

Tests and interpretation

The testing and interpretation of ferret urine is very similar to that of cat urine. Herbivorous small mammals differ in the following ways:

- Their urine is normally alkaline
- Grossly, it may vary greatly between individuals and even day-to-day in the same individual. Normal urine may be red in rabbits (Figure 10.25) or sludgy in rabbits and guinea pigs
- Crystalluria is normal in all herbivorous rodents and lagomorphs. Typically, crystals will be calcium oxalate or calcium carbonate.

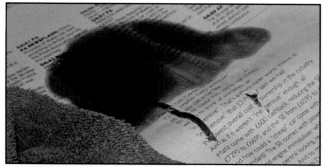

10.25 Normal red pigmented urine from a rabbit. (© John Chitty)

In all species, cytology is of great importance, especially when interpreting bacteriology results. To avoid autolysis of cells during transit to the laboratory it is advisable to submit (in addition to plain and boric acid urine samples) either freshly prepared air-dried smears of urine sediment or a fixed sample (Figure 10.26). The presence of white cells will indicate an immune response to a possible pathogen. Cytological evidence of red cells will differentiate haematuria from red pigment in urine.

Specific gravity should be assessed in all small mammals; isosthenuria (SG 1.008–1.012) is a sensitive, though not specific, indicator of renal dysfunction.

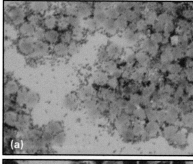

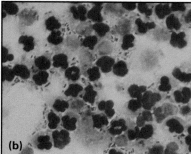

10.26 **(a)** Unfixed urine 24 hours old (original magnification x500). While bacteria are present, cells are too autolysed to be identified. **(b)** Fixed urine. Same urine sample fixed with buffered formalin 2 drops/ml, 24 hours old (original magnification x500). Note: the lobulated nuclei of neutrophils are clearly preserved, allowing the cells to be identified. (© Nick Carmichael)

Birds and reptiles

Urine testing is less useful in these species as there is cloacal mixing of urine and faeces. Finding glucose in urine does not therefore necessarily indicate true glucosuria unless there are very high levels.

In birds and reptiles, blood may be seen through the liquid part of the dropping. It should be determined whether this is:

■ Of renal origin (or bladder origin if the species has one) – blood is seen throughout the urine (Figure 10.27a)
■ Due to distinct haemorrhage (often of cloacal or reproductive tract origin) – blood is seen in the urine as a result of cloacal mixing.

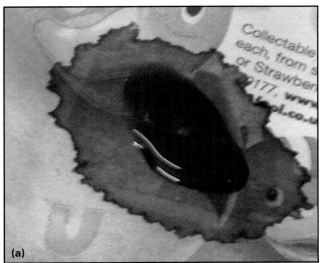

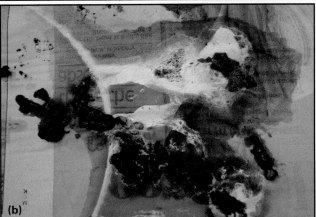

10.27 (a) Haematuria in a sun conure, caused by lead toxicosis. Frank, haemorrhage-free blood is mixed with normal urine. (b) Haematuria should not be confused with melaena, as seen in this hawk dropping. Here, the faecal portion contains dark digested blood from a proventricular ulcer and the blood staining emanates from this. (© John Chitty)

Bird droppings may be collected on paper and urine can be aspirated from here if done very quickly. Specific gravity and cytology can then be performed on this sample. Cytology can be useful with respect to inflammatory cells and renal casts. In some species (not captive parrots), renal coccidia may be an issue.

In reptiles, it is hard to obtain liquid urine samples. Those reptiles that produce liquid urine will normally only do so in bath water.

Reptiles with bladders (e.g. chelonians and some lizards) can have urine samples taken by cystocentesis.

■ In lizards, the bladder can be entered just cranial to the pelvic girdle in the ventral midline.
■ In chelonians, the bladder can be located in the ventral portion of the body, which can be entered via the prefemoral fossa.

Urine collected in this manner can be submitted for culture and cytology/parasitology; renal coccidia are more common in reptiles than in mammals or birds.

Faeces

Small mammals

Gross appearance

Carnivorous species (e.g. ferrets) have looser stools than herbivorous species. In herbivorous species, faeces must be distinguished from caecotrophs, and true diarrhoea must be distinguished from some of the more sludgy urine. It is also important to understand what is normal for individual rodents and rabbits, as any change in faecal output (size, consistency, number of pellets) may be an indicator of ill health, e.g. pain and gut stasis.

Collection

Faeces may be collected from an animal's living quarters; it should ideally be collected on clean paper and should be as fresh as possible.

Birds

Gross appearance

The gross appearance of the dropping (or 'mute' in raptors) provides a lot of information about the bird. The dropping consists of faeces plus soluble and insoluble urine. 'Loose droppings' may therefore represent diarrhoea (Figure 10.28a) or polyuria (see Figure 10.29a). In cage birds, substrates such as sandpaper and grit are of little use for adequate examination of the dropping (Figure 10.29). Owners should therefore be advised to collect a day's droppings on to newspaper or kitchen roll, thus allowing proper examination of the relative constituents of the dropping, including the colour and appearance of each constituent (Figure 10.30).

PRACTICAL TIP
It should be remembered that:

■ Droppings produced during travelling may be a lot looser than normal
■ There is a lot of variation between bird species, e.g. seed-eating parrots and pigeons have a smaller, drier dropping than raptors and nectar-eating parrots (lories and lorikeets).

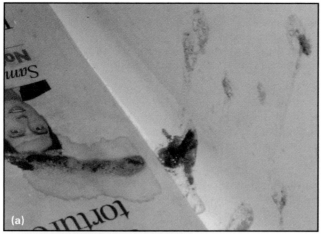

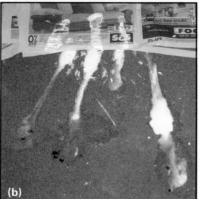

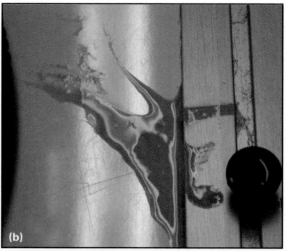

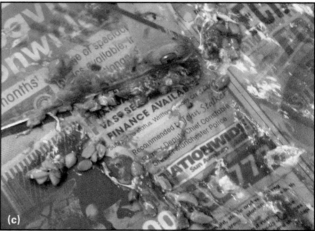

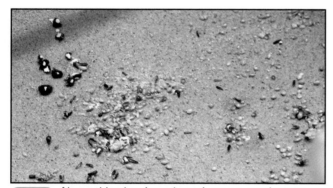

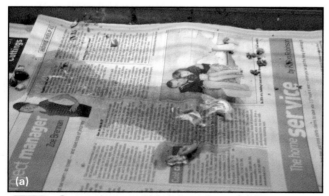

10.28 (a) Droppings from a parrot with enteritis. Contrast with (b), a normal mute from a falcon. Note the effect caused by normal (healthy) ejection of the mute. This is referred to as 'slicing'. (© John Chitty)

10.29 Normal budgerigar droppings on sandpaper. While these are clearly normal, it is hard to distinguish abnormalities unless droppings are collected on paper. (© John Chitty)

10.30 Some abnormal bird droppings. (a) From an African grey parrot with polyuria. (continues)

10.30 (continued) Some abnormal bird droppings (b) Biliverdinuria in a falcon. (c) Undigested seed in droppings is a sign of upper gastrointestinal disturbance. This must be distinguished from loose droppings landing on discarded seed. (© John Chitty)

Collection

Fresh droppings may be collected from the floor of the cage. The freshest samples, collected on to clean paper, should ideally be used. In some cases (e.g. assessment for a *Chlamydophila* PCR or for *Giardia*) it may be appropriate to collect a pooled sample over 3 days. For faecal Gram stains or avian bornavirus PCR, a cloacal swab may be more appropriate.

Gram staining

Gram staining (Figure 10.31) is a rapid and sensitive test and can be used, for example, in a parrot with diarrhoea, to identify the microorganisms in a faecal smear that are likely to be causing the diarrhoea. In the healthy bird, there should be a moderate number of microorganisms, comprising approximately 70% Gram-positive rods, 25% Gram-positive cocci and a few yeasts and Gram-negative rods.

Gram stains have been used as part of a 'well bird' check in parrots, though their use is controversial in this respect. The test is not appropriate in other bird species, e.g. raptors, where the faecal flora consists predominantly of Gram-negative rods.

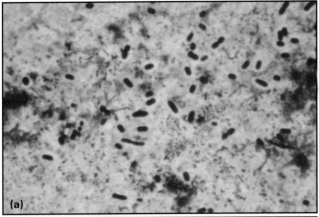

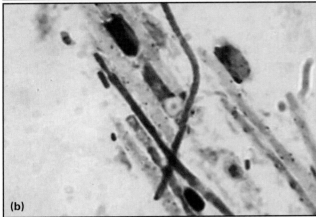

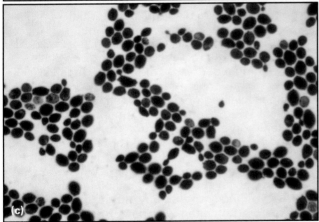

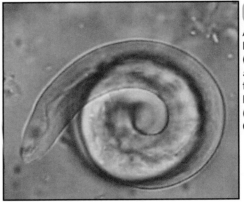

Collection

The animal should be watched closely so that a sample can be collected as soon as possible after it has been produced. Faeces left in the vivarium overnight tend to dry out and so become useless for testing.

A faecal sample is particularly useful when investigating cases of anorexia; however, in these patients there is usually reduced or non-existent faecal output. A sample may be obtained in one of two ways:

- Bathing reptiles will often induce defecation
- Cloacal washes may be useful, whereby warmed saline (2–5 ml/200 g bodyweight) is carefully syringed into the cloaca and the caudal abdomen is then gently massaged so that saline and faeces can be pushed out of the cloaca into a receptacle.

Parasitology

Standard faecal flotation methods are appropriate for exotic pets and wildlife. Where lungworm is suspected, Baermann techniques should be used; however, this parasite is rarely found in the species discussed in this Manual, with wild hedgehogs being the only exception (Figure 10.32).

10.32 A lungworm larva (*Crenosoma striatum*) from a hedgehog. (© John Chitty)

10.31 Gram staining. **(a)** *Clostridium* proliferation; large Gram-positive (dark blue) rods noted on a background containing smaller bacteria and debris in a faecal smear from a penguin (original magnification ×1000). **(b)** *Macrorhabdus ornithogaster* from a wasting budgerigar (original magnification ×400). (© John Chitty) **(c)** *Candida* showing typical narrow-based budding and morphology from the gastrointestinal tract of a vulture (original magnification ×1000). (© Nick Carmichael)

Reptiles

Gross appearance

As in birds, the 'faeces' actually consist of a mixture of faeces with soluble and insoluble urine. There is usually less liquid in reptile faeces than in those of birds, and the urine is more mixed through. Conversely, the actual dropping is usually looser than that of birds, especially in carnivorous lizards.

Where only small amounts of faeces can be obtained, a simple wet preparation for viewing with a microscope may be more appropriate than flotation as this will at least give an indication as to whether parasites are present and will provide a qualitative guide to numbers. It is important to appreciate the parasite species that are found in individual exotic pet species, and their relative pathogenicities. In raptors, it is important to distinguish secondary parasitism from primary parasitism – e.g. raptors will have inadvertently ingested any parasites carried by their prey.

In herbivorous rodents and rabbits (Figure 10.33), it is important to distinguish coccidial oocysts (potentially pathogenic) from non-pathogenic *Saccharomyces* yeasts.

In birds and reptiles it is sometimes necessary to look for motile protozoans (e.g. trichomonads in gamebirds; Figure 10.34). In these cases, a very fresh sample (<20 minutes) should be used and a wet preparation examined. This technique can also be used to identify other endoparasites such as worms and their eggs (Figure 10.35).

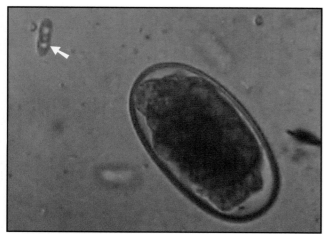

10.33 A nematode (*Trichostrongylus* spp.) egg in a faecal sample from a rabbit (×400 original magnification). A *Saccharomyces* yeast cell can be seen to the left (arrowed). (© John Chitty)

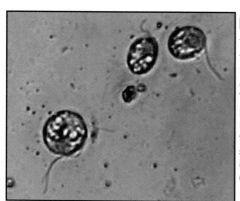

10.34 Trichomonads from a budgerigar crop wash. These parasites may also be found in faecal samples. (© John Chitty)

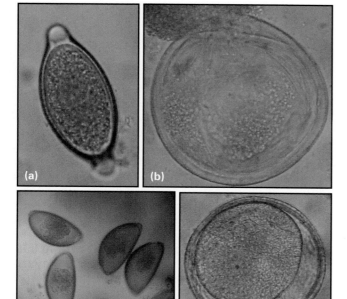

(a) (b)
(c) (d)

10.35 Bird and reptile endoparasite eggs (all at ×400 original magnification). **(a)** Avian *Capillaria*. **(b)** Avian cestode. **(c)** Oxyurids (*Pharyngodon* spp.) (pinworm) from a bearded dragon. **(d)** Tortoise ascarid (*Angusticaecum* sp.) (© John Chitty)

Bacteriology

Antibiotic 'failure' is a common feature of exotic animal practice. This may be due to:

- Failure to use a correct dose rate
- Failure to use a drug that will penetrate the infected area
- Failure to correct the underlying causes of infection
- Failure of the bacteriology testing to show the pathogenic bacterial species and hence the correct sensitivity pattern.

Some of these problems will be enhanced by poor sample taking and so may be avoided by asking the following questions.

Questions that must be asked when taking bacteriology samples

- **Are you likely to find pathogens?** Might this be a bacterial lesion? If so, does it look to be of the type that may be associated with a particular pathogen?
- **Are you likely to find commensal bacteria?** All areas of the body can be associated with commensal bacterial species. These may invade damaged tissue (or may be facultative pathogens) or may simply be normal 'passengers' in sampling. In this respect, you must be able to distinguish potential commensal bacteria from potential pathogens.
- **Are you likely to get contamination?** If sampling a deep area of the body, it is very easy to get contamination from more superficial regions – e.g. when taking deep nasal swabs from rabbits there is a strong likelihood of contamination from the nares and rostral nasal cavity. In reptiles in particular, there is often contamination from surface environmental bacteria when, for example, swabbing skin or shell lesions.
- **Are you likely to find anything?** Some lesions are not associated with bacteria. In some cases there may be sufficient inhibitory factors (e.g. sampling from the centre of an abscess) that there is little chance of any bacterial growth from a swab.

The following may assist in obtaining more meaningful results:

- Swabbing from deeper lesions after superficial debris and contamination have been cleaned away (e.g. in the case of shell rot, after physical debridement of the damaged scute)
- Submitting biopsy specimens for culture (e.g. infected bone or abscess wall)
- Utilizing both anaerobic and aerobic culture, especially in abscess specimens
- In reptiles, performing culture at both 37°C and 22°C. Many reptile bacterial infections are associated with low environmental temperatures

- Cytology: Smearing aspirates on slides or examining direct impression smears of open lesions. Ideally, both a Gram stain and a trichrome stain (e.g. Diff-Quik) should be used. The finding of inflammatory cells is always suggestive of infection, and bacteria may be directly visualized. A sparse mixed population of bacteria suggests contamination or commensal organisms, whereas the presence of many monomorphic forms is likely to be of greater significance. This enables a rapid provisional diagnosis and prompt empirical antibiosis based on bacterial morphology
- Histopathology: Examining stained tissue samples can reveal organisms and the cellular responses to them, which may help to distinguish infection from contamination.

Above all, a thorough understanding of the animal's needs and of the underlying factors that may predispose to bacterial infection are required; otherwise even excellent sampling technique and correct choice of antibacterial therapy will not succeed.

Handling pathological samples

Once the samples have been obtained, the principles of handling them are essentially similar to those for dogs and cats.

Sample handling requirements

- *In vitro* degenerative changes need to be minimized.
- Patient details must be clearly recorded on the samples.
- Samples should be in suitable containers to reach the laboratory safely.
- Samples must be packaged to comply with the International Air Transport Association (IATA) and postal regulations for diagnostic specimens.
- The laboratory request form is completed clearly and correctly and enclosed with the samples.

Minimizing *in vitro* changes

All biological samples start to degenerate once collected from the patient; to maximize the diagnostic yield from a sample it is important to minimize these *in vitro* changes. For haematology and cytology samples where intact cells are present, it is important that air-dried smears are made as soon as possible after sample collection, as these prevent any further degeneration of cells in the material. Further information on making smears from blood and fluid samples is given in Figure 10.36.

Anticoagulants

(See also Figure 10.1.)

EDTA

While EDTA (ethylene diamine tetra-acetic acid) is an appropriate anticoagulant for blood samples from all

Blood smear preparation, using either fresh heparinized whole blood or a drop of fresh blood from the tip of a syringe:

Technique
1. Place a small drop of blood on to a clean, grease-free glass slide.

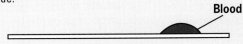

2. Take another clean glass slide as a spreader (preferably one with a bevelled edge) and draw this back into the blood drop, allowing the blood to flow across the spreader surface.

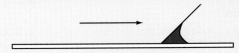

3. Holding the spreader at an angle of approximately 30 degrees to the sample slide, move the spreader gently forward in a single smooth action.

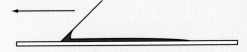

4. Slide the spreader to the end of the slide – do not lift the spreader from the slide
5. Label the smear and allow to air dry – do not heat.

All fresh blood films are useful but a perfect blood smear should have a smooth rounded tail approximately one cell thick at its end, and cover approximately two-thirds of the length of the slide. This is the same technique as described for blood smears in the dog and cat.

Tips and common problems
- If the blood film 'falls off' the end of the slide, try using less blood and/or moving the spreader more quickly.
- If the blood film is too short or too thin, try using slightly more blood and/or spreading more slowly.
- The presence of 'smudged' white cells is often associated with pressing too hard with the spreader.
- Red cells that overlap at the tail indicate that too much blood was used and/or that it was spread too slowly.
- An absence of white cells in the body and many white cells at the tail indicate that blood was spread too slowly or that the spreader was lifted before smear completion.

10.36 Techniques for preparing smears from blood and fluid samples.

mammal species, it is unsuitable for blood from many bird species and for all reptile species as it can cause cells to disrupt and lyse, making the sample unsuitable for analysis. The susceptibility to lysis varies between bird species (e.g. EDTA can be used for most parrot species); lysis is generally most marked in birds with webbed feet.

Heparin

Heparin is the preferred anticoagulant for two reasons:

- There is no risk of lysis
- The plasma collected from centrifuged samples

is suitable for biochemical analysis, which means that a single sample can be used for a full profile of haematology and chemistry.

One disadvantage of using heparin, however, is that continued cell metabolism and breakdown within the sample can affect the results of some biochemical tests, principally potassium and phosphate assays. To avoid this problem in larger species, where the total sample size is >0.75 ml, approximately 0.3 ml of blood and a smear can be submitted for haematology, with the remainder of the sample centrifuged and the separated plasma submitted for biochemistry.

Fixatives

For fluid cytology submissions such as washings, aspirated fluids and urine, the use of some form of cell fixation may be required in addition to the preparation of smears. It is advisable to check the requirements of the laboratory. Figure 10.26 shows how the use of small amounts of buffered formalin can dramatically improve the preservation of neutrophils in urine, which would be unrecognizable if only urine without the formalin were submitted.

Recording patient details

Problems of confusion regarding the identity of samples either in the practice or at the laboratory can be avoided if samples are labelled immediately after collection. For blood tubes it is advisable to use an indelible fine marker pen, while slides should be labelled either with a diamond-tipped pen, which etches the glass, or with pencil if using slides with a frosted end. Ink markings on slides can be washed off when the slides are fixed before staining, rendering them vulnerable to misidentification.

Using suitable containers

Laboratories provide polypropylene containers that are designed not only to optimize the sample quality but also to withstand normal handling during post or courier transit. For this reason it is not necessary to add supplementary bandaging, etc., to sample containers. Glass slides must be sent to the laboratory in rigid plastic slide containers or they run the risk of breaking in transit, which would both render them useless and pose a health and safety risk to postal and laboratory staff. All sample container lids should be checked before dispatch to avoid the possibility of leakage; however, the application of tape is unnecessary and can cause problems at the laboratory receiving the samples.

Packaging samples to comply with postal regulations

Within the UK, pathological material can be sent through Royal Mail, provided it is packaged in accordance with specific requirements set out in the regulations (Packing Instructions 650 for category B substances). The requirements set out in these regulations are given in Figure 10.37. While the tubes and postal materials supplied by the laboratory will comply with these regulations, it is the responsibility of

---

Sample packaging
The primary sample container must be leak-proof, wrapped in sufficient absorbent material to absorb any spillage and placed in a sample bag with the request form in the pouch. The sample bag should then be placed in a leak-proof secondary package for posting.

Labelling of packages
Any package containing infectious substances must be marked with:

- The sender's name, address and phone number
- The receiver's name and address
- UN number 3373
- The shipping name ('infectious substances') if appropriate
- 'Diagnostic Specimens' or' Biological Substance, Category B'.

 Packing Instructions 650 for diagnostic specimens in the UK.

the practice submitting the samples to comply with the packaging and labelling requirements. Royal Mail regulations in the UK prohibit the use of normal mail to send diagnostic samples outside the UK and to send whole animals for post-mortem examination.

Completing the laboratory request form correctly

In addition to ensuring that the details of the patient, practice and date of sampling are clearly recorded on the submission form, it is important to ensure that the tests required are clearly indicated, together with any test codes that are appropriate to the laboratory undertaking the analysis. As the tests used for exotic species are often less familiar than those used for dogs and cats, it is advisable to speak to the laboratory directly before samples are dispatched if there is any doubt regarding which test or groups of tests are required.

Health and safety considerations

- All samples must be dealt with appropriately with regard to ensuring the health and safety of individuals collecting, handling or transporting pathological material.
- Healthy reptiles commonly excrete *Salmonella* and healthy birds may excrete *Chlamydophila*, the causal agent of psittacosis in humans. Whenever faecal samples are to be collected by owners or members of the practice staff, they should be made fully aware that the material could potentially pose a risk to their health and they should be told to handle material appropriately. Gloves should be worn and hands must be washed after sample collection.
- Unfixed tissue samples (e.g. biopsy samples) and cytology samples may contain a variety of pathogenic organisms and should be handled in a similar manner.
- Particular care should be taken when sample containers are open and there is a possibility of spillage and contamination. Appropriate disinfection procedures and materials should be in place to cover this eventuality.

References and further reading

Campbell TW and Ellis C (2007) *Avian and exotic animal hematology.* Blackwell Professional Publishing, Iowa

Clark P, Boardmann W and Raidal S (2009) *Atlas of Avian Clinical Hematology.* Wiley, Chichester

Dorrestein GM (2008) Clinical pathology and post-mortem examination. In: *BSAVA Manual of Raptors, Pigeons and Passerine Birds,* ed. J Chitty and M Lierz, pp. 73–96. BSAVA Publications, Gloucester

Dorrestein GM and de Wit M (2005) Clinical pathology and necropsy. In: *BSAVA Manual of Psittacine Birds, 2nd edn,* ed. N Harcourt-Brown and J Chitty, pp. 60–86. BSAVA Publications, Gloucester

Heard D, Harr K and Wellehan J (2004) Diagnostic sampling and laboratory tests. In: *BSAVA Manual of Reptiles, 2nd edn,* ed. SJ Girling and P Raiti, pp. 71–86. BSAVA Publications, Gloucester

Jenkins J (2006) Clinical pathology. In: *BSAVA Manual of Rabbit Medicine and Surgery, 2nd edn,* ed. A Meredith and P Flecknell, pp. 45–51. BSAVA Publications, Gloucester

Lennox A (2009) Ferrets: clinical pathology. In: *BSAVA Manual of Rodents and Ferrets,* ed. E Keeble and A Meredith, pp. 230–236. BSAVA Publications Gloucester

Ward ML (2006) Physical examination and clinical techniques. In: *BSAVA Manual of Rabbit Medicine and Surgery, 2nd edn,* ed. A Meredith and P Flecknell, pp. 18–37. BSAVA Publications, Gloucester

Wesche P (2009) Rodents: clinical pathology. In: *BSAVA Manual of Rodents and Ferrets,* ed. E Keeble and A Meredith, pp. 42–51. BSAVA Publications Gloucester

Self-assessment questions

1. Which of these is a parasite of the rat?
   a. *Ctenocephalides felis*
   b. *Polyplax spinulosa*
   c. Trombiculid mite
   d. *Eimeria* spp.
2. List the venepuncture sites that may be utilized in a large (180 cm) adult male iguana and the method of restraint.
3. Which of these is not a granulocyte?
   a. Heterophil
   b. Eosinophil
   c. Monocyte
   d. Basophil
4. In which species is jugular venepuncture particularly difficult?
   a. Adult female Harris' hawk
   b. Ferret
   c. Female rabbit
   d. Guinea pig
5. Into which anticoagulant would you collect bird or reptile blood for haematological examination?
   a. Citrate
   b. Lithium heparin
   c. EDTA
   d. Fluoride-oxalate
6. The superficial ulnar/basilic vein would be least suitable for blood collection in which of the following species?
   a. Goshawk
   b. Electus parrot
   c. Zebra finch
   d. Rhode Island red hen

11

Outpatient care and nurse-led clinics

Molly Varga and Lucy Gott

This chapter is designed to give information on:

- Lifestage considerations; hand-rearing; vaccination; neutering; geriatric care
- Practical advice on nutrition, weight management and behavioural problems
- Medical and surgical patient discharge and follow-up consultations
- Examples of client leaflets.

Introduction

The importance of initial and ongoing contact with patients cannot be overstated. This contact is often maintained by the nursing staff through nurse-led clinics, creating a strong patient–client–practice bond that benefits everybody and allows nursing staff to work to their full potential.

The RCVS Code of Professional Conduct for Veterinary Nurses (2012) states that:

- Veterinary nurses must make animal health and welfare their first consideration when attending to animals
- Veterinary nurses must keep within their own area of competence and refer cases responsibly.

Veterinary nurses must not undertake a task unless they have the knowledge, skills and competence to complete it, and it must be performed in a way that carries no risk of harm to patients and protects the interests of the public. While many of the procedures detailed in this chapter are within the competence of the qualified veterinary nurse, it must be acknowledged that – due to species differences, difficulty in handling or requirements for sedation – modification of the scope of the veterinary nurse's involvement may be necessary. It is the responsibility of the veterinary surgeon in charge and the veterinary nurse involved to undertake only those tasks for which they have

been properly trained. With respect to nurse-led clinics this may mean referring a patient on to a veterinary surgeon, or declining to perform services for which the nurse feels he or she is not appropriately trained. It should be noted that the Registered Veterinary Nurse (RVN) now bears professional responsibility for his or her actions. The constraints of the Veterinary Surgeons Act 1966 (Schedule 3 Amendment) Order 2002 are discussed in Chapter 9.

Nurse-led clinics

- By addressing general healthcare, clinics are important for maintaining contact with clients whose pets are generally well and where clinical intervention is not warranted. It is often sensible to combine these clinics with ongoing client education (see examples of handouts at the end of this chapter).
- Specific clinics may be concerned with issues such as lifestage, behaviour or weight management. They allow decision-making to be undertaken by professional veterinary staff rather than placing responsibility on the owner.
- Clinics may also be pre-empted by previous medical or surgical care. These clinically oriented nurse-led clinics allow for evaluation of the success of the nursing care plan, re-assessment of clinical progress and prompt nursing or veterinary intervention if needed.

Information on setting up and running nurse-led clinics is given in the *BSAVA Manual of Canine and Feline Advanced Veterinary Nursing*. Consideration should be given to specific requirements for handling and examining exotic pets and wildlife, as detailed in earlier chapters.

General procedures and healthcare

In addition to the species-specific information given later and in client handout examples, the following general points should be borne in mind. It is important to be able to spot potential problems while undertaking seemingly routine procedures. The ability to recognize problems, and to communicate their significance to an owner, is paramount in obtaining the correct care for the animal.

Ear cleaning

Dirty ears in rabbits may indicate that they are unable to get their feet far enough forward to clean their ears themselves, or that they are not able to balance well enough to do so. Underlying causes such as middle ear disease, encephalitozoonosis, arthritis and back pain can all contribute to this problem. Diagnosis and treatment of the underlying cause is necessary; any animal presented with a request for ear cleaning must therefore be checked by a veterinary surgeon prior to cleaning taking place.

> ⚠ **WARNING**
> **Rabbits with ear mites should not have their ears cleaned until treatment has been initiated, as the ears will be excruciatingly painful and itchy.**

Proprietary ear cleaners may be used, although most of these are not authorized for small mammals. In most cases, using a suitably sized cotton wool ball to clean the external ear is all that is required, and ear cleaner should not be directly instilled into the ear. Should more extensive cleaning be needed, sedation may be required.

Fur trimming

Trimming fur is a common request for rabbits and guinea pigs, often prompted by a failure to eat caecotrophs (rabbits) or a general failure to groom. These behaviours – as well as urine scalding of fur in the perineal region – may be caused by medical problems, which should be recognized and addressed at the time of grooming. Diagnosis of the underlying problems and their treatment will promote the wellbeing of that patient, and a veterinary check-up should be advised.

Rabbits and guinea pigs

Rabbits and guinea pigs, particularly those breeds with longer fur (e.g. angora or angora-cross rabbits), will occasionally require fur to be clipped where it is matted or soiled.

- Because rabbit skin in particular can be thin and fragile, restraint of the patient must be adequate and the clippers used should be in good condition and sharp (see Chapter 9).
- The skin should be gently stretched until taut and the fur clipped in the direction of its growth with the blades nearly parallel to the skin.
- In individuals that become very stressed, or where the underlying skin is damaged, sedation may be required and veterinary advice should be sought.

Wildlife

Wild mammals with skin wounds will often benefit from having the fur around the wound clipped. This allows remote visualization of the wound (removing the necessity for frequent capture and restraint) as well as easier cleaning. Most wild mammals will require some form of chemical restraint for clipping.

Nail or claw trimming

Nail or claw trimming is frequently requested by owners. Attention needs to be paid to whether it is appropriate; for example, arboreal species should not have their nails trimmed as it can affect their ability to climb and may cause them to fall. Overgrown nails may indicate a medical problem, such as a reduction in mobility (e.g. due to arthritis); or over-long nails on one limb might be secondary to traumatic damage.

Mammals

Claws or nails of mammals can be clipped in a similar manner as for cats and dogs. The aim is to reduce the length while avoiding cutting into the quick.

- Rabbits and ferrets can be restrained as described in Chapter 1, and usually tolerate the procedure well.
- Guinea pig claws often curl around and are more easily clipped using nail clippers made for humans rather than those for dogs or cats.
- Less familiar species such as skunks and raccoons may require sedation.
- In most cases there is no reason to clip the claws of any wild mammal.
- Should bleeding occur, this can be stopped by the application of a styptic pencil or wound powder (see Chapter 9).

Birds

The trimming of birds' nails often requires two people, but using the owner to help with restraint is not ideal. Two nurses experienced in handling birds, or a veterinary surgeon and nurse working together, can clip the nails of even the largest birds appropriately. It is rarely necessary to clip the nails of a raptor, and this is perhaps best done with veterinary advice. It is also rarely necessary to clip the nails of a wild bird, especially if the individual is to be released.

- Prior to catching the bird, all doors and windows should be closed. For diurnal species, switching off the light so that the room is dark makes capture easier.

- Birds should be restrained as described in Chapter 1, being very careful not to compromise the movement of the chest (as this will stop the bird being able to breathe).
- Each nail can be clipped using appropriately sized nail clippers or, in the case of parrots, filed down using an electrical craft burr (e.g. Dremel).
- Should bleeding occur, this can be stopped by the application of a styptic pencil or wound powder. Any excess styptic should be rinsed off once bleeding has stopped.

Reptiles

- Larger chelonians may need sedation in order enable access to the claws. In such cases veterinary supervision is mandatory.
- The claws of larger specimens are best shortened using a craft burr.
- The claws of arboreal species should not be clipped unless absolutely necessary, as this will affect their ability to climb.
- Should bleeding occur it can be stopped by the application of a styptic pencil or wound powder.

Beak trimming

Beak trimming is often requested for both tortoises and birds. An overgrown beak may suggest that there is not enough opportunity for normal wear provided by the diet or environment, or that there is a medical problem (liver disease in birds) or physical problem (jaw misalignment), causing overgrowth.

Birds

Bird beaks can be trimmed/shaped using a craft drill. This procedure should only be undertaken by nurses that have been trained appropriately; otherwise the nurse should restrain the bird while the veterinary surgeon in charge of the case performs the procedure. If the bird has not been recently examined by a veterinary surgeon, or has evidence of a beak deformity such as 'scissor beak' (lower beak extends to one side and the upper beak to the opposite side), then involvement of the veterinary surgeon is required.

- The bird should be restrained as described in Chapter 1, making certain all doors and windows are shut prior to attempted capture; it is unwise to rely on an owner for restraint. In some cases a general anaesthetic may be advised.

- The beak should be trimmed so that it is symmetrical and a normal physiological length.
- On occasion, bleeding during beak trimming can occur, and this may be stopped as described above for claw clipping. Veterinary advice should be sought if bleeding occurs.

Tortoises

Tortoise beaks may be trimmed using sharp clippers or a craft drill. This procedure should only be undertaken by nurses that have been appropriately trained.

- The head of the tortoise is extended and held still, while the edges of the beak are shortened to a normal physiological length.
- Larger specimens or those that can fully retract their heads and close their shells (e.g. African spurred tortoise) may require sedation.

Routine dental checks

Incisor checks can easily be accomplished within a nurse-led clinic. The front teeth of small mammals (rabbits, guinea pigs, chinchillas, rats, hamsters, etc.) can be examined by gently pulling back the top lips. The nurse should look for length, symmetry, quality of visible enamel, and hair or food trapped.

Burring of the incisors is best undertaken with advice from the veterinary surgeon, as it is likely that the patient will also have underlying problems with the cheek teeth, which will not be resolved by reducing incisor length. Incisors should *never* be clipped using nail clippers.

Wing trimming

While wing trimming is a regularly requested procedure it should not be thought of as routine. Clients often have unrealistic expectations of wing trimming, and may request it inappropriately. The bird should be examined by a veterinary surgeon prior to considering a wing trim. It would be unwise for a veterinary nurse to undertake wing trimming without having a good familiarity with birds and prior training.

Checking or implanting microchips

Veterinary nurses may be asked to implant microchips in many less familiar species. The principles are the same as for cats and dogs. Common sites for microchip implantation are listed in Figure 11.1.

	British Veterinary Zoological Society	**Federation of Zoological Gardens of Great Britain and Ireland** [a]	**Conservation Breeding Specialist Group**
Small mammals	Between scapulae	Between scapulae	Between scapulae, left of centre
Birds	Left pectoral muscle	Left pectoral muscle or left thigh	Left pectoral muscle
Reptiles	Lizards: left quadriceps muscle or subcutaneously in this area Snakes: left nape of neck, twice the head length caudally from tip of nose Chelonians: subcutaneously in front of left hindleg, intramuscularly in thin-skinned species	Lizards and snakes: dorsal side of tail base Chelonians: left shoulder	Lizards: >12.5 cm left inguinal region; <12.5 cm in coelomic cavity Snakes: subcutaneously on left-hand side of body Chelonians: left hindlimb socket

11.1 Microchip implantation sites (from www.bvzs.org). [a] Now the British and Irish Association of Zoos and Aquariums.

Mammals

Mammals such as rabbits, ferrets, skunks and raccoons can have microchips implanted subcutaneously between the shoulder blades in the same way as a cat or dog.

Restraint is dependent on the species:

- Rabbits generally present no problems
- Ferrets should be held by a nurse using one hand as a brace around the neck (this is safer than scruffing) and the other to hold around the pelvis, allowing the implanter access to the back of the neck (Figure 11.2)
- Raccoons and skunks, and native wildlife may require sedation.

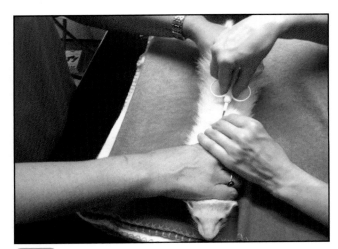

11.2 Restraint of a ferret for microchipping.

Birds

The microchip is implanted into the left breast muscle. Many birds require sedation/anaesthesia for this, and significant bleeding may occur after implantation, so this is a veterinary procedure.

Reptiles

Microchips can be placed in a variety of sites, depending on size and species. Some bleeding may occur after microchipping, and haemostasis can usually be achieved by applying pressure on the area.

Because reptile skin is less elastic than that of mammals or birds, tissue adhesive is often used to close the hole made by the microchip after implantation. Larger specimens, valuable specimens (where skin damage may affect their value) or those that are aggressive may require sedation prior to microchipping, and veterinary involvement is required.

Hibernation

Hibernation is a period of cooling required by many species of reptile in the wild (not just tortoises) to prepare them for breeding. Most species of non-tropical reptile undergo some form of hibernation. In captivity, while some keepers will cool down their snakes in order to prepare them for breeding, the most commonly hibernated animals are tortoises.

It is very important that the species has been correctly identified (see Chapter 4), as not all are suitable for hibernation. If identification is not certain, or if the animal is suspected to be of a tropical species, hibernation should not be attempted.

Common hibernating chelonians:

- Box turtle
- Hermann's tortoise
- Horsfield's tortoise
- Marginated tortoise
- Spur-thighed tortoise.

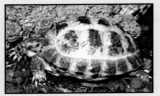

Horsfield's tortoise

Non-hibernating chelonians include:

- African spurred tortoise
- Hingeback tortoises
- Indian star tortoise
- Leopard tortoise
- Radiated tortoise
- Red-footed tortoise
- Yellow-footed tortoise.

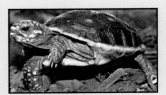

Red-footed tortoise

A physical examination should be performed prior to hibernation, as well as a faecal examination to check for the presence of gastrointestinal parasites. A parasite infestation can be fatal to the tortoise if present in the gastrointestinal tract during hibernation. Tortoises should be in good health with a good body condition (see below and Chapter 6 for ways to assess this.) Unwell, recovering or underweight tortoises should not be hibernated. It is advisable not to hibernate a tortoise until it is 2–3 years old and more than 200 g in weight, although a lot depends on the experience of the owner, and a very short period of hibernation might be considered (Mader, 2006).

Body condition assessment

General principles for assessing body condition in mammals, birds and reptiles are summarized in Figure 11.3. **These principles are not a substitute for accurate weighing on appropriate scales.** Chapter 6 provides more species-specific guidance regarding body condition scoring.

Mammals

Backbone:
- The dorsal spinous process should be palpable but not 'visible'.
- If the muscles on either side of the spine are concave and the processes easily appreciated, the animal is thin or underweight.
- If the muscles are convex and the spinous processes difficult to feel, the animal is overweight.

Ribs:
- The ribs should be able to be felt but not 'seen'.
- If ribs cannot be felt, the animal is likely to be overweight.
- If the outline of the ribs is visible, the animal is likely to be underweight.

Rump:
- Fat is stored over the rump in many species. The pelvic bones should be palpable but not 'visible'.

Birds

Keel muscles:
- The muscles on either side of the keel (sternum) can be used to assess body condition in most species of bird. The activity of the bird in question must, however, be remembered: birds that are active will have leaner pectoral muscles than those that are sedentary or not flown.
- If the keel is very prominent and the muscles on each side are concave, the bird is likely to be thin or underweight.
- If the muscle bellies are flush with the keel, the bird is in good body condition.
- If the pectoral muscles protrude above the level of the keel and the keel bone is difficult to feel, the bird is likely to be overweight.

Subcutaneous fat:
- Fat is laid down under the skin and can be 'visualized' in many species if the feathers are dampened down with water. Large amounts of subcutaneous fat indicate a bird in good to heavy body condition.

Reptiles

Lumbar musculature:
- The body condition of snakes may be assessed by feeling the lumbar muscles on each side of the dorsal spinous processes.
- Snakes in poor body condition will have prominent spinous processes and an almost triangular cross-section.
- In snakes that are overweight it may be difficult to palpate the spine, and the muscle groups on each side may form an almost heart-shaped cross-section.

Tail fat:
- In species that have tails, the amount of fat at the tail base can give an idea of the body condition. Geckos, in particular, store fat in the tail.
- Where body condition is good, the tail base will be plump and the pelvic bones difficult to 'see' or feel.
- Where body condition is poor, the tail base will be thin and bony, with the pelvic bones prominent.

Coelomic fat bodies:
- These are a mechanism for storing fat inside the body cavity and can be felt, with practice, in most lizards.
- In animals in poor body condition, the coelomic fat pads are reduced in size as the fat is used up.
- Animals that are overweight have large prominent coelomic fat pads.

Jackson's ratio:
- This is a calculation used to assess the bodyweight of Mediterranean spur-thighed tortoises and Hermann's tortoises. The straight carapace length is compared to the bodyweight to determine whether the individual tortoise is overweight, normal or underweight. Similar calculations have been used for other chelonian species; the calculations are species-specific and so must be used appropriately. The ratio should not be used in individuals with shell deformities. It is important to remember that there are medical conditions that can affect bodyweight, e.g. hepatic lipidosis and follicular stasis; this assessment tool should therefore only be used and interpreted with care.

11.3 Assessment of body condition in mammals, birds and reptiles. These are methods of first principle for evaluating the bodyweight of a wide variety of species. They are necessarily general and exceptions may occur. These principles are not a substitute for accurate weighing on appropriate scales. See Chapter 6 for further details on body condition scoring.

Lifestage considerations

Mammals

The average lifespan of a pet rabbit is 7–10 years. Ferrets can live 8–12 years, guinea pigs up to 9 years, and chinchillas up to 15 years. Common age-related changes seen in mammals are discussed in Figure 11.4, along with suggestions for treatments and supportive measures. **All these patients should be regularly checked by a veterinary surgeon.**

Birds

Life expectancy and key lifestages of psittacine birds are shown in Figure 11.5.

Significant physiological changes occur at puberty, related to egg production. Many female birds benefit from a moderate increase in calcium and vitamin D3 for egg shell formation and the prevention of post-ovulatory stasis (egg binding).

All species of bird become less active with advancing age (Figure 11.6), leaving them more

Condition	Species of mammal affected	Clinical signs and consequences	Veterinary treatments and lifestyle changes required
Renal failure	All	Polydipsia/polyuria; weight loss and possible attendant reduction in mobility, leading to pressure sores; reduced appetite; vomiting (ferrets)	Water intake should be monitored and supported (feeding wet food, spraying greens with water); fluid therapy may be required. Weight and appetite should be monitored regularly (the smaller the animal, the more frequently weight should be checked). Medications commonly used in other species can be used (e.g. phosphate binder, ACE inhibitors, anabolic steroids)
Congestive heart failure	All Rabbits: acquired valvular disease and various structural defects Guinea pigs: cardiomyopathy and pericardial effusion Chinchillas: acquired valvular defects Ferrets: acquired valvular disease and cardiomyopathy	Reduction in appetite; weight loss; reduction in mobility; inability to complete normal exercise tasks (including eating); open-mouth breathing; coughing. Guinea pigs in particular may develop dependent oedema	Drug treatment may include furosemide, pimobendan and ACE inhibitors. Patients presenting collapsed should be examined immediately by a veterinary surgeon. The animal should be placed in an oxygen tent and monitored constantly, until it is stabilized
Osteoarthritis	All	Reduction in mobility; lameness; inability to groom; inability to consume caecotrophs (rabbits) or faecal pellets (chinchillas and guinea pigs); increased aggression to owners and conspecifics.	NSAIDs often used for long-term pain relief. Supplements (e.g. glucosamine, chondroitin) may be helpful. Soft bedding and assistance grooming
Cataracts	All Rabbits: may be related to encephalitozoonosis Guinea pigs: may be hereditary or related to diabetes mellitus	Reluctance to move, bumping into objects in the environment; increased reliance on cage companions	Maintain a consistent environment and do not move objects or furniture around
Weight loss	All species	Reluctance or inability to move; pressure sores (decubital ulcers)	Cause of weight loss should be investigated by a veterinary surgeon. Supportive care, fluid therapy and assisted feeding (including within the home environment) may be helpful. Dietary modification may be required
Dental disease	Rabbits, guinea pigs, chinchillas: acquired dental disease Ferrets: periodontal disease	Drooling; weight loss and reluctance/inability to eat; masses around the face; pawing at face	Appropriate dentistry. Long-term pain relief may be required. Assisted feeding techniques should be demonstrated to owners and appropriate circumstances under which to use them should be discussed
Uterine adenocarcinoma	Rabbits	Abdominal enlargement; gut stasis; mammary cysts/growths; dyspnoea/open-mouth breathing	Surgical neutering should be discussed with owner at an early stage. Once disease has progressed, long-term outlook is poor. Palliative treatment (pain relief, assistance with grooming or eating caecotrophs) may be considered

11.4   Common age-related changes seen in mammals. Some of these conditions may arise in adulthood rather than in old age in some cases.

Species	Age at fledging	Age at weaning	Age at puberty	Age at sexual maturity	Life expectancy
Small (e.g. budgerigar, cockatiel)	3–4 weeks	6–11 weeks	4–6 months	1 year	Budgerigar: 9–11 years Cockatiel: 12–15 years
Medium-sized (e.g. African grey, Amazon parrots)	10–12 weeks	12–16 weeks	3–4 years	6–7 years	African grey: 50 years Amazons: up to 80 years
Large (e.g. macaws)	12–15 weeks	16–20 weeks	4–5 years	5–10 years (varies with species)	50 years

11.5   Lifestages of psittacine birds.

Problem	Consequences	Potential solutions
Reduced activity and mobility	More prone to obesity; atherosclerosis; pressure sores on feet; joint pain; dyspnoea due to increased fat in coelomic cavity; cardiac disease (hypertension)	Reduce cholesterol in diet; slight reduction in dietary sodium. Provide perches of differing widths to distribute weight pressure on feet; surgical and medical management of pressure sores; may require ongoing anti-inflammatory pain relief
Articular gout	Swollen, painful joints; secondary to poor renal function or acute dehydration. Secondary reduction in mobility	Slight reduction in dietary protein and phosphorus. Pain relief may be required. Allopurinol may reduce ongoing gout problems by reducing uric acid levels
Age-related cataracts	Poor eyesight can lead to an even more sedentary bird	
Arthritis	Pain can affect behaviour and appetite	NSAIDs
Tumours	Clinical signs will depend on site and type of tumour	Surgical excision if possible. Symptomatic treatment, including analgesia

11.6 Common problems that can affect older birds.

prone to obesity and the problems associated with this (e.g. atherosclerosis). As with other animals, aged birds can also have reduced organ function and reduced immunity to infection. As the captive geriatric population increases, with documentation of physical and behavioural changes, more knowledge will be gained to treat future generations of pet birds in old age.

Reptiles

The age at which reptiles reach maturity varies greatly, as maturity is linked more to size than age. Growth and size are influenced by many factors, including temperature, diet and environment. Sexual maturity may coincide with behavioural changes, which may have serious consequences for owners and handlers, particularly in the case of offensive aggression in male iguanas (see later).

Reptiles either lay eggs (oviparous) or bear live young. Those bearing live young may be ovoviviparous, where some degree of egg production occurs in the oviduct and the egg hatches before delivery, or viviparous, where a placenta-like membrane provides some nutrition to the developing embryo (see Chapter 4).

Many female animals will produce eggs seasonally, regardless of whether a male is present or not. Suitable conditions should be provided for laying in this situation; often a hide box with damp substrate (e.g. sand or vermiculite) is appreciated. However, specific requirements may vary. Female reptiles often reduce their food intake or stop eating in the later stages of pregnancy (or gravidity), with viviparous species fasting for longer periods than oviparous species.

Owners should watch for subtle changes in behaviour, appetite, weight, mobility and reproduction that could indicate the onset of old age.

Annual veterinary checks and blood tests should be recommended from maturity onwards. Older reptiles may show signs of renal disease, articular or visceral gout and tumours. Changes could be secondary to other disease processes or may follow long-term dietary or environmental deficiencies.

Hand-rearing

Requests for information on hand-rearing of various species are fairly common. The goals of hand-rearing are similar, independent of the species involved.

- Hand-rearing is not ideal; it should be viewed as a last resort if parental rearing is not possible.
- Animals being hand-reared should be provided with suitable nutrition at suitable intervals to allow normal growth and development.
- Hand-rearing should be undertaken in such a way that animals do not become imprinted on human carers.
- Many animals are better cared for in a rehabilitation situation and not in a veterinary practice. Early transfer to a wildlife rehabilitation centre is strongly recommended.

Mammals

Rabbits

Rabbits are altricial (born with little fur and closed eyes, requiring maternal care) and hand-rearing of kits is often unsuccessful. The younger the kits are when hand-rearing starts, the poorer the chance of success. Rabbit kits are usually only fed by the doe for approximately 5–10 minutes, once or twice a day. They emerge from the nest at around 18 days, usually start to nibble grass or hay at 3 weeks, and are fully weaned at around 25 days.

It is very important to determine whether the kits have been truly abandoned before attempting hand-rearing. It is also worth trying to hold the doe and place the kits to her teats to encourage feeding, although the doe's milk may dry up if she finds this stressful. Ideally, newly orphaned kits should be placed with another litter born around the same time and the new doe encouraged to accept them as her own. Rescue centres may be able to help in finding a new mother.

Rabbit milk contains 13–15% protein, 10–12% fat and 2% carbohydrate. This can be difficult to replicate. Some examples of rabbit milk replacer products are shown in Figure 11.7. Homemade formulas may

Product examples	Protein content	Fat content	Fibre content	Salt (sodium) content
Cimicat (Petlife International)	33%	22%	0%	0.4%
Lactol Puppy Milk (Sherley's, Beaphar)	24% (crude)	24% oils and fats	0%	0.5%
Esbilac (Pet Ag Inc)	35% (minimum, crude)	40% (minimum, crude)	0%	No information
Wombaroo Rabbit Milk Replacer (Wombaroo Food Products Australia)	37% (minimum, crude)	42% (minimum, crude)	0%	0.8% maximum

11.7 Examples of rabbit milk replacers.

also be used (e.g. one part evaporated milk to one part water (boiled then cooled), with one egg yolk and one tablespoon of cornstarch added to each cup of mixture). Use of a probiotic (e.g. Avipro, Vetark) or feeding of caecotrophs from other healthy rabbits is recommended to allow the gut to be colonized by suitable bacteria. Good hygiene is vitally important to avoid the gut being overrun with pathogenic bacteria; all equipment should be kept clean, and the formula should be made up freshly for each feed.

- Kits should be fed three or four times a day. Care should be taken to avoid aspiration pneumonia, which is a common cause of fatality in young kits. The best way to achieve this is to feed small volumes and then allow swallowing. Baby rabbits will nurse from the mother on their backs, so this is an appropriate position in which to feed them.
- Rabbits are usually completely reliant on the doe's milk for the first 21 days. They can be encouraged to nibble hay or freeze-dried grass at 3 weeks. Greens should be introduced with care at 4 weeks, offering thumbnail-sized pieces only for the first few feeds and increasing very gradually to prevent enterotoxaemia, which can result in fatal diarrhoea. Milk feeds should be continued until kits are fully weaned, at between 5 and 8 weeks of age.

As with puppies and kittens, rabbit kits should be encouraged to urinate and defecate by wiping the perineal area with a damp cloth. All kits should be weighed daily throughout the hand-rearing process, and those either failing to gain or losing weight should be examined by a veterinary surgeon.

Ferrets

Baby ferrets (kits) are born with little fur and closed eyes. They are reliant on maternal care for the first 4 weeks of life. Kits can be fostered on to a new mother successfully, preferably one with kits of approximately the same age. It is wise to mix the new kits with the existing ones and to make certain the scent of the mother is on the new kit, by rubbing some bedding over its body.

Should hand-rearing be required, kitten or puppy milk replacer can form the basis of the diet.

Ferret milk contains 34% fat and 26% protein. This is a much higher fat content than puppy or kitten milk, so one additional egg yolk can be added to each 250 ml of the replacer to increase the fat content. NB The egg yolk is not cooked and therefore the milk cannot be stored.

- Ferret kits should be fed every 2 hours for the first 2 weeks, slowly increasing the volume at each feed. When the kit has had enough milk it will usually appear very sleepy and will slow down its sucking dramatically.
- By 14 days of age, the volume at each feed should be enough to allow less frequent feeding and by 21 days, when solid foods can be introduced, the feeding should be approximately four times a day, evenly spaced out.
- Suitable solid feeds to introduce include proprietary dry ferret diets, kitten food and minced up fresh meat.

Kits should be stimulated to 'toilet' by gently rubbing the perineal area with a moistened cotton bud or cloth. All kits should be weighed daily throughout hand-rearing and if they are failing to gain weight, or are losing weight, they should be examined by a veterinary surgeon.

Wild mammals

It is very important to transfer orphaned wildlife to a rehabilitation centre as soon as possible after discovery. Hand-rearing juvenile wild animals can result in individuals losing their fear of humans and being unable to be returned to the wild. For short periods, while transfer is being arranged, foxes, badgers and otters can be reared on puppy or kitten milk replacer. Toiletting should be stimulated by rubbing the perineum with a moistened cotton bud or a damp cloth.

If kept in captivity for longer periods, otter cubs will need a more specialized milk. Otter milk is very high in fat and protein but very low in lactose. The following recipe is suggested:

- 1 part Esbilac
- 2 parts water
- 1 part Multimilk
- 1 part whipping cream
- With cod liver oil and Mazuri fisheater tablets.

Birds

Psittacine birds

Hand-rearing of chicks may be required:

- If the parents are not able to rear the chicks or are ignoring a chick
- To allow parent birds to breed again; in this case it is preferable to leave chicks with their parents until their eyes start to open before removing them for hand-rearing.

The brooder

The brooder in which the chick is to be kept for the first 3 weeks or so should be constructed from materials that are easy to clean and disinfect. It should have a thermostat and thermometer. The substrate on the bottom should be easy to change/clean, absorbent and non-slip (to prevent 'splay leg' and other developmental abnormalities); good examples include paper-based cat litter, kitchen towel and soft towels.

Most newly hatched parrot chicks should be kept in an incubator/brooder at 35–37°C for the first 7 days, at 33–34°C for the next 7 days, and the temperature then reduced to 32°C. Exact requirements will vary according to breed, size and number of chicks in the brooder.

Once the pin feathers are unfurling and the chick has a good covering of down, it can be taken from the brooder and kept at an ambient temperature of 22–25°C in a suitable container (e.g. a clean plastic box, without a lid, containing the same substrate as the brooder). Areas for hiding, darkness and privacy should be provided, as well as toys, etc., for mental and emotional stimulation. Many psychological and physical needs must be addressed and met during the development of the neonate (see Further reading).

Feeding

Feeding on demand is best for proper physical and psychological development but the following guidelines can be applied.

Feeding guidelines for psittacine chicks

- 0–7 days: six to eight meals per day (usually over around 17 hours; it should only be necessary to feed weak chicks overnight).
- 7–14 days: four to six meals per day.
- After 14 days: three to four meals per day until fully weaned.

The very young and the smaller species will require the most frequent feeding, as it is preferable to feed smaller meals more frequently than to overfill the crop. It should normally take around 4 hours for the crop to empty. However, this may be affected by factors such as food consistency or illness and so should be closely monitored; it should not necessarily be a time guide for frequency of feeds.

Hand-rearing formulas are available for most psittacine species; some examples are given in Figure 11.8. A fresh mixture should be made up for each feed, using boiled and cooled water, according to the manufacturer's instructions.

- The ratio of solids to water will typically be around 1:3. It is vital to achieve the correct consistency: if the food is too runny the chick will be hungry and gain weight poorly; if the food is too thick this can result in delayed crop emptying with a thick residue, which may lead to bacterial infection ('sour crop').
- The ideal temperature for the feed is around 41°C. Food <37°C may be rejected by the chick as too cold. Food >43°C can cause crop burns.
- Feeds can be administered by spoon, syringe or a crop tube. Syringe-feeding poses the greatest risk of aspiration; tube feeding carries least risk if carried out by trained personnel.

Chicks should be weighed daily, first thing in the morning before feeds commence. A guideline for weight gain is around 1–2 g/day (species-dependent)

Product	Nutrients	Suitable for
Harrison's (Bird Foods UK) Neonate Formula	Protein 26% minimum Fat 14% minimum Fibre 0% minimum Moisture 10% minimum	Parrots: hatching to 7 days Cockatiels: hatching to 21 days Passerine birds: hatching to weaning
Harrison's (Bird Foods UK) Juvenile Hand Feeding Formula	Protein 18% minimum Fat 11% minimum Fibre 4% minimum Moisture 10% minimum	Macaws, cockatoos, African grey parrots, Amazons, conures, pionus: from day 1 Cockatiels: 21 days to weaning Other parrots: 7 days to weaning
Kaytee Exact Hand Feeding Baby Bird	Crude protein 22% minimum Crude fat 9% minimum Fibre 5% maximum Moisture 10% maximum	Formulated for all baby birds
PrettyBird (International, Inc)	All 10% maximum moisture	
	19/8: Protein 19%; Fat 8%	Lories, cockatoos, most Amazons
	19/12: Protein 19%, Fat 12%	African grey, macaws, pionus, conures, cockatiels, lovebirds
	22/10: Protein 22%; Fat 10%	African grey, eclectus, Asian parakeets

11.8   Examples of some popular hand-rearing formulas available for psittacine bird species.

until around day 10, when weight gain should increase (by as much as 10–20 g/day in larger species at peak growth).

Weaning

Weaning should begin when chicks start to explore their surroundings and look for food. A small amount of a variety of foods should be offered 'buffet style' for the chick to try. Around three different types of soft vegetables should be included, such as squash, sweet potato, broccoli, grated/cooked carrot or parsnip (no added salt), with softened pellets and a few pulses. A very limited amount of seeds and nuts can also be given but should be stopped after weaning. As more solid foods are taken, the frequency of hand-feeding should gradually decrease, while weight is closely monitored. It is not unusual for some weight loss to occur during the early stages of weaning.

Garden birds

- Most of the garden birds presented will be passerine species. A sample client handout on hand-rearing such garden birds can be found at the end of this chapter.
- Should any unusual species be presented, they should be identified and information sought regarding correct hand-rearing techniques.

It must be emphasized that most baby birds that appear to have been abandoned have not actually been so, and their parents will be around somewhere watching them. In an ideal situation these baby birds should be returned to the nest, or placed in a suitable container (e.g. a small clean plastic box) which can then be placed in such a position (e.g. within the branches of a tree) that the chick is safe from predation but accessible to its parents. Chicks in this situation should be watched for several hours before confirming there is no parental contact and removing them for hand-rearing.

All passerine birds eat grains and insects. They produce altricial (nidifugous) young, i.e. chicks are born bald and require significant maternal care. The breeding strategy of most passerine birds is to produce enough young to support a high mortality rate. This means that in normal circumstances many juveniles die each year. Chicks that present without full feather cover will still be dependent on parental care.

For seed- and insect-eating species (e.g. tits, dunnocks, sparrows and finches) commercial soft-bill or insectivore diets complemented by small-seed mixes may be used for hand-rearing.

Food can be offered from above the head to trigger a gaping response, using blunt forceps or a thin blunt spatula. Chicks should be fed until the crop is full; this can be easily assessed visually, or by palpation if feathers have developed. They should not be fed again until the crop is empty or nearly empty. Some chicks will continue to gape for food even though the crop is full, risking overfeeding.

All chicks should be weighed daily and weight gain documented.

Feeding guidelines for passerine chicks

- Very young chicks (1–4 days old) require very regular feeding, every 15 minutes for at least 12 hours (matching the hours of daylight during which they would be fed in the wild).
- From day 4 onwards, the frequency of feeding can be reduced to every 30–60 minutes and self-feeding should be encouraged.
- By day 14 feeding should be every 2–3 hours.
- Full self-feeding should be achieved by around 28 days.

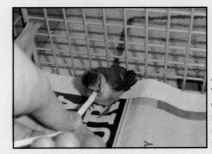

A baby blue tit being fed chopped mealworms. (Courtesy of Sarah Flack)

Raptors

In the wild, raptor chicks are parent-reared and only the strongest and most dominant chicks survive. Hand-rearing an orphaned wild raptor is a specialized endeavour and attempts to locate a suitable rehabilitation centre should be made.

It is crucial to provide correct nutrition to raptor chicks in order to promote healthy growth. The food offered should be digestible and contain sufficient protein, energy and nutrients for growth. The nutritional needs of chicks vary with age.

Newly hatched chicks will often beg for food within 8–12 hours of hatching. The yolk sac will continue to be resorbed over the first 48 hours of life; however, feeding should begin straight away. Fresh muscle meat from day-old chicks (fresh or thawed) is a suitable food and should be offered using forceps. Chicks should only be fed when the crop is empty, which can be assessed visually or by gentle palpation. Each chick should be weighed daily and should be gaining weight daily.

- From 2–3 days of age, muscle meat or portions of 'pinkie' mice can be given four to six times per day, as soon as the crop is empty (Figure 11.9). At this stage, a balanced avian vitamin and calcium supplement should also be added to the diet (e.g. Nutrobal, Vetark) to avoid nutritional osteodystrophy.
- By the end of the first week, raptor chicks can be offered cut-up portions of whole chicks (i.e. not just muscle meat) and they may be able to self-feed from a dish.
- At 14 days, chicks should be self-feeding from a dish.
- Fledging times vary depending on the species but, in general, fledging has usually occurred by 5–6 weeks of age.

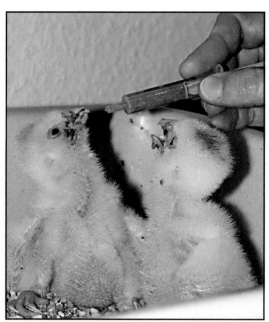

11.9 Minced day-old rats can be fed to raptor chicks using a syringe. The amount of food can easily be adjusted for each bird. Food remnants should be removed. (© Michael Lierz)

Reptiles

Most reptiles are born fully independent, with no assistance provided by the parents after hatching (i.e. they are precocial). Most problems encountered when rearing reptiles are due to inappropriate feeding or environmental conditions, combined with the very small size of young, whose condition can change rapidly.

Vaccination

Mammals

Vaccinations available and protocols for commonly seen small mammals are given in Figure 11.10.

Neutering

Mammals

Rabbits

Neutering of both male and female rabbits is strongly recommended. Surgical neutering of females is undertaken from 4 months of age, depending on the size and maturity of the individual. Some authors feel that neutering after puberty has occurred is preferable; however, the author (MV) has found that neutering younger females is much less technically difficult and results in smaller surgical wounds and more rapid healing. It is not known whether neutering rabbits prepubertally will result in an increased incidence of adrenal disease. Female rabbits that remain un-neutered are at significant risk of developing uterine adenocarcinoma as they age. Indeed, a high proportion of intact females will display pre-cancerous changes in their uterus at 2 years of age.

Male rabbits are neutered from 4 months of age, as long as the testes have descended.

Ferrets

Neutering can reduce the scent of males, reduce hormone-related aggression and prevent unwanted pregnancies. Where multiple ferrets are kept together, keeping a vasectomized male with intact females is

Species	Vaccination	Age of animal at first vaccination	Frequency
Rabbits	Combined myxomatosis/VHD	From 6 weeks	Every 12 months
	Viral haemorrhagic disease (VHD)	From 5 weeks. There is some maternal immunity but kits are susceptible from 6–8 weeks	Every 12 months
	Myxomatosis: there is currently no authorized myxomatosis-only vaccine in the UK		
Ferrets	Canine distemper	8 weeks	At 8 and 12 weeks, then annually
	Rabies	4 months	Annually; check requirements with Defra if required for a Pet Passport
Raccoons	Canine distemper	8 weeks; boosters at 12 and 16 weeks	Annually
	Feline panleucopenia (FIE)	8 weeks; boosters at 12 and 16 weeks	Annually
	Rabies	4 months	Varies
Skunks	Canine distemper	8 weeks	Annually
	Rabies	8 weeks	Varies

11.10 Vaccinations available and protocols for commonly seen small mammals.

a management option; although this may not be suitable for pets and show animals, this system allows non-fertile matings to occur, which bring cycling females out of oestrus.

Surgical neutering

In the female (jill), neutering has historically been recommended to prevent fatal post-ovulatory anaemia (POA), which occurs if a jill is unmated during a season. However, research has linked surgical neutering to increased incidences of ferret adrenal disease: although most common in middle-aged or older ferrets, adrenal disease can also be seen in neutered ferrets under 1 year old. Elevated oestradiol and other sex hormones produced by the adrenal gland cause the clinical signs, which include: hair loss, sometimes with pruritus; a swollen vulva; thin dry skin; a distended abdomen; muscle atrophy; and hindlimb weakness.

The male (hob) may develop prostatic cysts and acute urinary retention after castration as a consequence of adrenal disease.

Hormone implants

Implants of a gonadotrophin-releasing hormone (GnRH) agonist, such as deslorelin, may be used as an alternative to surgical neutering. Deslorelin is a slow-release formulation (lasts around 24 months), which can also be used in surgically neutered ferrets as a preventive measure against adrenal disease. The implant is most effective if fitted during the winter non-breeding season (November to March in the northern hemisphere), starting from the first winter after 6 months of age. The implant is fitted under anaesthesia and is placed subcutaneously between the shoulder blades. The jill may develop some vulval swelling and signs of oestrus around 4 days after implantation, lasting up to 2 weeks.

Rodents

On occasion owners may request that chinchillas or guinea pigs are neutered in order to simplify keeping groups of animals. Surgically it is much easier to neuter males, and this is associated with a much lower complication rate. In all cases the males should be old enough to have descended testes (this can be confirmed by palpation). Males should be kept separate from females of breeding age for 1 month after neutering.

Female guinea pigs may require neutering for medical reasons, such as the development of large ovarian cysts. These patients should be examined by a veterinary surgeon.

Skunks and raccoons

Animals such as skunks and raccoons may be neutered when kept in captivity. Much less is known about the optimum time to do this and the consequences of doing it too early or too late. This uncertainty must be made clear to an owner when discussing neutering of these species. It is preferable to refer owners for a veterinary consultation, where all the possible issues can be discussed in detail.

Wild mammals

In most cases there are no indications for neutering wildlife species, and specialist advice should be sought prior to considering neutering as an option.

Practical dietary advice and weight management

The provision of a poor diet is by far the most important cause of disease in exotic pets. It is useful for a veterinary nurse to be familiar with suitable diets and with strategies for dietary change, and to possess resources for the acquisition of dietary items and information. Specific information on normal dietary requirements of various species may be found later in this chapter and also in Chapters 2, 3, 4 and 5.

Selective eating can be a significant problem and can allow nutritional deficiencies to occur, even when a balanced diet is offered. This is especially true when the diet offered is made up of a variety of ingredients, as not all ingredients will be eaten and the diet will therefore not be balanced. One easy way around this, which is applicable to most species, is to feed a good quality monocomponent feed as the basis of the diet (pelleted diets are now available for most species), and supplement this with natural or favourite food items. This at least ensures that most of the nutritional needs are met. In the longer term, dietary advice can be refined and tailored to the owner's situation.

Different ways of presenting food can encourage exotic pets and wild animals in captivity to show natural behaviours when searching for and prehending food items. Foraging for food is a behaviour that takes up many hours a day in the wild. This can be replicated in captivity using a number of techniques, including scatter feeding and puzzles.

Food as environmental enrichment

Most animals in the wild spend a significant amount of their time searching for and then eating food. In a captive situation food is provided, usually in a bowl, and the time spent eating it is minimal. The rest of the time that would have been spent looking for food is now unoccupied; for intelligent animals such as parrots, boredom can cause significant clinical problems. The way food is presented can go some way towards alleviating this problem. There are several strategies that can be employed:

- Scatter feeding: spreading small pieces of food through the substrate, making the animal work to find them
- 'Treat wraps': small treat foods wrapped in pieces of paper (not newspaper) or placed in small cardboard boxes so that these must be found and retrieved
- Forage perches: small holes are drilled into a perch, into which food items can be pushed
- Wrapping a bird's food bowl in paper or cardboard that it can rip open in order to feed.

For all species, provision of water is a basic requirement. It is also important to consider the method of provision and the quality of the water. For example, chameleons drink only from water droplets on leaves and so water must be provided in this manner, either by using a waterfall or drip system or by misting plants within the enclosure.

Mammals

Rabbits

Further information on diet for healthy rabbits is given in Chapter 5.

Fibre

Fibre is essential both for normal tooth wear and for promoting gut motility. An ideal diet would therefore comprise 85% grass (including hay) and 15% leafy greens. Providing *ad libitum* hay, with a small amount of good quality pelleted food (approximately a tablespoonful per day) and fresh vegetables, is a more practical alternative. Commercially cultivated vegetables do not provide the same nutritional content as those found in the wild; home-grown vegetables and weeds are therefore preferable, although pelleted food will provide the vitamins, minerals and fibre that may be lacking in cultivated vegetables, as well as improving owner compliance and ease of feeding.

Importance of dietary fibre to rabbits

Indigestible fibre:

- Is essential for normal gut motility
- Promotes normal tooth occlusion (due to silicates)
- Decreases food retention in the caecum, which could affect normal gut flora and encourage an increase in pathogenic bacteria
- Decreases the risk of trichobezoars (hairballs)
- Has no nutritional value.

Digestible (fermentable) fibre:
- Provides a substrate for microflora in the caecum
- Gives caecotrophs a firmer consistency
- Provides optimal pH and volatile fatty acid production in the caecum.

Carbohydrates

Carbohydrates appear to be digested more efficiently by older rabbits than by young rabbits. A high-carbohydrate low-fibre diet has been linked with enterotoxaemia in susceptible rabbits that have been recently weaned.

Calcium

Calcium in the diet is important for bone calcification, and a constant source is necessary for the continual growth of teeth. Calcium absorption is controlled by parathyroid hormone. In rabbits, unlike other mammals, this absorption is directly related to the amount of calcium in the diet and is not limited to the requirements at the time. The main route for calcium excretion is the kidneys. Too much calcium in the diet can cause urine sludging, urolithiasis and renal mineralization. Alfalfa hay is very high in calcium, containing around three times the amount found in grass hays (e.g. Timothy or oat), and so the feeding of this should be restricted. Intake of alfalfa-rich pelleted diets should also be reduced. Calcium-rich greens such as kale, spinach and spring greens form a very valuable part of the diet and so should not be excluded, but should be fed in moderation. If calcium reduction is required, suitable greens should be offered such as broccoli, celery leaf, Brussels sprouts and dandelions. Greens can be sprayed with water prior to feeding, as increased water intake is necessary to help prevent urine sludging.

Water

Fresh water should be available to all animals at all times. During periods of very hot weather, water bowls and bottles should be checked at least twice daily as consumption may increase. During periods of cold weather, the nozzles of water bottles may freeze, making water unavailable, even if the bottle appears to be full. Water bottles should therefore also be checked twice daily in very cold weather. Changes in water intake should be noted and reported to the veterinary surgeon in charge of the particular patient.

Weight management

Average normal weights for common rabbit breeds are given in Figure 11.11. Obesity has a number of detrimental effects on health (Figure 11.12) and a weight management programme may be required.

It can be difficult to reduce calorie intake in rabbits as they are so efficient at dealing with seemingly indigestible food matter. Because the microflora in the caecum breaks down fibre to fatty acids and fat, only the least digestible fibre (e.g. hay and very tough vegetation) will pass through the gut unchanged and help with weight loss (Harcourt-Brown, 2002). The most effective diet for weight reduction would therefore be grass or hay plus water, with small quantities (15% of total diet) of fibrous green vegetables offered as a treat. Rabbits should be weaned off pellet/cereal mix diets gradually, while increasing the amount of grass, hay and fibrous vegetables provided, aiming to cut out all pellets from 2 weeks. This may take longer to achieve depending on the individual's response to change.

Rabbit breed	Average adult weight
Beveran	3.5–5.5 kg
Dutch	1.6–2.5 kg
Flemish giant	10 kg or more
Himalayan	1–2 kg
Lops	Mini: 1.5 kg; dwarf 2.5 kg; French: 5 kg
Netherland dwarf	Approximately 1.1 kg
New Zealand white	Approximately 5 kg
Rex	3–4.5 kg

11.11 Rabbit breed-specific normal average weights.

Effect of obesity	Consequences
Inability to reach anus to eat caecotrophs	Reduced absorption of important nutrients; build-up of caecotrophs around the perineum, leading to skin infections and possibly fly strike
Excessive dewlap and skin folds around perineum	Urine scalding and skin fold dermatitis/pyoderma
Increased work on cardiovascular system	Hypertension and cardiac hypertrophy
Reduced exercise	Less calorie expenditure; more weight gain
Increased pressure on bony protuberances and joints	Pressure sores and exacerbation of arthritis, especially in older rabbits
Inability to groom effectively	Increase in population of *Cheyletiella yasguri* mites or other external parasites to a degree that causes clinical signs

11.12 Effects of obesity on the health of rabbits.

Rabbits should be weighed weekly during a weight loss programme. There is a serious risk of hepatic lipidosis if an obese rabbit has a period of reduced food intake or loses weight too quickly. It is therefore of vital importance to monitor actual amounts of food consumed and to perform regular weight checks. Close monitoring of droppings produced (i.e. size and numbers) can also be an indicator of food intake, as reduced intake will result in reduced gut motility – another important factor to take into account when considering a weight reduction diet. Weight loss should be gradual, with a reduction in bodyweight of no more than 1.5% per week.

Ferrets

Ferrets require an all-meat high-protein diet. They need highly digestible food due to their rapid gut transit time (approximately 4 hours). They are commonly fed commercial pelleted ferret food, which is well balanced and has a suitable protein content. Kitten food can be used as part of a balanced diet, as long as high-protein items such as chicken wings, chicks or eggs are also offered. It should be emphasized that kitten food is not high enough in protein and contains too much carbohydrate to be a suitable diet alone or for the long term. Cat and dog food should be avoided, as should treats that are high in carbohydrates or sugars.

Obesity is more common in ferrets housed in cages, due to lack of exercise. Obesity may also be

Approximate normal weight ranges for ferrets:

- Adult male (hob): 1–2 kg
- Adult female (jill): 0.5–1 kg.

There is a natural weight gain during the winter non-breeding season (particularly in the hob) of up to 30%.

due to leaving food (especially dried biscuits) with the ferret all day or offering high-calorie treats. Exercise should be increased by allowing the ferret to spend more time out of the cage or by using a harness and lead to walk the ferret outdoors. The owner should concentrate on feeding the higher protein components of the diet, cutting out biscuits or other high-carbohydrate items.

Birds

Psittacine birds

Several nutritionally complete parrot diets are commercially available, in the form of a muesli-type mix or as pellets. These diets are designed either as a base to which fresh foods suitable for the specific species may be added, or are formulated for an individual species/group. Ther e are also several commercial nectar-based diets available for birds such as lories and lorikeets.

In spite of the availability of such diets, most parrots in the UK are given a seed-based diet that is unlike what they would eat in the wild. Seeds are high in fat and are nutritionally imbalanced; they lack calcium, vitamin A, zinc and chromium. In many cases these birds do not receive additional vitamin or mineral supplementation. Calcium deficiency, hypovitaminosis A and obesity are therefore all relatively common (and preventable) nutritional diseases seen in pet parrots. Other items must be added to a seed-based diet in order for it to become more balanced; although even if a wide variety of foods, including pulses, fruits, vegetables and seeds, is offered, this only provides a balanced diet if everything is consumed. When given the choice, birds will often pick out their favourite foods, usually selecting those high in fat but low in vitamins and minerals. Offering a monocomponent diet avoids selective eating; monocomponent diets are made from ingredients that are bound together and formulated to produce a nutritionally balanced diet in a pellet or biscuit form. Common components of parrot diets are summarized in Figure 11.13.

Converting parrots from a seed-based to a pellet-based diet

A bird that has always received a seed-based diet may initially show reluctance to change and so will require some degree of patience and enthusiasm from the owner. Parrots are neophobic (afraid of new things or experiences) and this contributes to the difficulty encountered when persuading them to try new foods. It should be stressed that the process of conversion could take as little as a few days but it can take weeks, or even months, to achieve.

Due to their high metabolism, birds must eat frequently throughout the day and they can become seriously weak in just 24 hours if not eating. When converting a parrot to a pellet diet, it is therefore very important to observe it carefully in order to check that the pellets are being eaten. The bird should ideally be weighed every couple of days to check that bodyweight is being maintained. As they may refuse even to try a novel food placed in their cage

Food type	Examples	Comments
Seeds	Millet, sunflower, safflower, hemp, sesame, rape, linseed	High in fat and low in calcium. Do not form a major portion of the diet for many types of psittacine bird in the wild. They should be kept in an air-tight container and checked for dust and moulds
Vegetables	Carrots, peppers, celery, pumpkin, sweet potato, squash, courgette, salad greens, kale, spring greens, broccoli, beans	Higher nutritional value than fruits. Vividly coloured green, red or yellow vegetables should be offered on a daily basis. Most vegetables can be offered either raw or cooked and in a variety of methods of presentation (whole, sliced, chopped, shredded, etc.)
Legumes/ sprouts	Peas, beans, commercial or home-produced seed sprouts	Sprouts are a good way to maximize the nutritional value of pulses. Care must, however, be taken as they will rapidly deteriorate when left at room temperature and commercially produced sprouts may carry *Salmonella*; they should therefore always be thoroughly washed prior to feeding and only left in the food bowl for a few hours if not eaten immediately
Fruits	Apples, pears, berries, citrus fruit (in moderation), bananas, pomegranate, grapes, kiwifruit, mango, papaya, guava, figs	Fruits are generally high in sugar and low in minerals and vitamins, so should be viewed as a treat food in most species. Eclectus and lories are exceptions to this rule; fruit and sugary nectar form a portion of their diet in the wild and therefore should be provided as part of the regular diet
Items of animal origin	Chicken bones, cuttlefish, meat and dairy products	Many owners feed cooked chicken bones to their parrots without problems and feel that they are a good source of calcium. However, chicken bones pose a risk of gastrointestinal perforation if they splinter during consumption, and the availability of the calcium within these bones is variable at best. Meat and dairy products are not a part of the natural diet of most parrot species so it is difficult to recommend their inclusion in a balanced diet, especially where the nutritional requirements of parrots can be fulfilled in other ways (there are many suitable commercial alternatives)
Grains	Oats, corn, wheat	Can be very high in carbohydrate. Caution is required as they may swell after feeding
Nuts	Peanuts, hazelnuts, Brazil nuts, almonds	High in fat, though are often part of the natural diet in species such as macaws. Nuts can harbour moulds such as *Aspergillus* spp., which can cause both infection and toxicity. Human-grade nuts should be offered and should be checked for moulds prior to feeding. Offering unshelled nuts can form part of a nutritional environmental enrichment programme

11.13 Common components of parrot diets.

or enclosure if they don't recognize it as food, it is vitally important that any bird showing no interest in a new diet is also given an opportunity to eat its usual diet. Pellets and seeds should not, however, be mixed in the same bowl as this can lead to selective eating, with the bird simply ignoring or discarding the pellets. Fruits and vegetables should also be offered as treats, to provide some nutritional supplementation as well as psychological and environmental enrichment. Given that some pellet diets are seed-based, the key components of a new diet must be checked.

If the bird's droppings become scant or dark green or black, this can be an indication that it is not eating sufficient amounts. However, it is quite common for droppings to change colour or consistency due to a new diet. This is normal, but owners should be advised to contact the practice if this is prolonged or they become concerned.

Weight management

Obesity is usually due to a high-fat, often seed-based diet and limited exercise. It should be noted that some species (e.g. Amazons, pionus) are more prone to obesity and high blood cholesterol, and that species such as the hyacinth macaw have a diet naturally higher in fat in the wild.

In obese animals, fat may be visible under the skin and the pectoral muscles will bulge past the level of the keel (see earlier). Overweight birds may display heat intolerance and reduced mobility.

> ### Obesity can lead to:
> - Hepatic lipidosis – fatty infiltration of hepatocytes; occurs especially after a period of inappetence in the obese bird. Bird shows clinical signs of liver disease including yellow/ green urates, possibly ascites and dyspnoea
> - Atherosclerosis – thickening of major arteries with cholesterol deposits; may lead to secondary renal failure
> - Dyspnoea – air sacs are restricted by excess fat
> - Lipomas
> - Calluses and pressure sores on feet
> - Reduced mobility.

Weight loss in birds can be achieved using the following advice:

- The amount and availability of seed in the diet should be reduced, and pulses and vegetables offered instead
- The bird should ideally be converted on to a pelleted diet (NB the key components of the

pelleted diet must be checked, as some are seed-based), supplemented with vegetables and fruit (see earlier)
- The bird should be weighed regularly, using the same scales each time
- Care must be taken with any change in diet to ensure that the bird is eating. Birds have a high metabolism and need a regular calorie intake; hepatic lipidosis would be a risk if a bird failed to eat
- The bird should be allowed to spend more time out of the cage if possible
- Other forms of enrichment for play should be provided to expend energy and to focus attention away from food, e.g. an Amazon parrot may spend a long time tearing up a telephone directory.

Raptors

Most raptors are fed whole vertebrate prey animals (fresh or frozen then thawed). These include day-old chicks, quails, turkey poults and, occasionally, rodents or rabbits. The younger the frozen chicks are, the lower their nutritional value will be and the higher the cholesterol content (from the yolk sacs). If a bird is to be fed very young chicks in the long term, the yolk sacs should first be removed. A diet of only muscle meat will be significantly deficient in calcium and may lead to rickets and pathological fractures. Growing birds may benefit from a commercial vitamin and mineral supplement placed inside the chicks on a regular basis. Commercially produced foods are likely to be free from disease and lead shot, whereas fresh food that the animal has taken in the hunt can be a source of lead shot, trichomoniasis, candidiasis, aspergillosis and other infections. It is therefore sensible to check freshly caught prey for signs of disease before allowing this to be eaten.

Reptiles

Common dietary items fed to reptiles are given in Figure 11.14 (see also Chapter 4). Many pet shops sell formulated pellet diets for a variety of reptile species. These are useful to provide the basis of the diet and can then be supplemented by fresh food to provide interest. However, many animals do not eat these pellets and some species require movement to stimulate feeding behaviours. In many cases, a dietary supplement is sensible to avoid nutritional deficiencies. Vitamin and mineral powders added to fresh vegetables are usually well accepted; however, some of the powder may fall off prior to eating. Supplement powders 'dusted' on to live food often falls off before the reptile eats it, so is of limited use as the only supplementation. Feeding or 'gut loading' of insect prey with a vitamin- and mineral-rich diet is much more effective. Proprietary foods are available for feeding to live prey before it is given to the reptile. Fresh greens should also be offered (fruit is less nutritionally valuable).

It should be borne in mind that a reptile's dietary requirements may change with age (Figure 11.15).

Vegetable group	Examples	Additional information
Cultivated green leaves	Kale, salad greens, rocket, spinach, spring greens, carrot tops, coriander, basil, mint, parsley, endive, chicory, bok choi, pak choi	Spinach contains oxalates that can bind to calcium and reduce its availability in the diet so should be given in moderation. All leaves should be washed prior to feeding; leaving them wet can be a good strategy for increasing water intake
Wild plants	Freshly picked grasses (not clippings as these ferment), dandelion leaves, plantain, nasturtiums, marigolds, raspberry leaves, hay, grape leaves, clover, vetch, blossoms and leaves from edible bushes and trees	Take care to identify plants correctly. Some organizations sell wildflower seed packs suitable for growing and feeding to tortoises. Wild plants will generally be lower in sugars and higher in fibre than cultivated plants
Other vegetables	Courgette, carrot (shredded or chopped), peppers, pumpkin, squash, beans and peas (fresh and sprouted), radish	Sprouted legumes can be contaminated with *Salmonella*, so washing these before use and using them promptly is recommended
Fruits	Reptiles from the tropics can be given fruits from a similar area, e.g. mango, guava, papaya. Other suitable fruits include figs, apple, kiwifruit, melon, pear, pineapple and berries	Fruits should be limited to a small amount twice a week for most species
Invertebrate prey	Crickets (juvenile and adult), mealworms, superworms, morio worms, waxworms, silkworms, cockroaches, beetles (see Figure 4.23)	Most invertebrate prey is commercially produced but wild-caught specimens can also be used as food. Different species vary in calcium, fat and protein content. Most invertebrate prey is fed live, to stimulate a feeding response in the reptile. Invertebrate prey is a potential source of internal parasites. It should be obtained from reputable sources
Vertebrate prey	Pinkies, fuzzies, mice, rat pups, whole rats, rabbits, goat, fish, chicks (see Figure 4.22)	Whole prey should be fed where possible, to provide a balanced diet. The health and age of the prey item affect its nutritional content. Very juvenile specimens may lack mineral content, while older prey may be obese. Vertebrate prey may be a source of internal parasites

11.14 Common items that feature in the diets of reptiles. All plants should be free from pesticides.

	Examples	Dietary balance (approximate)	Juveniles	Adults
Feeding frequency			Most species should be fed once or twice daily	Varies with species and size: from every second day (e.g. green iguana) to every second month (e.g. Burmese python)
Carnivorous/ insectivorous species	Some aquatic turtles; snakes; alligators; caiman; many lizards, e.g. bearded dragons	Protein 50% Carbohydrate 5% Fat 45%		Larger prey possible. For snakes, prey can be of a similar size to the diameter of the snake
Omnivorous species	Many lizards; some aquatic turtles; wood turtles; forest tortoises	Protein 25% Carbohydrate 50% Fat 25%	Tend to eat more protein and fat when young than when they mature	Some species' dietary preferences change with age, e.g. bearded dragons become less reliant on protein and more reliant on vegetable matter as they get older
Herbivorous species	Many tortoises; some lizards, e.g. green iguana, uromastyx, prehensile-tailed skinks	Protein 20% Carbohydrate 75% Fat 5%		Species that are herbivorous as juveniles will usually remain so throughout life

11.15 Changes in the dietary requirements of reptiles that occur with maturity.

When giving dietary advice to reptile-keepers, it must be stressed that, in the absence of a suitable housing environment, a good diet will not be enough to keep a reptile in good condition. As discussed in Chapter 5, the correct temperature gradient and lighting for the species must be provided. This includes the provision of ultraviolet light for some species (see Figure 5.8). Correct husbandry is essential for the health and wellbeing of reptile pets.

Captive reptiles are susceptible to a range of nutritional disorders, including starvation, malnutrition and obesity. Specific vitamin and mineral deficiencies or excesses may give rise to conditions such as metabolic bone disease (Figure 11.16).

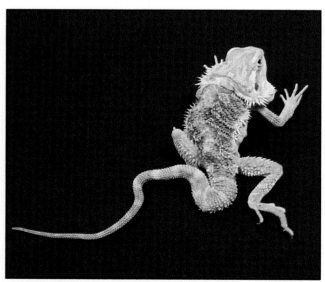

11.16 This bearded dragon shows signs consistent with secondary nutritional hyperparathyroidism (also known as metabolic bone disease, MBD). (© Dave Matthews)

Behavioural advice

Pet behaviour is a very complex issue into which there has been, and continues to be, extensive research; some suggestions for further reading are given at the end of the chapter. The behaviour of some exotic species can be difficult to interpret; it is therefore important to acknowledge any changes and to have an appreciation of normal *versus* abnormal behaviour. Signs of aggression and potential problem-solving strategies in rabbits, ferrets and parrots are given later in the chapter.

Mammals

Rabbits

Bonding

Rabbits are social animals and appear to benefit from companionship when kept as pets. It is not possible just to introduce a new animal and expect the existing pet to accept this, as rabbits are also territorial and have a defined social hierarchy in the wild. Letting a new rabbit into an existing rabbit's territory is likely to lead to aggression and probably fighting, and can result in serious injury both to the rabbits and to any human attempting to separate them. Introductions between rabbits need to be made slowly, a process known as 'bonding', with the expectation that a strong relationship that is beneficial to both rabbits is achieved. An example of a client handout on this is provided at the end of the chapter.

- The rabbits should initially be housed in separate cages in close proximity to each other. Visual and olfactory contact should be allowed before physical contact: they should be allowed out into the surrounding area one at a time, so they can take in each other's scents. Bedding from each cage can be swapped into the other rabbit's cage, to get them used to the scent of a new individual. Feeding the rabbits near to the barrier between them is useful, as eating is a communal activity in the wild. The rabbits' litter trays should be positioned away from the barrier to reduce stress.

■ It is best if rabbits are introduced on neutral territory (so neither will feel the need to defend their territory, and they may even seek assurance from each other). A bath tub is often recommended; however, a small pen in a different room or area of the garden is also suitable.

■ Scattering food is also recommended, to give the rabbits an opportunity to forage and eat together without having to fight over a single food bowl.

■ Opportunities for the rabbits to escape from each other should be provided, along with plenty of areas to find cover. In general at least one hide per rabbit (plus one additional hide, to allow them to run from one to another) is necessary. The hides should initially only be big enough to fit a single rabbit, so they can act as refuges from aggression.

■ It may be necessary to repeat the introductions on neutral territory numerous times before bonding is successful.

■ Bonding should always be attempted under adult supervision; owners should be prepared to separate fighting rabbits, taking care not to get injured themselves. Some fighting is to be expected while the initial 'pecking order' is established. Examination for bite marks, etc., after introductions is advised.

Unfortunately, attempts at bonding are not always successful and some rabbits will always have to be housed alone (these may be 'bonded' to a soft toy). While rabbits of the same gender can live successfully together, the most successful pairings are between neutered rabbits of opposite sexes.

Sexual behaviour

In male rabbits, sexual behaviour includes chasing, tail-flagging, mounting (other rabbits, inanimate objects, owners, etc.), urine spraying and nipping. Behavioural changes from decreased hormone influence are often not apparent for 30 days or more after neutering. Sexual behaviour may still be exhibited in some cases for several months after neutering, particularly in bucks with prior breeding experience (Bradley-Bays et al., 2006). It will still be necessary to keep newly neutered males separate from females for at least 4–6 weeks, as they may still produce viable sperm in this time.

Aggression

Aggressive behaviour may arise for a number of reasons (Figure 11.17). Aggression in rabbits can become a problem if the medical and psychological causes are not addressed. Aggression can result in physical damage to other rabbits within the environment, but also to owners. It is a leading cause of rabbits being placed into a rehoming situation.

Ferrets

Aggression

Ferrets may bite or nip as a sign of aggression. Reasons for this aggressive behaviour and strategies for mitigation are shown in Figure 11.18.

Signs	Reason for aggressive behaviour	Potential strategies to mitigate the aggressive behaviour
Growling, chasing, biting (especially genitals)	Dominance: occurs especially if a new rabbit is introduced; can also occur during the breeding season (February/March to September in UK)	See bonding suggestions in text. Ideally pair a male and female (both neutered). If two entire males, castrate the subordinate or both
Growling, lunging, biting, ears upright	Territorial aggression: more pronounced during breeding season or if cage/hutch is too confined	Determine and resolve underlying cause, e.g. cage/hutch size
Tail flagging, nipping, chasing, mounting	Sexual maturity: males at 4–5 months; females at 3–4 months	Neutering
Fighting, particularly among females	Hormonal/maternal in females: in 2–3-week cycles over breeding season	Neutering outside of breeding season
Aggression directed at objects or other animals, not at the actual source	Redirected aggression: the real cause may be a perceived threat or source of fear	Determine and address underlying cause
Crouched flat position, ears flat against head, eyes may be bulging, avoids being picked up, kicking and biting during handling	Fear: often due to a lack of, or inappropriate, handling	Prevention: handling rabbits from a young age; if older, a gradual process whereby the rabbit will need to form positive associations with being handled
	Pain: may cause aggression in a usually docile rabbit	Determine and address underlying cause

11.17   Approaches to aggression in rabbits.

Reason for aggressive behaviour	Potential strategies to mitigate the agressive behaviour
Play aggression: the handler is seen as a playmate. Biting is normal behaviour among young playing ferrets, similar to puppies	Avoid aggressive play such as tugging toys and wrestling. Handler can make a high-pitched sound when nipped (especially in the case of play-related aggression); this signals that play has gone too far
Fear: due to poor socialization or if startled	Frequent handling from a young age. Handler should make their presence obvious before approaching or handling
Pain	Diagnosis and treatment of the source of pain
Sexual aggression: can be normal among conspecifics during mating behaviour	

11.18 Approaches to aggression in ferrets.

Birds

Psittacine birds

Captivity reduces independence to some degree. The pet bird does not need to find food, which in the wild may necessitate travelling great distances. It also no longer has to fear predation, defend territory or find a partner or nest site. Mental and physical stimulation through interaction and environmental enrichment are therefore of great importance. The age at which puberty occurs varies greatly (see Figure 11.5). Increasing levels of sexual hormones may lead to the first signs of territorial behaviour and perceived aggression, and can be quite alarming to owners. This is an important time at which to begin training and to increase exercise and play in order to use up high levels of energy.

Training

Using training to establish a healthy relationship between owner and parrot takes time and commitment from the owner and other family members, and can be challenging – but also very rewarding. It can result in a well stimulated and socially stable bird with happy owners. Parrots respond well to positive reinforcement that rewards desired behaviour with praise, attention, physical contact such as head scratching, or a food treat. The reward will differ depending on what the individual bird considers to be worth obtaining. Training sessions should be short, upbeat and preferably carried out in an area away from the cage or the bird's perceived territory. Consistency is key; the same commands and training methods should ideally be used in all training sessions.

Useful commands include:

- 'Step up' on to a hand (Figure 11.19)
- 'Step down' on to a perch from the hand
- 'Present wing/foot'.

The bird should be observed during the training sessions and adjustments made accordingly. For example, is the bird more likely to step up/down if the perch/hand to be stepped on to is higher or lower than the level stepping from? What are the circumstances in which the bird behaves more desirably? It should also be borne in mind that birds respond differently to different colours and so may 'perform' more desirably if the trainer wears a particular colour.

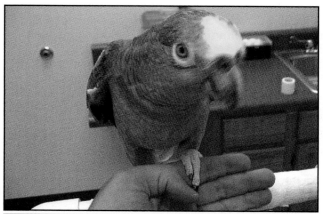

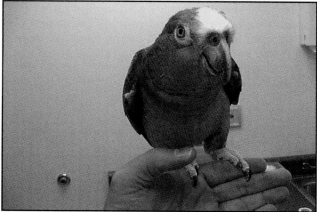

11.19 The 'step up' command can be taught to parrots.

An example of a client handout on training parrots is given at the end of this chapter.

Aggression

Unnatural behaviour such as biting or lunging may be triggered by fear or a perceived need to defend themselves or their territory. Careful assessment of the circumstances in which the aggressive behaviour is shown is vital, as only when the underlying cause is determined can strategies to modify the behaviour be implemented.

Feather plucking or mutilation

This is a complex condition that always warrants a veterinary consultation and medical work-up. It is not merely due to boredom.

Causes of feather plucking include:

- Heavy metal poisoning
- *Chlamydophila* infection
- Environmental contamination, e.g. aerosol or plug-in air fresheners, nicotine from cigarettes
- Environmental factors, e.g. low humidity
- Metabolic diseases, e.g. hepatopathy
- Primary skin conditions
- Parasites.

As well as ruling out medical conditions, taking a full history is very important, including the bird's diet, environment, cage position, daylight hours, owner's routine, etc., before a behavioural condition can be diagnosed. The nurse's role is in the reassessment of feather loss, continuation of dietary and behavioural strategies, and re-evaluation of wounds and redressing as necessary.

Reptiles

Stress in reptiles can lead to behavioural changes, immunosuppression and increased susceptibility to disease. Causes include:

- Over-handling of the more shy, solitary species, e.g. chameleons and adult green iguanas
- Housing a naturally more sociable species alone, e.g. bearded dragons and leopard geckos; it is best to house one male with a group of females
- The presence of a mirror or other reflective surface in the enclosure; the reflection could be perceived as a threat, causing striking and nose/facial injury
- Leaving prey animals in the enclosure for long periods, especially if the reptile is uninterested
- Visual and/or physical contact with other species, e.g. a cat or dog
- Visual contact between adult males of the same species.

Aggression

Lizards

Aggression in lizards is summarized in Figure 11.20. Behaviours such as standing erect, body inflation and head bobbing are designed to make the reptile appear larger and more of a threat. Thrashing, whipping the tail, striking and biting are also common signs of aggression.

Aggression in male iguanas is linked to increased levels of testosterone during the breeding season (generally November to April). Male iguanas may chase and bite female owners and handlers during this time, and unprovoked attacks on female owners during their menstrual period have been noted, possibly due to a response to pheromones (Mader, 2006). Certain colours of clothing could also be triggers and, if a pattern emerges between colours and aggression, these colours should be avoided. Male owners can be seen as competition by the iguana, leading to head bobbing, tail lashing and sometimes biting behaviour. Castration of the iguana can be useful in these cases and is most effective if performed before the start of the breeding season. Reducing daylight hours or provision of a soft toy for the male to mate with may also reduce the frequency of attacks.

Signs of aggression	Reason for aggressive behaviour	Potential strategies to mitigate the aggressive behaviour
Body inflation Standing very erect on all four legs Broadside posturing Dewlap extension Open-mouthed threat (particularly chameleons) Head bobbing Possibly biting, striking and tail-whipping (especially in sexually mature iguanas during breeding season)	Defensive aggression is usually caused by stress	Ensure correct handling; approaching too quickly or incorrect handling can cause stress and aggressive behaviour
	Territorial defence, particularly between males housed together	Ideally house naturally solitary species alone, e.g. adult male iguanas, many species of chameleon. Groups of leopard geckos or bearded dragons show less aggression when there are multiple females with one male. Chameleons should be housed in such a way that visual contact between males is not possible
	Sexually motivated aggression, e.g. in male iguanas. This is a normal, expected behaviour but poses a serious safety hazard to owners and veterinary staff	Castration before sexual maturity can be useful; if performed before sexual maturity, secondary sexual characteristics may be decreased or absent. It may be necessary for menstruating women to avoid contact with the iguana during its breeding season. Reduction in daylight hours. No exposure to other male iguanas and female conspecifics. Certain colours can be a trigger, e.g. handler's clothing; once the colours or patterns have been pinpointed they should be avoided. Could consider deslorelin implant to reduce hormonally stimulated behaviours

11.20 Approaches to aggression in lizards.

Snakes

Snakes quickly establish territorial markers in their enclosures; too much movement of cage furniture or cleaning too often may therefore increase stress. Some species are naturally more aggressive by nature, or aggression can be a fear response.

Snakes may strike the handler if they are mistaken for food or get 'caught in the crossfire'. Long tongs should be used to introduce food items.

Discharge advice

A written discharge plan is advisable, and this should include a scheduled recheck appointment (Figure 11.21). In all cases, owners should be advised on methods of:

- Administering medication (this should be demonstrated and areas of concern discussed or practiced)
- Assisted feeding
- Targets of food volume to give
- Weight loss comfort zones (i.e. amounts of loss that are tolerable)
- Circumstances in which a re-check should be scheduled (if earlier than originally planned).

Medication

Methods of administering medications to small mammals, birds and reptiles are summarized in Figure 11.22. Many owners are very nervous about giving medication and it is sensible to demonstrate this to them and confirm their capability to carry out the technique unassisted.

Date of discharge...

Animal's name..

Owner's address...

Condition...

Medications prescribed: drug, dose, duration   Method demonstrated

1. ....   ☐

2. ....   ☐

3. ....   ☐

Is supported feeding required?

No   ☐

Yes   ☐

- Food required:
- Method of feeding advised: ....Demonstrated ☐
- Volume of food:...Frequency of feeding:..
- Current bodyweight:...Target bodyweight:..

Call the practice:

- If your pet:
  - Does not tolerate the support feeding
  - Vomits
  - Regurgitates or otherwise fails to swallow food or medication
  - Appears weak or unable to move
- If you are otherwise concerned about their condition

If your pet has had surgery:
Check the surgical wound daily and **contact the practice if it seems red, swollen or is seeping fluid**

Monitor the stitches; these are due to be removed on:..
Watch for signs of pain or discomfort. These can include: aggressive behaviour, lack of mobility, vocalization, reduction in food intake. If any of these occur, **contact the practice immediately**.
If your pet has a dressing, please make certain this remains dry and is not being chewed by your pet. If the dressing gets wet, appears to smell or has been chewed, **please contact the practice immediately**.

Re-check required?

No   ☐
Yes   ☐   Date ....

11.21   An example of a discharge sheet for handing to clients.

Oral	Injection	Nebulization
Many medicines come in liquid form, making dosing and administering easier	Standard precautions should be observed, as for injecting dogs and cats Owners should be trained in suitable restraint, as well as injection techniques. In all cases they should be advised to draw back to confirm placement prior to injecting, i.e. no blood entering the needle hub or syringe. There should be a small amount of negative pressure on pulling back	This is the provision of medication in a form that can be inhaled. It is usually achieved using a commercial nebulizer, such as those made for human patients with asthma. The apparatus is fixed to the side of the cage or carrier, with tubing and wiring covered in tape to prevent chewing by the patient. The cage is then usually covered with a towel or plastic sheeting to keep the vapour inside
Small mammals		
Liquid medicines can be given directly into the mouth from a syringe, with care taken not to overwhelm the animal and cause choking. In some cases, medicine may be concealed in food, especially if it is palatable Some larger mammals may accept tablet formulations, either directly or in food items	Injections may be given either subcutaneously or intramuscularly. The technique is similar to that used for dogs and cats. See Chapter 6 for injection sites	Most mammals tolerate nebulization well, although they should be observed for signs of distress. In particular, those species that do not tolerate heat well (rabbits, guinea pigs, chinchillas) should be closely monitored, as heat may build up under a cover. Shorter, more frequent periods of nebulization should be employed if necessary
Birds		
Birds should be gently restrained in order to receive liquid medicines. They should ideally be held upright and the beak gently opened, with the medicine dripped or squirted into the lower beak below the tongue. This allows the bird to swallow without choking. Restraining the head gently will stop the bird shaking its head and spitting out the liquid Birds of prey can be given tablets and liquids concealed in food items Some bird medications are provided in drinking water, but this is unreliable as sick birds will not drink predictably There are tablet formulations marketed for pigeons	In most bird species injectable medications are best given into the breast muscle. Due to the thinness of bird skin, subcutaneous injections can prove difficult. The top two-thirds of the breast muscles on either side of the keel can be used Owners should be shown how to palpate the area, clean it with an appropriate antiseptic and insert the needle	Nebulization is commonly used in bird medicine and is usually well tolerated. All birds should be observed for signs of distress; if these are noted, the bird should be removed from a temporary cage or carrier or, if in its own cage, the nebulization stopped and the apparatus removed
Reptiles		
Almost all oral medicines for reptiles are in liquid form. Provision of medication in the drinking water is not reliable The reptile should be restrained and the head held still. In most species the mouth can be opened using a piece of cardboard (or an old credit card) inserted between the lips/beak edges. The medicine can then be dribbled into the mouth, taking care not to overwhelm the animal and cause choking	Most injectable medications are given intramuscularly to reptiles. Suitable areas include the muscle masses in the proximal fore- or hindlimbs. Where there is concern regarding the renal portal system (where injected drugs go straight to the kidney and are either excreted or cause kidney damage) the forelimbs should be used. This could include cases where the patient has been dehydrated or where the drug to be administered is known to be toxic to the kidneys Snakes are usually injected into the muscle masses on either side of the dorsal processes of the spine, in the middle third of the body. Owners should be made aware that liquid will occasionally seep back out of the skin after injection, as the skin of reptiles does not close as quickly as that of other species. It is sometimes difficult for owners to tell whether they have injected the drug into the muscle or under the skin; occasionally a blob of swelling will be noted under the skin after injection. This should resolve rapidly as the drug is taken up by the body	While nebulization is potentially useful in reptiles, it is less commonly used than in the other species groups. This is because many species are able to hold their breath for prolonged periods (longer than the time they might be placed in a nebulization chamber). However, in cases where it would be beneficial, such as for the treatment of respiratory disease, the animal should be monitored for breathing as well as for signs of distress

11.22   Methods of administering medication that can be employed by owners at home.

Monitoring and assisting feeding

> ⚠️ **WARNING**
> **Appropriate cautions should be taken prior to allowing owners to crop feed birds at home, as the procedure is very risky. Owners that have never crop fed previously should not be advised to do this at home. Under certain circumstances, where appropriate training has been undertaken, crop feeding at home may be possible; however, at the discharge appointment the veterinary nurse must make certain that the owner is competent to undertake the task. If in doubt, advice should be sought from the veterinary surgeon in charge of the case.**

For many exotic species it is better to discharge them, so that they can return to their normal environment, before they are able to feed completely independently. Methods of assisted feeding in the practice hospital are described in Chapter 5. Methods of assisted feeding for small mammals, birds and reptiles that can be employed at home are summarized in Figure 11.23. It is important that any kind of forced or assisted feeding is done safely, with minimal risk to both animal and owner, and demonstration is advised.

Post-hospitalization checks

Definite plans for re-examination of the patient at suitable intervals should be made. The interval will be determined by both the species involved and the condition being treated.

Goals for regaining independence should be set for each of the activities of living in the nursing care plan, including mobility, feeding, grooming, elimination and playing (see Chapter 6). There should be a documented improvement in each of these at every

Monitoring self-feeding	Hand-feeding	Assisted feeding
Small mammals		
Many rabbits and rodents will take hay/other food into their mouths as if eating, but will then just 'mouth' it before dropping it. Watching feeding carefully is therefore important In critical cases, food should be weighed before it goes into the cage and again when it is taken out. Pellets of monocomponent diets can be counted in and out	Many mammals are accustomed to taking treats from the owner's hand and will continue to do so even if they are not interested in eating their normal diet. In some instances where mobility is a problem, simply putting the food in an accessible position may be sufficient	Rodents can be fed using the oral syringe method, whereby food is squirted into the mouth. Food must be of a slurry consistency and the volumes given each time should not overwhelm the mouth, to avoid causing choking or aspiration. This means that the syringe must be inserted into the mouth multiple times Nasogastric tubes are also used, as are pharyngeal tubes in certain cases
Birds		
Prehending food, processing it and then swallowing it should be observed and confirmed. Some birds will still de-husk seeds even if they are not eating them and will simply throw food around, which will disguise the fact they are not eating In critical cases, food should be weighed before it goes into the cage and again when it is taken out. Pellets of monocomponent diets can be counted in and out	Many hand-reared psittacine birds will take familiar foods from the owner's hand or a spoon. Positive reinforcement and feeding little and often will provide encouragement but success relies on the animal having a degree of appetite	Crop feeding is the ideal method for most birds (although some species of bird do not have crops). See Chapters 1 and 6 for details. Some experienced owners may be capable of crop feeding, however careful discharge advice must be given. *If there is any doubt as to whether an owner is capable of tube feeding then it should not be recommended*
Reptiles		
When feeding live foods, stalking and catching should be confirmed as well as chewing and swallowing. Insects can easily hide, giving the impression that an animal is eating when it is not. Where individuals are given dead prey or vegetable matter, eating should be confirmed by observation. Dead prey is unlikely to be concealed within a vivarium so it is obvious whether it has been eaten or not. With vegetable matter, weighing the food in and out is less useful as it dehydrates in the warm environment of a vivarium. Counting the number of leaves/pieces offered/left may be more practical. Pellets of monocomponent diets can be counted in and out	Lizards may be hand-fed by placing food items into the back of the mouth, from where they are often swallowed. A similar method can be used in snakes (smaller than normal food items should be used). Some chelonians will take preferred food items from the owner's hand; however, this is not very reliable. Placing the food items in the mouth can be more effective, if it is possible to open it	Stomach tubing using a stainless steel gavage (crop) tube is the most efficient method for most pet reptiles. Liquid diets can be used initially, progressing to more concentrated herbivore or carnivore slurries. Pharyngostomy tubes are commonly employed in chelonians and may be left in place for long periods of time. They can also be placed in larger lizards and snakes, although this is less common

11.23   Methods of assisted feeding of exotic pets that can be employed by owners at home. Owners may be nervous about tube feeding and must be confident in carrying out these techniques prior to discharging the patient.

stage. If there is not, a re-evaluation and re-assessment of the medical and nursing plans should be undertaken. A failure to improve in each of these areas may in itself cause further damage and distress to the patient (e.g. pressure sores in animals that are not mobile, or fatty liver in animals that fail to eat).

Checks for medical patients should include:

■ A review of medical treatment and the client's ability to administer it: Has the medication been given? Has it been given correctly? Has the animal accepted the medication? Has the course been completed?
■ A review of feeding: Is the owner able to perform assisted feeding? Does the patient accept food? How much food is offered/eaten? Is a normal diet also being offered? Is any physical damage occurring secondary to feeding, e.g. oral damage?
■ Weight gain/loss: Is the animal gaining weight at an expected rate? Or has it, in fact, lost weight? If so, why (e.g. inadequate feeding, inappropriate food provided, feeding not accepted, deterioration or progression of clinical condition)?
■ All changes should be documented.

Checks for surgical patients should include:

■ Weight assessment: Every individual should be weighed at every postoperative check
■ Pain assessment: Behavioural and physiological markers can be used to assess pain postoperatively. There is a definite variation between species, but likely indicators of pain include: reduced activity; hunched posture; vocalization; reduced appetite; closed eyes; and reduced alertness. Physiological parameters, such as elevated heart rate, elevated respiratory rate and elevated body temperature in endothermic species, can also suggest pain. These should prompt re-evaluation and veterinary examination. (See Chapter 7 for discussion of analgesia protocols)
■ Assessment of feeding behaviour:
  – Mammals should eat at normal feeding intervals as long as pain relief is sufficient. Smaller mammals with high metabolic rates should have been observed eating prior to discharge
  – Birds should have been eating and maintaining bodyweight prior to discharge. Due to their high metabolic rate there is little leeway for error if a bird is not eating, and re-evaluation and assisted feeding should be commenced as soon as possible. However, crop feeding birds is a risky procedure for most owners to attempt at home (see above)
  – Reptiles should eat at normal feeding intervals, as long as they are mobile enough and pain relief is sufficient. Snakes with surgical wounds should be given small prey that will not increase their girth and so stretch the wound. Reptiles that have

undergone gastrointestinal surgery should be given an increasing plane of nutrition, with small species commencing feeding after 5 days and larger species after 10–15 days.

Wound healing

Postoperative wound healing in a tortoise is illustrated in Figure 11.24. Stages of wound healing in small mammals, birds and reptiles are outlined in Figure 11.25 (see also Chapter 9).

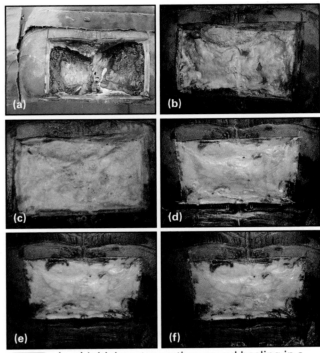

11.24 (a–c) Initial postoperative wound healing in a tortoise. (d–f) Subsequent healing following revision surgery on day 215. (© Kevin Eatwell)

Promoting wound healing

■ Methods of limiting patient interference with wounds include soft/hard collars, splints or dressings, bitter sprays, fake sutures, local anaesthetic ointment/infiltration, and good pain relief.
■ Reptiles should be kept within their preferred optimum temperature range (POTR) for the best chance of wound healing. It should be remembered that reptiles with reduced mobility may not be able to move well enough to thermoregulate and so may overheat if left too near a heat source.
■ All animals with external skin wounds should be provided with a clean, non-adherent, soft substrate.
■ Activity should be restricted to allow healing to occur. This may mean confining the patient to a smaller enclosure than normal, and limiting the potential for jumping, flying, climbing and any other form of unrestricted mobility.

Small mammals	Birds	Reptiles
Healing proceeds in a manner similar to that in cats and dogs	Skin heals rapidly but with much less formation of granulation tissue and less potential for scarring	Rate of healing can be very variable, depending on species, nutritional provision and environment. Craniocaudally orientated wounds heal more quickly than transverse wounds
At 3 days		
Stable scab is present with migration of granulation tissue occurring underneath	Scab may be present and wound discoloration may be noted. Greenish bruising is quite normal	Scab formed and stable
At 7 days		
Granulation tissue or early fibrous healing may be visible. Scab may have fallen off. *Swelling, discharge or skin discoloration all prompt review by the veterinary surgeon*	Fibroblasts already migrating under the scab, which may have already fallen off. *Swelling, discharge or skin discoloration all prompt review by the veterinary surgeon*	Scab still visible and stable. *Swelling, discharge or skin discoloration all prompt review by the veterinary surgeon*
At 14 days		
Wound healing should be sufficiently progressed to allow suture removal. A thin line of scarring may be visible. *Swelling, discharge or skin discoloration all prompt review by the veterinary surgeon*	Epithelialization has occurred; macrophages and heterophils have cleared infection from underneath the scab, which is likely to have fallen off. *Swelling, discharge or skin discoloration all prompt review by the veterinary surgeon*	Epithelial cells have started to migrate under the scab (the timing of this can depend on the stage of shed the animal is at). The scab may still remain attached. *Swelling, discharge or skin discoloration all prompt review by the veterinary surgeon*
At 30 days		
Healing should be complete, with faint scarring still visible	Wound healing complete. Bird skin does not scar in the same way as mammalian skin so this will not be evident; however, adhesions to the underlying muscle may be noticeable	Wound healing is not yet complete, but a stable healing scab or area of granulation tissue should be visible. Healing progresses faster at the times just before and after shedding, so healing may not be a linear process compared with other species
Time to suture removal		
10–14 days (similar to dogs and cats)	Absorbable sutures are often placed, which will dissolve over a 60–120-day period	42 days (may be left until next shed)

11.25 Stages of postoperative wound healing.

References and further reading

Bradley-Bays T, Lightfoot TL and Mayer J (2006) *Exotic Pet Behaviour: Birds Reptiles and Small Mammals*. Elsevier, St. Louis

British Veterinary Zoological Society (2012) *Guidelines for microchip transponder sites*: www.bvzs.org/publications/guidelines/microchip.html

Brown S (2006) *Bladder stones and bladder sludge in rabbits*: www.rabbit.org

Burkett (2007) *Switching birds to pellets is possible*: www.parrotandconureworld.com

Chitty J and Lierz M (2008) *BSAVA Manual of Raptors, Pigeons and Passerine Birds*. BSAVA Publications, Gloucester

Cooper B, Mullineaux E and Turner L (2011) *BSAVA Textbook of Veterinary Nursing, 5th edn*. BSAVA Publications, Gloucester

Ford SL (2009) *Balancing your parrot's lifestyle*. Client Information Sheet: www.vin.com

Fowler ME and Miller RE (2003) *Zoo and Wild Animal Medicine, 5th edition*. Saunders, St. Louis

Gentz E (2008) *Vaccination schedules for skunks*. Client Information Sheet: www.vin.com

Girling SJ (2003) *Veterinary Nursing of Exotic Pets*. Blackwell Publishing, Oxford

Girling SJ and Raiti P (2004) *BSAVA Manual of Reptiles, 2nd edn*. BSAVA Publications, Gloucester

Hall CJ (2010) Obesity in parrots: killing with kindness. *Parrots International Magazine*, volume **1**

Harrison GJ and Lightfoot TL (2006) *Clinical Avian Medicine*. Spix Publishing, Florida

Harcourt-Brown F (2002) *Textbook of Rabbit Medicine*. Butterworth Heinemann, Edinburgh

Harcourt-Brown F and Chitty J (in preparation) *BSAVA Manual of Rabbit Imaging, Surgery and Dentistry*. BSAVA Publications, Gloucester

Harcourt-Brown N and Chitty J (2005) *BSAVA Manual of Psittacine Birds, 2nd edn*. BSAVA Publications, Gloucester

Highfield AC (1998) *Safer hibernation and your tortoise*: www.tortoisetrust.org (updated 2011)

Hillyer EV and Quesenberry KE (1997) *Ferrets, Rabbits and Rodents*: Clinical Medicine and Surgery. WB Saunders, Philadelphia

Keeble E and Meredith A (2009) *BSAVA Manual of Rodents and Ferrets*. BSAVA Publications, Gloucester

Mader DR (2006) *Reptile Medicine and Surgery, 2nd edn*. Saunders Elsevier, St Louis

Magnus E (2005) Behaviour of the pet rabbit: what is normal and why do problems develop? *In Practice* **27**(10) 531–535

Magnus E, McBride A and Hearne G (2005) Aspects of rabbit behaviour. *Veterinary Review* **99**, 28–29

McBride A (2000) *Why Does My Rabbit....?* Souvenir Press, London

Meredith A and Flecknell P (2006) *BSAVA Manual of Rabbit Medicine and Surgery, 2nd edn.* BSAVA Publications, Gloucester

Meredith A and Johnson-Delaney C (2010) *BSAVA Manual of Exotic Pets, 5th edn.* BSAVA Publications, Gloucester

Mitchell MA and Tully TN (2009) *Manual of Exotic Pet Practice.* Saunders Elsevier, St. Louis

Mullineaux E, Best R and Cooper JE (2003) *BSAVA Manual of Wildlife Casualties.* BSAVA Publications, Gloucester

Sandford JC (1996) *The Domestic Rabbit.* Blackwell, Oxford

Saunders RA and Rees-Davies R (2005) *Notes on Rabbit Internal Medicine.* Blackwell Publishing, Oxford

Stanford M (2010) *Significance of cholesterol assays in the investigation of hepatic lipidosis and atherosclerosis*: www.harrisonsbirdfoods.com/avmed/articles/7-3cholesterol.pdf

UV Guide: www.uvguide.co.uk

Styles DK (2005) Avian neonatology and nursery management for the practitioner. *Proceedings, North American Veterinary Conference*, pp.1228–1231

Client handout examples follow. Please go to www.bsava.com/EPWN-extra for more ▶

Introducing a new pet rabbit

Molly Varga

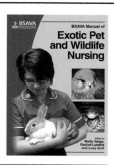

Preparation

- Introducing a new rabbit to your established pet needs to be approached carefully and can be a time-consuming process. Rabbits are territorial in the wild and have a defined social structure so they will need to 'work this out' in the home.
- Before introducing the new rabbit, your existing rabbit should be well and fully up to date with vaccinations. A check-up with your veterinary surgeon is recommended.
- Some pairings work better than others and this will depend on the individual rabbits. A neutered male with a neutered female is ideal, but other combinations can work.
- Before introduction both rabbits should have recovered from their neutering surgery.

First steps

- The first step is to keep both rabbits within sight and smell of each other. Bedding from each cage can be moved into the other cage regularly, so that each rabbit gets used to the smell of the other rabbit within its territory.
- It is also a good idea to feed the rabbits within sight of each other, preferably near the barrier between them. This is because eating is a social activity and it gets the rabbits used to being part of a social grouping.
- Once the rabbits are showing positive interest in each other (having non-aggressive interactions through the barrier, lying down near to each other) then physical introduction can start.

Putting them together

- The rabbits must be introduced to each other on neutral territory, such as in a room where neither rabbit has been previously. A bathroom (or even a bath!) or a pen in a new room is suitable. For rabbits that live outdoors, an area that is neutral must still be chosen. Bringing the rabbits indoors can work, or you can use outside space that neither has had previous access to.
- It is a good idea to scatter food around the area in which the rabbits are to meet. This avoids them having to fight over a single food bowl, and encourages them to forage, an activity they would perform in the wild socially.
- The meeting must be supervised by an adult who is prepared to physically separate the rabbits if they fight. Care must be taken, as rabbits in the middle of a fight will often bite indiscriminately and human injury can occur.
- A short meeting – 5 to 10 minutes – is suitable for the first time. There should be some sniffing and chasing, but the meeting should be stopped if fighting occurs. A good outcome is both rabbits lying down and apparently ignoring each other.
- If fighting does occur, both rabbits should be checked for wounds and must be treated if wounds are found.
- Meetings can be repeated daily for increasing lengths of time.
- Once the rabbits are grooming each other, eating together and lying down peacefully with one another, they can be put together in their original territories (where they are living when they are not being bonded). If this goes well, and the rabbits are behaving positively for hours at a time, then they can be allowed to share a sleeping area and to live together permanently.
- If bonding does not progress as expected, contact your veterinary surgeon who will be able to refer you to a rabbit behavioural specialist.

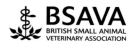

Basic training for your parrot

Molly Varga

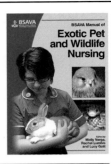

Why should I train my parrot?

- Parrots are intelligent animals but they can be aggressive or destructive if they become bored.
- Regular training sessions can bond you and your parrot, as well as allowing them to use their natural intelligence to perform useful tasks, such as stepping up on to a hand when it is time to be placed back into the cage, or allowing examination of their wings.

Where and for how long?

- The training should take place in a different room from where the parrot lives and plays. This will reinforce the fact that when they are taken there, training is planned.
- Training sessions should be brief to start with and should not be longer than your parrot's attention span (often as little as 5 minutes to start with).
- The amount of training required is determined by how you and your parrot live together.

How should I train my parrot?

- For each behaviour you are trying to promote, you will need a vocal command. For example, 'step up' to tell the parrot to step on to your hand.
- Each behaviour needs to be split up into tiny stages that can be achieved easily. For example, training your parrot to 'step up' might involve first getting them comfortable with your hand in the cage, then allowing them to investigate your hand, before they eventually climb on to it. The final stage is to encourage the parrot to step up in the cage on command.
- Successful completion of each stage should be rewarded with praise or a food treat. This is known as 'postive reinforcement'.
- The behaviour can then be attempted in a different setting, still using positive reinforcement. Once your parrot understands the command and consistently performs the behaviour, the positive reinforcement can gradually become less frequent and less predictable, so they do not know when a treat is coming. This will reinforce the behaviour more strongly.
- 'Negative reinforcement', such as hitting your pet, should NEVER be used.
- It is often tempting to shout at a bird that is behaving incorrectly, but most parrots see this as attention and therefore good. It is better to completely ignore incorrect or 'bad' behaviour. Parrots generally hate to be ignored!

Problem behaviours

- If you parrot becomes suddenly aggressive or destructive, they should be examined by your veterinary surgeon.
- If medical conditions are ruled out, training is likely to be the root of the solution for behavioural problems.
- For severe problems, your vet will be able to refer you to a specialist in bird behaviour problems.

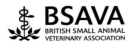

BSAVA
BRITISH SMALL ANIMAL
VETERINARY ASSOCIATION

BSAVA CLIENT HANDOUTS: EXOTIC PET AND WILDLIFE SERIES

Hand-rearing garden birds

Molly Varga

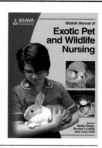

Finding a baby bird

- Most nestlings that are found on the ground are not abandoned, but have fallen out of the nest before they can fly properly.
- If the chick appears injured, it should be examined by a veterinary surgeon.
- As long as the chick appears to be uninjured, it should be placed in a small container (a plastic or cardboard box with the lid open) and the container placed in a safe position elevated above the ground. A tree branch under cover of leaves is suitable. This allows the parents access to the chick for feeding until it fledges.
- If there is no sign of the parents after several hours of watching from a safe distance, the chick may have been truly abandoned and hand-rearing should be considered.
- There are many wildlife rehabilitation centres in the UK that specialize in hand-rearing chicks and returning them to the wild. A list of various centres may be found at www.bwrc.co.uk.

Housing an orphan

- A chick being hand-reared should be kept warm and out of draughts.
- The chick can be kept in a small plastic cup lined with kitchen towel, which mimics the security and shape of a nest. These are easy to keep clean and small enough to move around so that the temperature can be kept constant.
- As a chick grows and becomes more independent, a small birdcage with low perches can be used.

Feeding an orphan

- Most garden birds eat seeds or insects. It is important to identify the species and age of the bird correctly in order to provide the correct diet.
- Commercial diets for insectivorous and seed-based diets are suitable for hand-rearing. Alternatively, Kaytee Exact Hand-rearing food (a parrot diet) can be used for grain eaters, while mealworms (or for short periods until better arrangements can be made, cat food) may be used for insectivorous birds.
- Chicks will often gape in response to movement above their heads, and food can be dropped into their mouths from blunt forceps (tweezers), a small syringe or a small spoon.
- Very young chicks must be fed very regularly (every 15 minutes or so while there is daylight) and will eat up to 20% of their bodyweight daily. Food should be offered in the form of a paste, so that it is less likely to be inhaled and cause choking.
- Feeding should continue until the crop is full. This can be monitored visually as a bulge at the base of the neck that gets bigger as you feed the chick.
- Once the crop is full, feeding should cease until the crop appears empty again.
- As chicks grow and become more mature they should be hand-fed less frequently, but should be given food items in the 'nest' that they can explore and so start to eat independently.
- Weighing the chick each day will show whether it is growing.

Cleaning the 'nest'

- After feeding the chick will pass faeces in a sticky mucus sac, which should be removed.
- Keeping the nest area clean to avoid the build-up of potentially harmful bacteria is very important.
- Some of these, like *E. coli* and *Salmonella*, can affect people too, so you should was your hands thoroughly after handling the chick and cleaning its nest.

Letting it go

- The time to fledging and independence varies from 14 days (blackbirds) to more than 30 days (crows).
- The method of release can vary with species, and it may be sensible to consider enlisting the help of a local wildlife centre who can release the fledgling with a group of other chicks of the same species.
- Otherwise, once the chick is large enough and well feathered enough to fly, it can be placed in a safe area in a garden (or similar sheltered outdoor space) and allowed to fly away.
- Supplementary food can be provided in a container elevated off the ground for a few days until the chick learns to fend for itself.

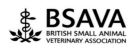

© BSAVA 2012
BSAVA Manual of Exotic Pet and Wildlife Nursing

Appendix

Common and scientific names

Common names have been used throughout this Manual for readability. This Appendix gives the equivalent taxonomic names.

Mammals

English name	Latin name
African pygmy hedgehog	*Atelerix albiventris*
Asian small-clawed otter	*Aonyx cinerea*
Bennett's wallaby	*Macropus rufogriseus rufogriseus*
Black rat	*Rattus rattus*
Brown rat	*Rattus norvegicus*
Chinchilla	*Chinchilla lanigera*
Chinese hamster	*Cricetulus griseus*
Common marmoset	*Callithrix jacchus*
Common mouse *see* House mouse	
Common rabbit *see* European rabbit	
Common rat *see* Brown rat	
Dama wallaby *see* Tammar wallaby	
Daubenton's bat	*Myotis daubentonii*
Degu	*Octodon degus*
Edible dormouse	*Myoxus (Glis) glis*
Eurasian (European) badger	*Meles meles*
Eurasian (European) otter	*Lutra lutra*
European (Domestic) rabbit	*Oryctolagus cuniculus*
European hedgehog	*Erinaceus europaeus*
Ferret	*Mustela putorius furo*
(Eastern) Grey squirrel	*Sciurus carolinensis*
Guinea pig	*Cavia porcellus*
Harvest mouse	*Micromys minutus*
House mouse	*Mus musculus*
Mongolian gerbil	*Meriones unguiculatus*
Noctule bat	*Nyctalus noctula*
Parma wallaby	*Macropus parma*
Pipistrelle bats	*Pipistrellus pipistrellus, P. pygmaeus*
Raccoon	*Procyon lotor*
Red (European) fox	*Vulpes vulpes*

English name	Latin name
Red-necked wallaby	*Macropus rufogriseus*
(Eurasian) Red squirrel	*Sciurus vulgaris*
Roborovski hamster	*Phodopus roborovskii*
Russian dwarf Campbell hamster	*Phodopus campbelli*
Russian dwarf winter white hamster	*Phodopus sungorus*
Siberian chipmunk	*Eutamias sibiricus* or *Tamias sibiricus*
Slender-tailed meerkat	*Suricata suricatta*
Stoat	*Mustela erminea*
Striped skunk	*Mephitis mephitis*
Sugar glider	*Petaurus breviceps*
Syrian hamster	*Mesocricetus auratus*
Tammar wallaby	*Macropus eugenii*
Water vole	*Arvicola terrestris*

Birds

[a] CITES Listed birds: the common names here do not conform entirely with those common names used by Defra; to be safe the Latin should be used.

English name	Latin name
African grey parrot	Psittacus erithacus
African spotted eagle owl	Bubo africanus
Australian king parrot	Alisterus scapularis
Bald eagle	Haliaeetus leucocephalus
Bali myna(h) (Rothschild's starling)	Leucospar rothschildi
Barn owl	Tyto alba
Barnacle goose	Branta leucopsis
Bengal eagle owl (Indian eagle owl)	Bubo bengalensis
Bengalese finch (society finch) – derived from the white-rumped munia (lonchura striata)	Sometimes referred to as Lonchura domestica
Black kite	Milvus migrans
Black swan	Cygnus atratus
Black vulture	Coragyps atratus
Blue and gold macaw	Ara ararauna
Blue-fronted Amazon	Amazona aestiva
Blue-headed pionus parrot	Pionus menstruus
Budgerigar	Melopsittacus undulatus
Canada goose	Branta canadensis
Chicken	Gallus gallus domesticus
Cockatiel	Nymphicus hollandicus
Common kestrel	Falco tinnunculus
Common wood pigeon	Columba palumbus
Diamond dove	Geopelia cuneata
Domestic (greylag) goose	Anser anser
Double yellow-headed Amazon	Amazona ochrocephala
Eclectus parrot	Eclectus roratus
Emu	Dromaius novaehollandiae
Eurasian buzzard (common buzzard)	Buteo buteo
Eurasian collared dove	Streptopelia decaocto
Eurasian hobby (hobby)	Falco subbuteo
Eurasian sparrowhawk (sparrowhawk)	Accipiter nisus
European bee-eater	Merops apiaster
European eagle owl	Bubo bubo
European honey buzzard	Pernis apivorus
Galah (roseate cockatoo)	Elophus roseicapilla
Golden eagle	Aquila chrysaetos
Gouldian finch	Erythrura gouldiae
Grande eclectus	Eclectus roratus roratus
Greater rhea	Rhea americana
Greenwing macaw	Ara chloropterus
Grey parrot see African grey parrot	
Griffon vulture	Gyps fulvus
Gyrfalcon	Falco rusticolus

English name	Latin name
Harris' hawk	Parabuteo unicinctus harrisi
Hill myna(h)	Gracula religiosa
Hyacinth macaw [a]	Anodorhynchus hyacinthus
Indian peafowl	Pavo cristatus
Island canary (canary)	Serinus canaria
Lanner falcon	Falco biarmicus
Lesser rhea	Rhea pennata
Lesser sulphur-crested cockatoo	Cacatua sulphurea
Little owl	Athene noctua
Madagascar lovebird	Agapornis cana
Mallard	Anas platyrhynchos
Maroon-bellied conure	Pyrrhura frontalis
Merlin	Falco columbarius
Mute swan	Cygnus olor
Northern goshawk (goshawk)	Accipiter gentilis
Ostrich	Struthio camelus
Peach-faced lovebird	Agapornis roseicollis
Peregrine falcon	Falco peregrinus
Quaker (monk) parakeet	Myiopsitta monachus
Rainbow lorikeet	Trichoglossus haematodus
Red and blue lory [a]	Eos histrio
Red kite	Milvus milvus
Red lory	Eos rubra
Red-bellied macaw	Orthopsittaca manilata
Red-tailed hawk	Buteo jamaicensis
Ringneck parakeet [a]	Psittacula krameri
Rock dove (domestic or racing pigeon)	Columba livia
Saker falcon	Falco cherrug
Scarlet macaw [a]	Ara macao
Secretary bird	Sagittarius serpentarius
Snowy owl	Bubo scandiaca
Spix's macaw [a]	Cyanopsitta spixii
Splendid parakeet	Neophema splendida
Steppe eagle	Aquila nipalensis
Sun conure	Aratinga solstitialis
Tawny eagle	Aquila rapax
Tawny owl	Strix aluco
Timneh grey parrot	Psittacus erithacus timneh
Turkey	Meleagris gallopavo
Umbrella cockatoo	Cacatua alba
White-bellied caique	Pionites leucogaster
White-capped pionus parrot	Pionus senilis
White-tailed sea eagle	Haliaeetus albicilla
Yellow-sided caique	Pionites leucogaster xanthomeria
Zebra finch	Taeniopygia guttata

Reptiles

Lizards

English name	Latin name
Anole lizards	*Anolis* spp.
Asian water dragon	*Physignathus cocincinus*
Asian water monitor	*Varanus salvator*
Australian water dragon	*Physignathus lesueurii*
Basilisk lizard *see* Common basilisk	
Bearded dragon *see* Inland bearded dragon	
Caiman lizard	*Dracaena guianensis*
Common basilisk	*Basiliscus basiliscus*
Common blue-tongued skink	*Teliqua scincoides*
Common lizard	*Zootoca vivipara*
Day geckos	*Phelsuma* spp.
Fat-tailed gecko	*Hemitheconyx caudicinctus*
Frilled lizard	*Chlamydosaurus kingii*
Giant day gecko	*Phelsuma madagascariensis grandis*
Gila monster	*Heloderma suspectum*
Green anole	*Anolis carolinensis*
Green iguana	*Iguana iguana*
Inland bearded dragon	*Pogona vitticeps*
Jackson's chameleon	*Chamaeleo jacksoni*
Leopard gecko	*Eublepharis macularius*
Madagascar day gecko	*Phelsuma madagascariensis*
Malaysian monitor lizard *see* Asian water monitor	
Monitor lizards	*Varanus* spp.
Panther chameleon	*Furcifer pardalis*
Prehensile-tailed skink	*Corucia zebrata*
Sand lizard	*Lacerta agilis*
Savannah monitor	*Varanus exanthematicus*
Slowworm	*Anguis fragilis*
Solomon island monkey-tailed skink *see* Prehensile-tailed skink	
Spiny-tailed lizards	*Uromastyx* spp.
Standing's day gecko	*Phelsuma standingi*
Thai water dragon *see* Asian water dragon	
Three-horned chameleon *see* Jackson's chameleon	
Tokay gecko	*Gekko gecko*
Variegated gecko	*Gehyra variegata*
Veiled chameleon	*Chamaeleo calyptratus*
Water dragon *see* Asian water dragon	
Yemen chameleon *see* Veiled chameleon	

Snakes

English name	Latin name
Anaconda	*Eunectes murinus*
Ball python *see* Royal python	
Boa constrictor *see* Common boa	
Boelen's python	*Morelia boeleni*
Burmese python	*Python molurus bivittatus*
Californian kingsnake	*Lampropeltis getula californiae*
Common boa	*Boa constrictor imperator*
Cornsnake	*Pantherophis guttatus guttatus*
Diamond python	*Morelia spilota spilota*
Emerald tree boa	*Corallus caninus*
Eurasian water snakes	*Natrix* spp.
European adder	*Vipera berus*
European viper *see* European adder	
Garter snake	*Thamnophis sirtalis*
Grass snake	*Natrix natrix*
Green tree python	*Morelia viridis*
Honduran milk snake	*Lampropeltis triangulum hondurensis*
Kenyan sand boa	*Eryx colubrinus loveridgei*
Kingsnakes	*Lampropeltis* spp.
Leopard snake	*Elaphe situla*
Mangrove snake	*Boiga dendrophila*
Oregon red-spotted garter snake	*Thamnophis sirtalis concinnus*
Rainbow boa	*Epicrates cenchria*
Red-tailed boa constrictor	*Boa constrictor constrictor*
Reticulated python	*Python reticulatus*
Royal python	*Python regius*
Sand boa	*Eryx colubrinus*
Smooth snake	*Coronella austriaca*
Tree python *see* Green tree python	

Chelonians

English name	Latin name
Afghan tortoise *see* Horsfield's tortoise	
African spurred tortoise	*Geochelone sulcata*
Alligator snapping turtle	*Macroclemys temminckii*
Asian box turtle *see* Malayan box turtle	
Box turtles	*Terrapene* spp.
Burmese star tortoise	*Geochelone platynota*
Central American river turtle	*Dermatemys mawii*
Galapagos tortoise	*Geochelone nigra*
Giant Amazon river turtle	*Podocnemis expansa*
Greek tortoise *see* Spur-thighed tortoise	
Hermann's tortoise	*Testudo hermanni*
Hingeback tortoises	*Kinixys* spp.
Horsfield's tortoise	*Testudo horsfieldii*
Indian star tortoise	*Geochelone elegans*
Leopard tortoise	*Geochelone pardalis*
Malayan box turtle	*Cuora amboinensis*
Marginated tortoise	*Testudo marginata*
Mediterranean spur-thighed tortoise *see* Spur-thighed tortoise	
Mobile terrapin *see* Red-eared terrapin	
Red-eared slider *see* Red-eared terrapin	
Red-eared terrapin	*Trachemys scripta elegans*
Red-footed tortoise	*Geochelone carbonaria*
Russian tortoise *see* Horsfield's tortoise	
Soft-shelled turtles	*Trionyx* spp.
Spur-thighed tortoise	*Testudo graeca*
Star tortoise *see* Indian star tortoise	
Yellow-footed tortoise	*Geochelone denticulata*

Amphibians

English name	Latin name
American green tree frog	*Hyla cinerea*
Axolotl	*Ambystoma mexicanum*
Great-crested newt	*Triturus cristatus*
Green and black poison dart frog	*Dendrobates auratus*
Horned frog (pacman frog)	*Ceratophrys* spp.
Natterjack toad	*Epidalea calamita*
Pool frog	*Pelophylax lessonae*
Red-eyed tree frog	*Agalychnis callidryas*
White's tree frog	*Litoria caerulea*

Index

Index